Practical Plastic Surgery for Nonsurgeons

NADINE B. SEMER, MD
Clinical Instructor
Division of Plastic Surgery
University of Southern California
   School of Medicine
Los Angeles, California

illustrations by
MARTHE ADLER-LAVAN, MD
Philadelphia, Pennsylvania

HANLEY & BELFUS, INC.   Philadelphia

Publisher: HANLEY & BELFUS, INC.
                Medical Publishers
                210 S. 13th Street
                Philadelphia, PA 19107
                (215) 546-4995
                FAX (215) 790-9330
                www.hanleyandbelfus.com

Library of Congress Cataloging-in-Publication Data

Practical plastic surgery for nonsurgeons / by Nadine B. Semer.
        p. ; cm.
     Includes bibliographical references and index.
     ISBN 1-56053-478-8 (alk. paper)
        1. Surgery, Plastic. 2. Rural health services. I. Semer, Nadine B, 1960–
     [DNLM: 1. Reconstructive Surgical Procedures. WO 600 P895 2001]
     RD118.P73 2001
     617.9'5—dc21

                                                        00-054179

**PRACTICAL PLASTIC SURGERY
FOR NONSURGEONS**   ISBN 1-56053-478-8

Last digit is the print number: 9 8 7 6 5 4 3 2 1

Dedication

To Chris and Jenny McConnachie, Cosimo Storniolo and Meredith Weir, and all health care providers worldwide who are working to bring quality medical care to people living in rural areas

And to David, who helped me to see that anything is possible

Table of Contents

International Medical Missions

The following is a short list of organizations that sponsor international medical missions. There are many more. The World Wide Web and local medical/professional societies are other sources of information. The minimum time commitment ranges from a few days to several months to years. Some are religious-based organizations. Listing here does not imply recommendation or endorsement of any of these organizations. If you are interested in international work, research the organization well.

The best advice I can offer to health professionals going to work in any rural area is to be open to anything, be as flexible as possible, and above all respect the people you are working with and the people you are serving.

Nadine B. Semer, MD
www.practicalplasticsurgery.org
nadine@ppsurg.org

Organization	U.S. Contact Information and Internet Address
American Medical Student Association	1902 Association Drive, Reston, VA 20191 (703) 620-6600; www.amsa.org
Catholic Medical Mission Board	10 West 17th Street, New York, NY 10011 (800) 678-5659; www.cmmb.org
CB International	1501 West Mineral Avenue, Littleton, CO 80120 (800) 487-4224; www.cbi.org
Doctors of the World-USA	375 West Broadway, 4th Floor, New York, NY 10012 (888) 817-HELP; www.dowusa.org
Doctors Without Borders, USA Médecins San Frontières	6 East 39th Street, 8th Floor, New York, NY 10016 (212) 679-6800; www.doctorswithoutborders.org
The Flying Hospital, Inc.	11836 Fishing Pointe Drive, Newport News, VA 23606 (757) 873-6794; www.flyinghospital.org
Global Volunteers	375 East Little Canada Road, St. Paul, MN 55117 (800) 487-1074; www.globalvolunteers.org
Health Volunteers Overseas	P.O. Box 65157, Washington, DC 20035 (202) 296-0928; www.hvousa.org
Himalayan HealthCare, Inc.	P.O. Box 737, Planetarium Station, New York, NY 10024 (212) 829-8691; www.himalayan-healthcare.org
International Medical Corps	11500 West Olympic Blvd., Suite 506, Los Angeles, CA 90064 (310) 826-7800; www.imc-la.com
International Rescue Committee	122 East 42nd Street, New York, NY 10168 (212) 551-3000; www.intrescom.org
Interplast, Inc.	300-B Pioneer Way, Mountain View, CA 94041 (650) 962-0123; www.interplast.org
Mercy Ships	P.O. Box 2020, Garden Valley, TX 75771 (800) 424-7447; http://mercyships.org/index.htm
Operation Smile	6435 Tidewater Drive, Norfolk, VA 23509 (757) 321-7645; www.operationsmile.org
Physicians for Peace	229 West Bute Street, Suite 900, Norfolk, VA 23510 (757) 625-7569; www.physicians-for-peace.org
Presbyterian Church (USA), Worldwide Ministries Division, Mission Service Recruitment Office	100 Witherspoon Street, Louisville, KY 40202 (800) 779-6779; www.pcusa.org/msr
Project Hope	255 Carter Hall Lane, Millwood, VA 22646 (800) 544-4673; www.projhope.org

Preface

The intent of this book is to bring relief to people who sustain commonly encountered injuries and wounds. Without corrective treatment, these problems can destroy livelihoods and families. Immediate, acute care often stabilizes the patient, but may leave the patient with a minor or major disability. Lacking the resources typical of wealthier populations, even minor disabilities can have a devastating economic and social impact.

Plastic surgeons have developed reconstructive surgical techniques that can restore the injured person to a productive and fulfilling life. Unfortunately, this type of surgery has frequently been obscured by a cloud of unawareness or perceived difficulty.

Practical Plastic Surgery for Nonsurgeons describes straightforward plastic surgical information and techniques. This book will be useful to health care providers with limited access to specialists, especially providers who serve in rural and non-industrial settings. Medical students, nurse practitioner students, and residents in a wide variety of specialties will also benefit from this knowledge.

This book is intended for an audience far different from that of most other plastic surgery texts. There are many remarkable books that describe advanced techniques commonplace in my home city of Los Angeles. These excellent volumes describe superb results obtained by elite surgeons working with expensive equipment.

This book describes practical techniques that may be easily learned by a variety of medical professionals who have access only to basic equipment. Plastic surgical procedures are described in a clear, concise, step-by-step fashion. Someone without advanced surgical skills can use this book and provide effective treatment. Illustrative cases are used to help the reader understand the importance of plastic surgery input in a variety of situations. Explanation is given as to when and why it may be prudent to transfer care to a specialist.

It is my hope that this book will provide a greater understanding of how plastic surgical techniques can contribute to improved patient outcomes. This, in turn, should allow many injured patients to regain normal function and their rightful place in the community.

Nadine B. Semer, MD
Los Angeles, California

Chapter 1

SUTURING: THE BASICS

Suturing is the joining of tissues with needle and "thread," so that the tissues bind together and heal. The "thread" is actually specialized suture material.

Health care providers frequently encounter wounds in need of suturing, and it is important to become proficient. You can practice your suturing skills on pigs' feet, available at a butcher shop. This chapter gives you all the necessary information to perform basic suturing, including:

• Types of needles and suture material

• Selection of material for various wounds and situations

• Techniques

Information about the proper use of local anesthetics for pain control while placing sutures is discussed in chapter 3.

Suture Needles

There are two broad classifications of needles: curved and straight. A straight needle can be used without instruments. A curved needle must be handled with forceps and a needle holder.

Although hand sewing with a straight needle does not require forceps, the technique is cumbersome and entails a much higher risk of accidentally sticking yourself. Hence, suturing with a straight needle is uncommon and not recommended if curved needles are available. Generally, forceps and needle holders are available, and a curved needle is used for suturing. There are two types of curved needles.

Cutting Needle.   A cutting needle is used primarily for suturing the skin. It has a very sharp tip with sharp edges, which are needed to pass through the skin. Since you will place primarily skin sutures, you generally will use a cutting needle.

Tapered Needle.   Tapered needles, or "round-bodied" needles, have a sharp tip with smooth edges and are less traumatic to the surrounding tissues. They are used primarily on the deeper, subcutaneous tissues, blood vessels, and intestinal anastomoses. A tapered needle is not good for simple skin suturing because it is difficult to pass the tapered needle through the skin.

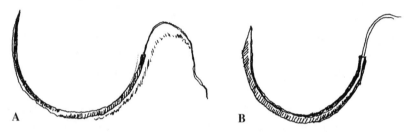

A, Tapered needle used for suturing subcutaneous tissue, fascia, and other deep structures. *B,* Cutting needle used for suturing skin. Note the difference specifically around the tip of each needle.

Suture Sizes

Sutures come in various sizes. The bigger the suture material, usually the bigger the needle. The sizing of sutures is similar to the sizing of needles for injection: the bigger the number, the smaller the size of the suture. Suture sizes range from 00 (very large, used to close the abdominal wall—about the size of large fishing line) to 10-0 (very tiny, used for microvascular anastomoses—as fine as a human hair). You generally will use sizes in the middle range: 3-0 to 5-0.

It is best to use small sutures on the face, such as 5-0 or 6-0. Smaller sutures are associated with decreased scarring, which is a concern with facial wounds. (See chapter 16, "Facial Lacerations," for more specific details.) On areas where cosmetic concerns are less important, 3-0 or 4-0 sutures are best, because the larger size makes the technique easier and the thicker sutures are stronger. The tendency is to use smaller sutures on children because of their more delicate skin. Rarely do you need anything larger than a 4-0 suture.

Suture Material

Many different suture materials are available. The main classifications are absorbable or nonabsorbable. A more subtle subclassification is whether the suture material is braided or nonbraided.

Unless there is a dire emergency, *never* use regular thread for sutures because of the risk of infection.

Nonabsorbable Sutures

Nonabsorbable sutures remain in place until they are removed. Because they are not dissolved by the body, they are less tissue-reactive and therefore leave less scarring as long as they are removed in a timely fashion. They are best used on the skin.

Absorbable Sutures

Absorbable sutures are dissolved by the body's tissues. The great advantage is that the sutures do not need to be removed. However, absorbable sutures tend to leave a more pronounced scar when used as skin sutures. Absorbable sutures are primarily used under the skin, where they are well hidden.

It is sometimes difficult to get patients to return for suture removal. If this is a concern, use an absorbable suture for skin closure. You should warn the patient that absorbable sutures probably will result in a more noticeable scar than nonabsorbable sutures with later removal.

Because it is often difficult to remove stitches from children (because of their crying and difficulty in staying still), absorbable materials should be used when suturing their wounds.

Braided Sutures

Braided sutures are made up of several thin strands of the suture material twisted together. Braided sutures are easier to tie than nonbraided sutures. However, braided sutures have little interstices in the suture material, which can be a place for bacteria to hide and grow, resulting in an increased risk of infection.

Nonbraided Sutures

Nonbraided sutures are simply a monofilament, a single strand. They are not made up of the little subunits found in a braided suture. Nonbraided sutures are recommended for most skin closures, especially wounds that may be at risk for infection.

Table 1.   Characteristics of the Most Commonly Used Suture Materials

Suture Material	Tissue Reaction	A or N	Braided	Non-Braided	Suture Strength	Primary Indication
Chromic catgut	+++	A	X		Lasts 3–4 wks at most	Facial wounds, lip/intraoral mucosa, children's wounds
Nylon	+	N		X	Loses 20% per year	Skin sutures
Polydioxa-none (PDS)	+	A		X	Lasts 4–6 mo	Intradermal sutures
Polyglycolic acid (Dexon)	++	A	X		Lasts about 1 mo	Intradermal sutures, sutures for fascia, muscle, mucosa, or subcutaneous tissue
Prolene	0	N		X	Lasts a long time	Skin sutures
Silk	+++	N	X		Loses strength within 1 yr	Very clean skin wounds, especially on eyelids

A = absorbable, N = nonabsorbable, 0 = no tissue reaction, +++ = highly reactive.

Suturing Techniques

When suturing the edges of a wound together, it is important to evert the skin edges—that is, to get the underlying dermis from both sides of the wound to touch. For the wound to heal, the dermal elements must meet and heal together. If the edges are inverted (the epidermis turns in and touches the epidermis of the other side), the wound will not heal as quickly or as well as you would like. The suture technique that you choose is important to achieve optimal wound healing.

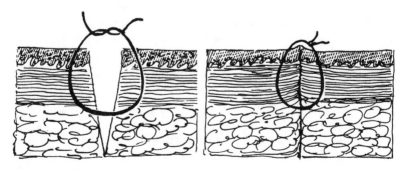

Sutures should be placed so that the skin edges are everted to ensure that the dermis is touching. This technique is important for proper healing. (From McCarthy JG (ed): Plastic Surgery. Philadelphia, W.B. Saunders, 1990, with permission.)

Instruments Needed

Needle holder: used to grab onto the suture needle

Forceps: used to hold the tissues gently and to grab the needle

Suture scissors: used to cut the stitch from the rest of the suture material

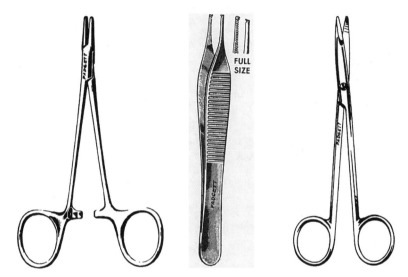

Left, Needle holder. *Center*, Forceps with teeth. *Right*, Suture scissors. (Courtesy of Padgett Instruments, Inc.)

How to Hold the Instruments

Whenever you use sharp instruments, you face the risk of accidentally sticking yourself. Needlesticks are especially hazardous because of the risk of serious infection (hepatitis, human immunodeficiency virus). To prevent needlesticks, get in the habit of using the instruments correctly. *Never handle the suture needle with your fingers.*

Scissors.   Place your thumb and ring finger in the holes. It is best to cut with the tips of the scissors so that you do not accidentally injure any surrounding structures or tissue (which may happen if you cut with the center part of the scissors).

Needle Holder.   Place your thumb and ring finger in the holes. When using the needle holder, be sure to grab the needle until you hear the clasp engage, ensuring that the needle is securely held. You grab the needle at its half-way point, with the tip pointing upward. Try not to grab the tip; it will become blunt if grabbed by the needle holder. Then it will be difficult to pass the tip through the skin.

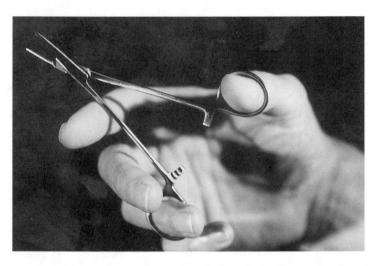

The needle holder and scissors are handled similarly. For maximal control, place the tips of your thumb and ring finger into the rings of the instrument. Your thumb does most of the work to open and close the instrument.

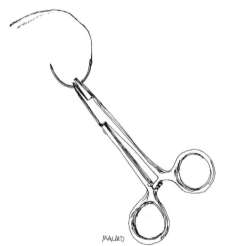

The needle should be held in the jaws of the needle holder at its midpoint (where the curve of the needle is relatively flat). This technique prevents you from bending the needle as it passes through the tissues.

Forceps.   Hold the forceps like a writing utensil. The forceps is used to support the skin edges when you place the sutures. Be careful not to grab the skin too hard, or you will leave marks that can lead to scarring. Ideally, you should grab the dermis or subcutaneous tissue—not the skin—with the forceps, but this technique takes practice. For suturing skin, try to use forceps with teeth, which are little pointed edges at the end of the forceps.

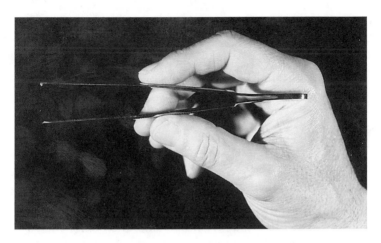

Hold the forceps as you would hold a writing instrument.

Placing the Sutures

For most areas of the body, except the face (see chapter 16, "Facial Lacerations"), the sutures should be placed in the skin 3–4 mm from the wound edge and 5–10 mm apart.

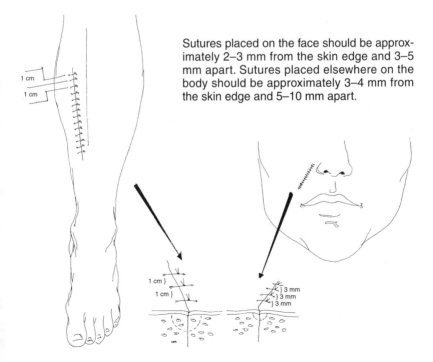

Sutures placed on the face should be approximately 2–3 mm from the skin edge and 3–5 mm apart. Sutures placed elsewhere on the body should be approximately 3–4 mm from the skin edge and 5–10 mm apart.

Start on the side of the wound opposite and farthest from you to ensure that you are always sewing toward yourself. By sewing toward yourself, the suturing process is made easier from a biomechanical standpoint.

Do not drive yourself crazy by placing too many sutures.

Simple Sutures

Indication.   This technique is the easiest to perform. It is used for most skin suturing.

Technique

1. Start from the outside of the skin, go through the epidermis into the subcutaneous tissue from one side, then enter the subcutaneous tissue on the opposite side, and come out the epidermis above.

2. To evert the edges, the needle tip should enter at a 90° angle to the skin. Then turn your wrist to get the needle through the tissues.

3. You can use simple sutures for a continuous or interrupted closure.

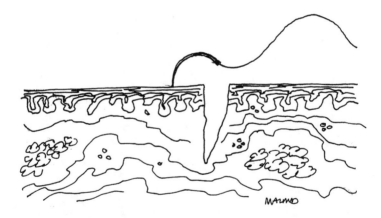

MALMO

The needle tip should enter the tissues perpendicular to the skin. Once the needle tip has penetrated through the top layers of the skin, twist your wrist so that the needle passes through the subcutaneous tissue and then comes out into the wound. This technique helps to ensure that skin edges will evert.

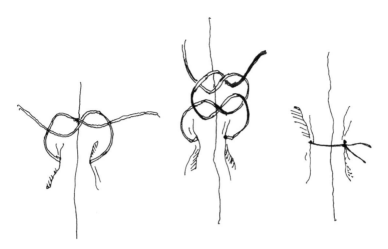

A simple suture.

Interrupted or Continuous Closure

Interrupted Sutures

- Interrupted sutures are individually placed and tied.

- They are the technique of choice if you are worried about the cleanliness of the wound.

- If the wound looks like it is becoming infected, a few sutures can be removed easily without disrupting the entire closure.

- Interrupted sutures can be used in all areas but may take longer to place than a continuous suture.

Continuous Closure

- Place the sutures again and again without tying each individual suture.

- If the wound is very clean and it is easy to bring the edges together, a continuous closure is adequate and quicker to perform.

- Continuous closure is the technique of choice to help stop bleeding from the skin edges, which is important, for example, in a scalp laceration.

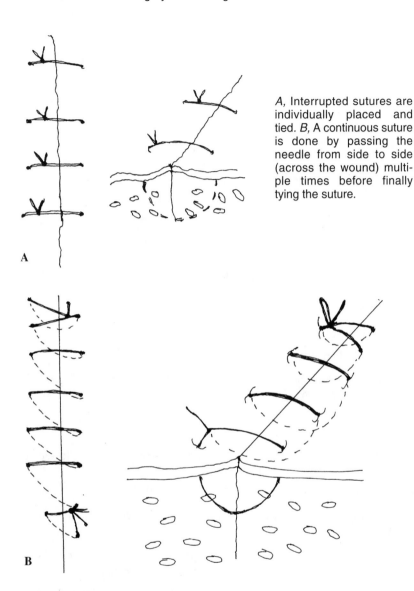

A, Interrupted sutures are individually placed and tied. *B*, A continuous suture is done by passing the needle from side to side (across the wound) multiple times before finally tying the suture.

Mattress Sutures

Indication.   Mattress sutures are a good choice when the skin edges are difficult to evert. Sometimes you may want to close a wound with a few scattered mattress sutures and place simple sutures between them. It is a bit more technically challenging to place mattress sutures, but it is often worth the effort because good dermis-to-dermis contact is achieved.

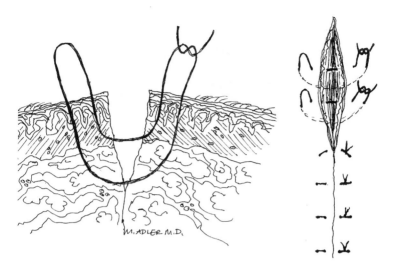

The vertical mattress suture.

Technique

1. Start like a simple suture, go from the outside of the skin through the epidermis into the subcutaneous tissue from one side, then enter the subcutaneous tissue on the opposite side, and come out the epidermis above.

2. Turn the needle in the opposite direction and go from outside the skin on the side that you just exited and come out the dermis below. Then enter the dermis on the opposite side and come out of the epidermis above.

3. Your suture is now back on the side on which you started.

Buried Intradermal Sutures

Indication.   This technique is useful for wide, gaping wounds and when it is difficult to evert the skin edges. When buried intradermal sutures are placed properly, they make skin closure much easier. The purpose of this stitch is to line up the dermis and thus enhance healing. The knot needs to be as deep into the tissues as possible (hence the term *buried*) so that it does not come up through the epidermis and cause irritation and pain.

Technique

1. Use a cutting needle and absorbable material.

2. Start just under the dermal layer and come out below the epidermis. You are going from deep to more superficial tissues.

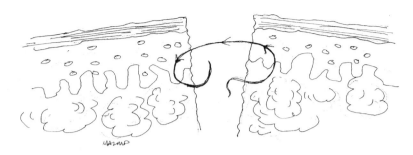

Buried intradermal suture.

3. Now the technique becomes a bit challenging. You need to enter the skin on the opposite side at a depth similar to where you exited the skin on the first side, just below the epidermis. To do so, you should position the needle with the tip pointing down and pronate your wrist to get the correct angle. It will help to use the forceps (in the other hand) to hold up the skin. The needle should come out of the tissues below the dermis. Try to get as little fat in the stitch as possible; it does not contribute to the suture.

4. Tie the suture.

Figure-of-eight Sutures

Indication.   This technique is useful for bringing together underlying tissues such as muscle, fascia, or extensor tendons. It is not commonly used for skin closure.

Technique

1. Usually a tapered needle and absorbable sutures are used.

2. Start on the side opposite from you. Go through the full thickness of tissues on that side, then finish the first half of the stitch by going from bottom to top on the opposite side. Advance just a little farther (1.0–1.5 cm) along the tissue. The needle should now be back on top of the tissue.

3. Now enter the first side (going from top to bottom) just across from the suture on the other side. Again go through the full thickness of the tissue and come out on the undersurface of the tissue.

4. Now enter the undersurface of the other side even with the first suture and come out on top.

5. The suture can now be easily tied.

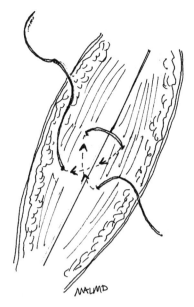

Figure-of-eight suture. This technique is used primarily to reapproximate deep tissues such as muscle or fascia.

Tying the Suture

The simplest way to tie the suture is by doing an "instrument tie," described below.

Simple Sutures

1. Pull the suture through the skin so that just a short amount of suture material (a few centimeters) is left out.

2. Take the needle out of the needle holder.

3. Place your needle holder in the center between the skin edges parallel to the wound. One end of the suture should be on each side of the wound without crossing in the middle.

4. Wrap the suture that is attached to the needle once or twice around the needle holder in a clockwise direction.

5. Grab the short end of the suture with the needle holder.

6. Pull it through the loops, and have the knot lie flat. The short end of the stitch should now be on the opposite side.

7. Let go of the short end.

8. Bring the needle holder back to the center, parallel to the wound edges.

9. Repeat steps 4–8 at least one or two times more.

10. Cut the suture ends about 1 cm from the knot.

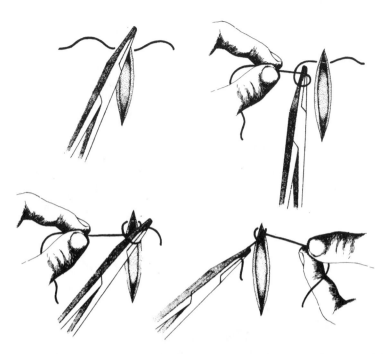

Instrument tie. Two loops of suture are wrapped around the distal portion of the needle holder, and the free end of the suture is then grasped and pulled through the loop thus formed. A third suture loop is wrapped around the needle holder in the opposite direction and pulled in a direction opposite to the first tie to form a square knot. Note that the short end of the suture switches sides as it is passed through the loop to create each knot. (From Simon RR, Brenner BE (eds): Emergency Procedures and Techniques, 3rd ed. Philadelphia, Lippincott Williams & Wilkins, 1994, with permission.)

Mattress Sutures

1. Pull the suture through the skin so that just a short amount of suture material (a few centimeters) is left out.
2. Take the needle out of the needle holder.
3. Both ends of the suture are on the same side. Place your needle holder between the ends of the suture.
4. Wrap the suture that is attached to the needle once or twice around the needle holder in a clockwise direction.
5. Grab the short end with the needle holder.
6. Pull it through the loops, and have the knot lie flat. The short end of the stitch should now be on the opposite side.
7. Let go of the short end.

8. Bring the needle holder back to the center, between the suture ends.

9. Repeat steps 4–8 at least one or two times more.

10. Cut the suture ends about 1 cm from the knot.

Continuous Suture

1. Do not pull the next to-the-last stitch all the way through; leave it as a loop.

2. Place your needle holder between the loop and the suture attached to the needle. The needle holder should be almost perpendicular to the wound.

3. Wrap the suture that is attached to the needle once or twice around the needle holder in a clockwise direction.

4. Grab the loop with the needle holder.

5. Pull it through, and have the knot lie flat. The short loop should now be on the opposite side.

6. Let go of the loop.

7. Bring the needle holder back to the center between the loop and the suture end.

8. Repeat steps 3–7 at least one or two times more.

9. Cut the suture ends about 1 cm from the knot.

Suture Removal

If the sutures are taken out within 7–10 days, suture removal is usually easy and should not cause more than a pinching sensation to the patient. (See chapter 11, "Primary Closure," for more details concerning the timing of suture removal.)

Simple Sutures

1. Cut the suture where it is exposed, crossing the wound edges.

2. Remove the entire stitch by grabbing the knot with a clamp or forceps and pulling gently.

Mattress Sutures

Removal of mattress sutures can be a little more difficult.

1. Grab the knot and try to lift it up a little; this should allow you to see a space between the suture strands.

2. Cut one strand of the suture under the knot.

3. Remove the entire stitch by grabbing the knot with a clamp or forceps and pulling gently. This suture will be a little harder to remove than a simple suture.

4. If you accidentally cut both ends of the suture, you will leave suture material behind.

5. Look on the opposite side of the skin for the suture. Grab it with a clamp or forceps, and gently remove the remaining suture material.

Continuous Sutures

1. Cut the suture in several places where it is exposed, crossing the wound edges.

2. Remove portions of the stitch by grabbing an end with a clamp or forceps and pulling gently.

3. The sutures to the knot must be cut in several places for removal.

Alternatives to Suturing

Other techniques can bring skin edges together to "suture" a wound closed without using sutures. These techniques require more expensive equipment than regular suturing.

Skin Stapler

Indication.   The skin stapler is a medical device that places metal staples across the skin edges to bring the skin together. The area must be anesthetized before placing the staples. The main advantage of staples over sutures is that they can be placed quickly. Speed may be an important advantage when you need to close a bleeding wound quickly (e.g., on the scalp) to decrease blood loss. Staples tend to leave more noticeable marks in the skin compared with sutures. They should not be used on the face.

Technique

1. The edges must be everted. Usually an assistant must help by using forceps to hold the skin edges so that the dermis on each side touches.

2. Place the center of the stapler (usually an arrow on the stapler marks the center) at the point where the skin edges come together.

3. Gently touch the stapler to the skin; you do not have to push it into the skin. Then grasp the handle to compress it; the compression releases the staple.

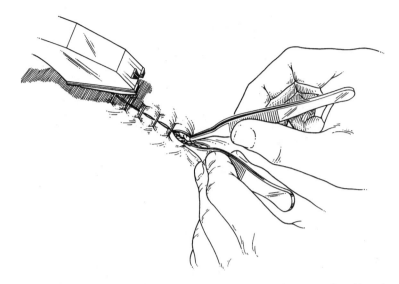

Close the skin with clips. The stapler should be centered over the skin edges before the staple is released. Be sure that the skin is everted. (From Skandala-kis JE, et al (eds): Hernia Surgical Anatomy and Technique. New York, McGraw-Hill, 1989, with permission.)

4. Release the handle, and move the stapler a few millimeters back to separate the staple from the stapling device.

5. The staples should be placed about 1 cm apart.

To Remove the Staples

A staple remover device can be used to remove the staples easily (see figures on next page). Put the jaws under the staple, and close the device. This bends the staple and allows it to be removed.

If you do not have a staple remover, a clamp can be placed under the staple. Then open the clamp to bend the staple so that it can be removed. Removing a staple in this fashion can be painful.

Adhesives

Specialized surgical adhesive materials allow the skin edges to be "glued" together. The advantage of adhesives is that the wound does not need to be anesthetized for closure. However, a traumatic wound must be thoroughly cleaned before closure, which often requires local anesthetic. Thus, this advantage may be only theoretical.

Adhesive compounds are quite expensive, and the quality of the resultant scar has still not been fully evaluated and compared with the scar

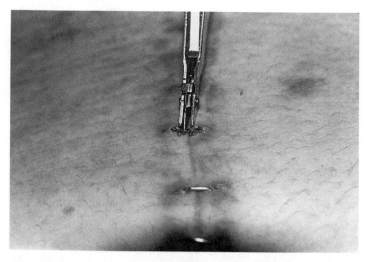

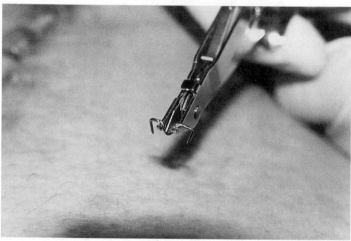

Removing a staple with a staple remover.

from a properly sutured wound. Thus only adhesive tapes are further discussed. *Never use regular household adhesives to try to close a wound.*

Adhesive Tapes

Adhesive tapes often are placed after sutures are removed to help keep the skin closure from separating. They also can be used as a means of closure for relatively small wounds whose edges easily come together.

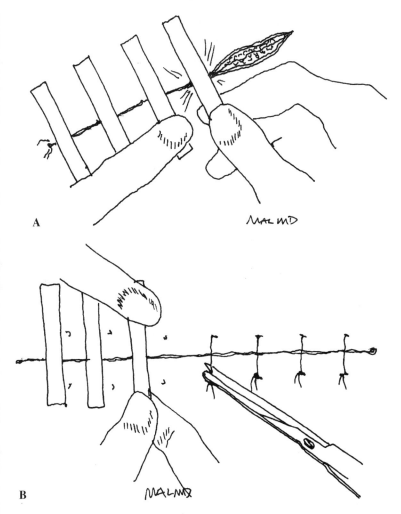

A, Closing the wound with adhesive strips. *B,* Placing adhesive strips to reinforce wound closure when sutures are removed.

After thoroughly cleansing the wound, gently hold the skin edges together with your fingers or a forceps. Cut the tape so that at least 2–3 cm are on each side of the skin edge once the tape is in place.

Place tape strips one at a time, several millimeters apart. The tapes should be placed across (perpendicular to) the long axis of the wound. Tapes stay in place for several days and should be allowed to fall off on their own. The patient can wash the area but should do so gently.

Bibliography

1. Edgerton M: The Art of Surgical Technique. Baltimore, Williams & Wilkins, 1988.
2. McCarthy JG: Introduction to plastic surgery. In McCarthy JG (ed): Plastic Surgery. Philadelphia, W.B. Saunders, 1990, pp 48–54.

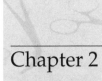

Chapter 2

BASIC SURGICAL TECHNIQUES

The previous chapter discussed suturing techniques. This chapter describes additional basic surgical skills. All rural healthcare providers should be proficient in these techniques.

Making an Incision

Many of the procedures explained in subsequent chapters of this book involve making incisions into the skin. Whether it be to remove a suspicious lesion or to create a flap for wound coverage, you must learn how to make an incision safely and efficiently. You will use a knife with a very sharp blade. It is important to know how to use the knife properly to prevent accidental injury to the patient or yourself.

Which Blade to Use

Knife blades come in various sizes (see figure below). There is no orderly scale to follow as with needle sizes. A no. 11 blade comes to a sharp point, whereas a no. 15 blade has a rounded end. A no. 10 blade is twice the size of the no. 15, and a no. 20 blade is bigger than the no. 10. It can be confusing, but most blades come with a picture on the packaging.

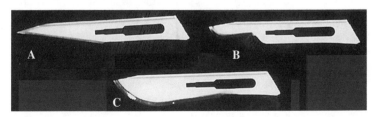

Commonly used knife blades. *A*, no. 11 blade; *B*, no. 15 blade; *C*, no. 10 blade.

Table 1. Deciding Which Blade to Use

Blade Size	Optimal Setting for Use*
No. 11	Draining an abscess, performing a shave biopsy
No. 15	Performing a biopsy, making incisions < 5 cm, any incisions on the face
Nos. 10, 20	Making incisions longer than 5 cm, debriding wounds

* This table describes the optimal knife blade to use if you have a choice of sizes. If you do not have the luxury of choice, any blade can be used for almost any situation.

Holding the Knife

For safety, use a blade only when it is attached to a handle. Some disposable knives come with the blade already attached to the handle. When they are not available, you may have to put the blade onto a knife handle yourself. Never touch the blade with your fingers; it is very sharp. Use a clamp or needle holder to grasp the blade, and position it onto the handle.

Hold the handle with your dominant hand, as if you were using a writing instrument. To have the best control over the instrument, hold the handle 3–4 cm away from where the blade meets the handle.

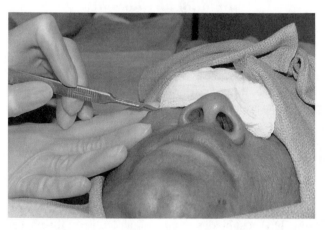

Hold the knife like a writing instrument 3–4 cm behind the point where the blade meets the handle.

Using the Knife

When you are about to make the incision, place the tissue under some tension. Use the index finger and thumb of your nondominant hand to push down on the skin, spread it apart, and make the skin taut. This technique makes the skin easier to incise.

Make the incision with the flat part of the knife, not the very tip. Push the blade down with just enough pressure to cut through the skin. You do not have to go exactly to the proper depth with the first cut. It is better to be too timid than too forceful. If you use too much force to make the incision, your knife may penetrate too deeply into the tissues and accidentally cut an important structure.

Which Side to Incise First

When you have to make two incisions (for example, to remove a suspicious skin lesion), look at their orientation. If they are to be made one above the other (for example, if you are working on the side of the leg), do the bottom skin incision first. If the top incision is made first, blood from the skin edges will drip down and obscure the area below. The presence of the blood makes it more difficult to perform the lower incision.

What to Do about Bleeding from the Skin Edges

1. **Apply pressure.** Most bleeding from skin edges stops on its own after pressure is applied over the area for a few minutes with a gauze pad.

2. **If you have access to an electrocautery device.** An electrocautery device applies an electrical current that coagulates the tissue and stops bleeding. When this device is used, the patient must be attached to a grounding pad. Wipe away the blood, and touch the bleeding spot with the cautery device. The bleeding usually stops. If you see bleeding from a small blood vessel, grab it with the tips of a metal clamp. Then touch the clamp with the cautery device. Be sure that the clamp is not touching any surrounding tissue. The current will pass through the clamp and burn the surrounding tissue as well.

Caution: Be sure that your gloves are intact before touching the clamp with the cautery device. If you have a hole in the glove on the hand holding the clamp, you will get zapped when you touch the clamp with the cautery device. You may experience a painful, small burn in your finger or even feel the electric current pass through your body.

3. **Close the wound with a continuous locking suture.** This technique places more tension on the skin edges than the usual continuous closure and often stops the bleeding. A continuous locking suture is often quite useful to control a bleeding scalp wound.

How to Place Continuous Locking Sutures

For the typical continuous suture technique, the thread should always remain *behind* the needle. With the locking technique, the thread lies *in front of* the needle as it comes out of the tissues. The suture, therefore, comes out of the tissues inside the loop. When the stitch is pulled through the loop, it places the suture material along the outside skin edge, putting pressure on the tissue. The pressure helps to control bleeding.

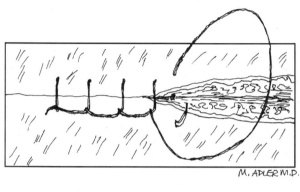

M. ADLER M.D.

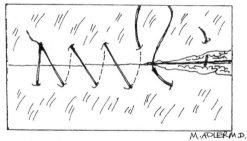

M. ADLER M.D.

Top, Continuous locking suture. *Bottom*, Continuous nonlocking suture. Note the differences in where the suture loop comes out of the skin relative to the needle as well as the appearance of the sutures on the skin.

How to Manage Bleeding from a Blood Vessel

1. **Apply pressure.** Application of pressure is always a good first choice. It prevents further blood loss and may allow the vessel to clot, thereby stopping the bleeding. Try this technique for at least 5–7 minutes. If it is unsuccessful, the following alternatives should be tried.

2. **If you have access to an electrocautery unit.** If the vessel is a vein or small (1–2 mm) artery, grab it with the tips of a metal clamp and touch the clamp with the cautery device. Be sure that your gloves are intact and that the clamp is applied only to the vessel.

3. **If you do not have access to an electrocautery unit or if the vessel is a larger vein or larger (3–4 mm) artery**, the end of the vessel should be tied off with a suture for secure hemostasis. There are two basic techniques for tying off a vessel (see figures on following pages).

Regular Tie

Regular ties are adequate for most veins and small (2–3 mm) arteries. Grasp the end of the vessel with a small clamp, and gently hold the vessel away from the surrounding tissues. Pass a piece of 3-0 or 4-0 silk or Vicryl suture material (the needle is not needed) around the vessel and under the clamp. Tie the suture securely, placing at least 3 or 4 knots.

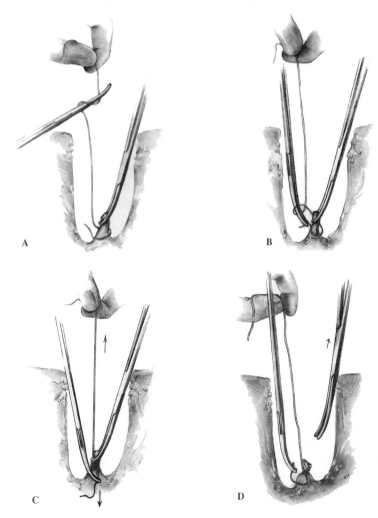

Four major steps *(A–D)* in tying off a vessel with the regular stitch. (From Edgerton M: The Art of Surgical Technique. Baltimore, Williams & Wilkins, 1988, with permission.)

Stick Tie

A stick tie is a more secure technique to control bleeding from a blood vessel. It is especially useful for arteries, because the thicker wall and increased interior pressure of an artery can cause a regular tie to come off of the vessel.

Grasp the end of the artery with a small clamp, and gently lift the vessel. Use a 3-0 or 4-0 silk or Vicryl suture with a needle (a tapered needle is best). Pass the needle through the center of the vessel just under the clamp. Bring both ends of the suture toward yourself (again, under the clamp), and tie the suture securely (just once).

Now take one of the suture ends and pass it completely around the vessel, making sure to pass the string under the clamp. Again, tie the suture. As you are tightening it, remove the clamp. Finish with 3–4 more knots.

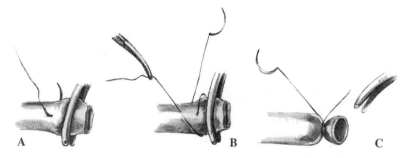

Stick tie: a more secure way to control bleeding from a blood vessel. (From Edgerton M: Art of Surgical Technique. Baltimore, Williams & Wilkins, 1988, with permission.)

Blunt Dissection

Blunt dissection is a technique for gently separating tissues while avoiding injury to important nearby structures such as blood vessels, nerves, or veins. Unless you use too much force, subcutaneous tissue and muscle will separate easily, while the surrounding nerves, vessels, and tendons will remain intact. For healthcare providers with limited surgical skills, blunt dissection is the technique of choice for separating tissues (for example, in exploring a wound or operating on a hand).

Blunt Dissection Technique

Insert the closed blunt tips of a scissors or the closed jaws of a clamp into the tissues (to a depth of approximately 1–2 cm). Then gently open the instrument. This action separates the tissues. Any fibrotic connections that are not important structures can then be safely cut with the scissors. Repeat these maneuvers as needed.

Alternatively, you can gently use your index finger covered with a gauze pad to separate tissues. This technique is especially useful for elevating a skin flap off an underlying muscle.

Sharp Dissection

Sharp dissection is a technique for separating the tissues using a knife or scissors. You must be careful not to cut accidentally an important structure. For healthcare providers without surgical expertise, sharp dissection should be used primarily in emergencies, for making a hole in the neck to create an airway, or for trying to enlarge a deep hole to control life-threatening bleeding. In addition, sharp dissection is used for undermining tissues (see below) or excising a lesion.

Undermining Skin Edges

To undermine skin edges, you cut beneath the skin along the edge of a wound to free the skin from its deep tissue attachments. The purpose is to increase skin mobility, which is important for a tension-free wound closure. It is also a necessary skill for performing local flaps.

Technique

Pinch the tissues around the edge of the wound with the forceps to ensure that the local anesthetic is still working. Give additional anesthetic as required. Lift the skin edge with the forceps, and with a knife or a scissors cut into the deep subcutaneous tissue along the length of the wound (try to stay at the same depth) until the skin has the required mobility.

An alternative method involves separating the skin and subcutaneous tissue from the underlying muscle. The plane of dissection is just above the fascia, the thin layer of connective tissue that overlies the muscle. By undermining the skin along this deeper plane, you may encounter less bleeding than if you cut directly into the subcutaneous tissue layer.

Bibliography

Edgerton M: The Art of Surgical Technique. Baltimore, Williams & Wilkins, 1988.

Chapter 3

LOCAL ANESTHESIA

Full surgical evaluation of a wound and suture placement can be quite painful. You must anesthetize the injured area to perform these procedures properly. The administration of a local anesthetic allows you to evaluate and treat wounds in the emergency department or clinic. If you are unable to attain adequate pain control, the patient should be taken to the operating room for exploration under general anesthesia.

Local anesthetics work by reversibly blocking nerve conduction. They primarily block the sensation of sharp pain; they do not block pressure sensation. Therefore, in an area that has been adequately anesthetized, the patient will not feel the sharp needle stick during suture placement but may feel a vague sensation of pressure. This information should be shared with the patient.

The duration of effect depends on how long the agent stays in the immediate working area before being absorbed into the circulation or broken down by the surrounding tissues.

Topical Agents

Topical agents (agents applied on top of the surrounding skin and absorbed into the area to provide anesthesia without injections) are now available. However, they are quite expensive and can be used only on the surface, not deep within an open wound. They can be quite effective for performing simple excisions or starting intravenous lines. Although topical agents may become important in the future, because of their expense and limited usefulness, they are not discussed further in this chapter.

Application of cold works for only a few minutes but may allow enough time to place one or two stitches. Cold also may help by decreasing the pain of local anesthetic injection. It can be especially useful in children. Have the patient hold ice over the area for 5 minutes before injection. Another way to apply cold is to spray the area with ethyl chloride solution.

Injectable Local Anesthetics

The easiest and most reliable way to anesthetize a wound is to inject a local anesthetic. There are two techniques: (1) direct injection of the local anesthetic agent into the area around the wound and (2) injection of the anesthetic agent around a sensory nerve that supplies sensation to the injured area. Both methods are addressed below, but first the two most commonly used anesthetic agents are discussed. Neither needs to be refrigerated, which is important in the rural setting.

Lidocaine (Lignocaine)

Lidocaine is the most commonly used and least expensive agent. The usual total dose that can safely be given is 3–5 mg/kg body weight. Do not give more than this amount at one time. The anesthesia becomes effective after 5–10 minutes and lasts, on average, from 45 minutes to 1 hour.

Bupivacaine (Marcaine)

Bupivacaine is a longer-acting agent than lidocaine, but it is also more expensive. The usual total dose that can safely be administered at one time is 2.0–3.0 mg/kg. Bupivacaine takes a few minutes longer to become effective than lidocaine (10–15 vs. 5–10 minutes), but its effect can last 2–4 hours.

The longer duration of effect can be valuable. Some wounds take more than 1 hour to clean and suture. In addition, bupivacaine gives residual pain control after the procedure is completed. Hand injuries are especially prone to pain, making bupivacaine a good choice for treating hand and finger injuries.

If both lidocaine and bupivacaine are available, they can be mixed together in equal parts and administered with one syringe. This combination gives the advantages of the quicker onset of anesthesia from the lidocaine with the longer duration of action of the bupivacaine.

Calculating the Amount to Administer

To calculate the mg dose, multiply the ml of solution that you plan to give by the concentration of the solution (mg/ml). The following table converts the commercially available anesthetic solutions to the mg/ml concentration of the anesthetic agent.

Concentration of Agent in Commercially Available Anesthetic Solutions

Agent	Commercial Solution (%)	Concentration (mg/ml)
Lidocaine	0.5	5
	1.0	10
	2.0	20
Bupivacaine	0.25	2.5
	0.50	5.0

Example: You expect to inject 30 ml of 1.0% lidocaine to anesthetize a relatively large wound:

$$30 \text{ ml} \times 10 \text{ mg/ml} = 300 \text{ mg of lidocaine}$$

The patient is a 70-kg man. A 70-kg man can receive 3–5 mg/kg or 210–350 mg of lidocaine. Your 30-ml dose is on the high end of the "safe" range.

Additives

It is sometimes useful to add additional drugs to the local anesthetic solutions to optimize their effect.

Bicarbonate

Both lidocaine and bupivacaine are acidic and therefore painful when injected. One way to lessen this pain is to add injectable sodium bicarbonate to the local anesthetic solution. Your patient will be grateful for this extra step. It is essential to use commercially prepared bicarbonate for injections. Do not try home-grown formulations. Be careful: adding too much bicarbonate to the anesthetic solution can lead to the formation of crystals. The proper mixtures are as follows:

- Lidocaine: add 1 ml of bicarbonate to each 9 ml of lidocaine before injection.
- Bupivacaine: add 1 ml of bicarbonate to each 19 ml of bupivacaine before injection.

Epinephrine

Epinephrine is a vasoconstrictor that shrinks blood vessels and thus reduces bleeding from the wound and surrounding skin edges. This makes wound examination and repair easier to perform. Epinephrine also decreases absorption of the anesthetic agent, which may allow safe injection of more than the usually recommended amount of anesthetic agent. Epinephrine requires 5–7 minutes to take effect. The maximal dosages of lidocaine and bupivacaine with epinephrine are as follows:

- Lidocaine with epinephrine increases to 7 mg/kg, and its effect lasts 1½–2 hours.

- Bupivacaine with epinephrine: dosing essentially stays the same at 2.0–3.0 mg/kg, and its effect still lasts 2–4 hours.

Lidocaine and bupivacaine are available in solutions premixed with epinephrine , but you can add it to the anesthetic solution yourself. Be very careful, however, because the amount of epinephrine to add is very small:

1. Add 0.25 ml of 1:1000 epinephrine to 50 ml of local agent (50 ml is the usual-sized vial). This will give a 1:200,000 dilution—safe for most procedures.

2. Err on the side of adding a little less rather than a little more if you are drawing the epinephrine with a syringe larger than 1 ml.

Contraindications to Adding Epinephrine

In certain circumstances the vasoconstricting effects of epinephrine can be detrimental and may lead to tissue loss. Examples include:

- Digital block (numbing the whole finger)
- On the tip of the nose
- On the penis
- Injury that results in a very ragged and irregular laceration. Epinephrine worsens the already compromised circulation of the skin edges.

Indications for Adding Epinephrine

- Straight cut with healthy-looking skin edges
- On the face, oral mucosa, and scalp, which have excellent blood circulation

Overview of Anesthetic Agents: Dosage and Duration of Action

Agents	Maximal dose (mg/kg)	Duration of Action
Lidocaine plain	3–5	45–60 min
Lidocaine with epinephrine*	5–7	1.5–2 hr
Marcaine plain	2.0–3.0	2–4 hr
Marcaine with epinephrine	2.0–3.0	2–4 hr

* You can add the same amount of bicarbonate to solutions with epinephrine as you add to plain solutions without epinephrine (see above for proper amounts).

Safety Hints

Caution about injections: It is quite dangerous to insert the syringe needle in the wrong place and inject the solution into an artery by mistake. A good habit to develop when giving any type of injection is to *draw back on the syringe (i.e., pull back on the plunger) before injecting the solution.* If you draw back and get blood, reposition the needle and draw back again. This technique prevents an accidental intra-arterial injection, which can cause serious complications. If you draw back blood with the initial insertion, you have not created a major problem. Because you are using a small needle, you should not do significant damage to the blood vessel, but you may need to hold pressure over the area for a few minutes to decrease bruising.

Caution about maximal safe dosage: Be aware of how much you are injecting to avoid exceeding the safe doses. Average-sized wounds (up to 4–5 cm) usually present no problem, but it is easy to forget about dosage concerns when you are working on larger wounds. All anesthetic agents have systemic as well as local effects. The safe dosage is based on the total weight of the patient (thus the maximal doses are given as mg of agent/kg of patient body weight). Overdose can lead to seizures and even cardiovascular collapse or death due to the myocardial depressant and vasodilator effects of these agents.

How to Administer the Local Anesthetic

Direct Infiltration Around the Wound

In many cases, injecting the anesthetic agent around the wound is an easy and reliable way to anesthetize the area. It is best to use as small a needle as possible. The bigger the number, the smaller the needle: use a 25- or 27-gauge needle, and inject slowly. Injection of the anesthetic agent can be painful, and a slower injection rate causes less pain.

You can inject directly into the wound to get the anesthetic into the surrounding skin if the wound is reasonably clean. Alternatively, inject in the noninjured skin along the outside of the wound. Inject until you see the skin start to swell.

One technique is to push the needle into the tissues completely to the hub, and then slowly infiltrate the anesthetic as you bring the needle out of the tissues. Be sure to allow enough time for the agent to take effect before starting your procedure (at least 5 minutes).

Nerve Blocks

In some areas of the body, discrete nerves that are responsible for sensation to the injured area are easy to locate. In these instances, local anesthesia can be infiltrated around (*not* into) the sensory nerve for pain control to the area around the wound. This approach is advantageous because the patient needs to undergo fewer injections than if you anesthetize the entire wound margins directly.

Nerve blocks are also a good choice when the wound is deep, because they often give a more complete block of the entire area, not just the skin. This approach is especially appropriate for larger wounds, because it usually requires less anesthetic agent than direct infiltration.

Whenever possible, use a relatively small needle (23- or 25-gauge) for the injection. *Always draw back on the syringe before injecting the anesthetic*. The nerves that you are blocking often are located near blood vessels.

Caution: You are probably injecting the anesthetic directly into the nerve if the patient complains of strong electric shocks or severe pain radiating along the distribution of the nerve. Stop the injection *immediately* and reposition the needle.

It usually takes a few minutes longer for the anesthetic to take effect than with direct wound injection. Often you must wait 10–15 minutes after giving a nerve block before proceeding with the procedure.

Nerve Blocks for Hand Injuries

Lidocaine, bupivacaine, or a combination of the two solutions can be used. Add bicarbonate if it is available. Epinephrine should *not* be used for anesthetizing the hand and fingers.

Digital Block

A digital block is the best way to evaluate and treat a wound on the finger. The digital nerves supply sensation to the volar and dorsal surfaces of the finger.

Anatomy.   Each finger and the thumb have two digital nerves that travel with the digital vessels along the lateral and medial sides of the digit. Look at your own finger from the side, bend it at the two joints (distal interphalangeal [DIP] and proximal interphalangeal [PIP] joints). The line that connects the joint creases is a good estimate of where each digital nerve runs.

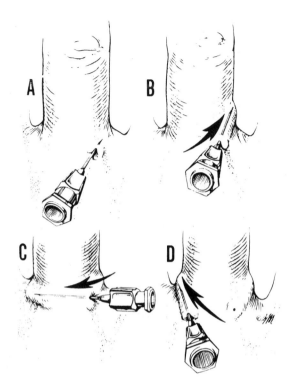

Digital nerve block, dorsal approach. Care must be taken to ensure that the anesthetic is not injected entirely circumferentially around the finger. (Illustration by Elizabeth Roselius. From Green DP, et al: Operative Hand Surgery, 4th ed. New York, Churchill Livingstone, 1999, with permission.)

Procedure

1. The injection is done from the dorsal (not volar) surface near the metacarpophalangeal (MCP) knuckle.

2. Insert the needle into the web space, when present (the thumb and little finger are not bordered on both sides by web spaces).

3. Aim the needle toward the MCP joint of the affected finger, moving in a volar direction.

4. Be careful not to inject too superficially on the volar side, or your injection will miss the area around the nerve.

5. Inject 2–3 ml of solution into each side of the affected finger.

6. Infiltrate 1–2 ml along the dorsal skin of the digit, just distal to the MCP knuckle.

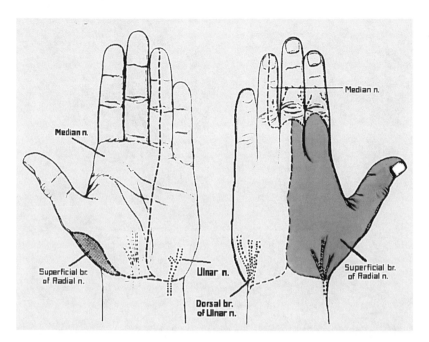

Pattern of sensory innervation of major peripheral nerves. (From Jurkiewicz MJ, et al (eds): Plastic Surgery: Principles and Practice. St. Louis, Mosby, 1990, with permission.)

Wrist Block

Three nerves supply sensation to the hand: the median nerve, ulnar nerve, and superficial branch of the radial nerve. If you infiltrate around all three nerves, you effectively anesthetize the entire hand. If an injury is within the distribution of any one or two nerves, simply infiltrate around the nerves that you need to anesthetize, based on the injury.

Median Nerve

The median nerve supplies sensation to the volar surface of the hand, from the lateral half of the ring finger to the thumb, and to the dorsal aspect of the fingers distal to the PIP joint, from the lateral half of the ring finger to the thumb.

Anatomy. At the wrist the median nerve lies between the palmaris longus (PL) and flexor carpi radialis (FCR) tendons. If the PL is absent (15% of the population), the landmark for injection is just medial to the FCR tendon.

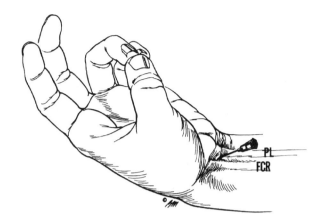

Wrist block, median nerve. PL = palmaris longus, FCR = flexor carpi radialis. (Illustration by Elizabeth Roselius. From Green DP, et al (eds): Operative Hand Surgery, 4th ed. New York, Churchill Livingstone, 1999, with permission.)

Procedure

1. Have the patient flex the wrist. The FCR and PL (if present) become noticeable in the distal forearm; the FCR is the more lateral of the two tendons.

2. Insert the needle just proximal to the wrist crease and medial to the FCR tendon.

3. *Draw back on the syringe and slowly inject 3–5 ml of anesthetic in the tissues deep to the skin.*

4. If the patient describes minor tingling, the needle is in the proper position. If the patient describes electric shocks or severe pain, the needle may be in the nerve. Stop injecting the anesthetic, and back the needle out a few mm before continuing to inject the anesthetic solution. *Do not inject the anesthetic directly into the nerve.*

Ulnar Nerve

The ulnar nerve supplies the remainder of the volar surface of the hand and the volar and dorsal surfaces of the ring and little fingers. The dorsal ulnar side of the hand is innervated by a branch of the ulnar nerve that comes off proximal to the wrist in the distal forearm.

Anatomy. At the wrist, the ulnar nerve lies with the ulnar artery lateral to the flexor carpi ulnaris (FCU) tendon. The artery is lateral to the nerve.

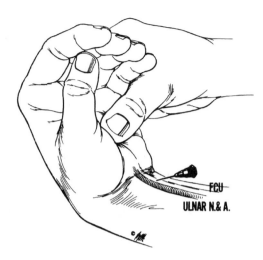

Wrist block, ulnar nerve. Note that the nerve lies between the artery and flexor carpi ulnaris (FCU) tendon. (Illustration by Elizabeth Roselius. From Green DP, et al (eds): Operative Hand Surgery, 4th ed. New York, Churchill Livingstone, 1999, with permission.)

Procedure

1. Have the patient flex the wrist. The FCU is palpable along the medial edge of the distal forearm.

2. Insert the needle just proximal to the wrist crease and just lateral to the FCU tendon.

3. *Draw back on the syringe before injecting the anesthetic to ensure that the needle is not in the ulnar artery.* If blood is drawn back, remove the needle and hold pressure over the area for several minutes.

4. Slowly inject 1–2 ml of local anesthetic.

5. To block the nerve branch that supplies sensation to the dorsal aspect of the hand, inject 1 ml of local anesthetic subcutaneously in the tissues overlying the ulnar nerve.

6. Advance the needle onto the dorsum of the wrist, and inject another 3–4 ml. Go about halfway around the wrist on the dorsal surface.

Superficial Branch of the Radial Nerve

The superficial branch of the radial nerve supplies sensation to the dorsum of the hand from the ring finger to the thumb; the dorsum of the thumb; and the dorsum of the index, middle, long, and ring fingers to the PIP joint.

Anatomy.   The superficial branch of the radial nerve often has several branches traveling in the tissues of the dorsolateral surface of the distal forearm and wrist.

Procedure

1. Feel for the radial artery pulse in the distal forearm, approximately 2 cm proximal to the wrist crease.

2. Insert the needle laterally to the point where you feel the pulse, and inject 1–2 ml of local anesthetic subcutaneously. *Draw back on the syringe before injection.*

3. Advance the needle into the tissues on the dorsum of the distal forearm.

4. Inject an additional 3–4 ml of solution halfway around the dorsal surface of the wrist.

Nerve Blocks for Facial Injuries

The nerves that supply sensation to the areas most commonly affected by facial trauma exit the skull along a line drawn perpendicular to the midpoint of the pupil. These nerves, designated as V_1, V_2, and V_3, are branches of the fifth cranial (trigeminal) nerve.

Lidocaine and/or bupivacaine can be used for facial nerve blocks. Add bicarbonate if it is available. Epinephrine is often a useful addition to the anesthetic solution.

V_1: Supraorbital Nerve Block

The supraorbital nerves supply sensation to the upper eyelid and overlying forehead. A supraorbital nerve is located on each side of the face.

Anatomy.   If you divide the supraorbital rim into thirds, the supraorbital nerve exits the skull at the point where the central and medial thirds meet.

Procedure

1. Insert the needle into the eyebrow overlying the point where the nerve exits the skull.

2. Inject 1 ml of anesthetic solution into the superficial tissues.

3. Advance the needle downward to the bone. You will feel the needle hitting against a hard surface when it meets the bone.

4. Back the needle 1–2 mm away from the bone, and inject another 2–3 ml of local anesthetic.

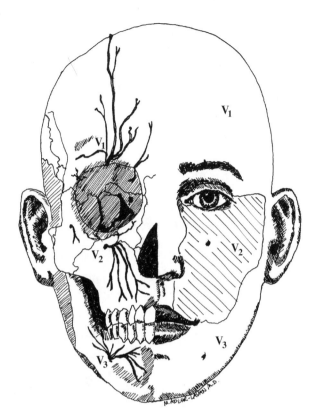

Anatomy of the trigeminal nerve branches (V_1, V_2, and V_3). These nerves provide sensation to the face and are amenable to nerve blocks.

V_1: Supratrochlear Nerve Block

The supratrochlear nerve supplies sensation to the medial upper eyelid, upper nose, and medial forehead.

Anatomy.   The supratrochlear nerve exits the skull along the medial aspect of the supraorbital rim just lateral to the area where the rim meets the nose.

Procedure

1. Insert the needle into the soft tissues overlying the point where you expect the nerve to exit the skull.

2. Inject 1 ml of anesthetic solution into the superficial tissues.

3. Advance the needle tip downward to the bone.

4. Back the needle 1–2 mm away from the bone, and inject another 1–2 ml of the solution.

Caution: For a forehead wound above the medial third of the eyebrow, both the supraorbital nerve and supratrochlear nerve probably need to be blocked on the side of the injury.

V_2: Infraorbital Nerve Block

The infraorbital nerves supply sensation to the upper lip, cheek, lateral aspect of the nose, and lower eyelid. There is one nerve on each side of the face.

Anatomy.   The infraorbital nerve comes out of the skull about ½ cm below the orbital rim along the vertical line drawn perpendicular to the midpoint of the pupil.

Procedure

1. Insert the needle into the cheek skin at the point where the vertical line drawn perpendicular to the midpoint of the pupil meets a horizontal line drawn from the bottom of the nose.

2. Advance the needle tip 2–3 mm into the tissues.

3. Inject 1 ml of solution.

4. Advance the needle tip further, going in a slightly superior direction as you pass through the tissues until you hit the underlying bone. The tip ultimately should travel superiorly about 1 cm.

5. Back the needle out 1–2 mm, and inject another 2–3 ml of the anesthetic.

V_3: Mental Nerve Block

The mental nerves supply sensation to the lower lip and the skin immediately below it. There is one mental nerve on each side of the face.

Anatomy.   The mental nerve exits from the mandible a few mm below and 5–10 mm lateral to the inferior aspect of the lower canine tooth root.

Procedure.

1. The mental nerve block is performed in the mouth.

2. Insert the needle into the mucosa a few mm below and 5–7 mm lateral to the root of the lower canine tooth.

3. Advance the needle tip until it hits the bone.

4. Inject 2–3 ml of solution.

Nerve Block Overview

Injury	Block
Finger	Digital block
Palm of hand	Median and ulnar nerve block
Multiple cuts on both surfaces of hands	Wrist block
Left inner cheek/upper lip	Left intraorbital nerve block
Right lower lip	Right mental nerve block
Center of forehead	Supraorbital and supratrochlear block on both sides of face

Sedation

Sedation can be a useful adjunct to local anesthetic. A sedative decreases the patient's anxiety about the upcoming procedure and increases the patient's cooperation. This, in turn, makes the procedure easier and safer to perform.

In the setting of exploring or closing a wound, the purpose of sedative medications is not to put the patient to sleep, but to make him or her somewhat drowsy and less anxious.

Caution: Sedative medications can cause respiratory depression. Always start with small doses, and gradually give additional medication until the desired amount of sedation is obtained. Patients should be monitored closely (blood pressure, heart rate, and respiratory rate) during and for at least 1 hour after the procedure is completed.

There are many sedatives from which to choose. The following table gives information about two commonly used benzodiazepines.

Useful Agents for Sedation

Agent	Route of Administration	Dose	Onset of Sedation (min)
Midazolam (Versed)	IV *Adult:* inject over 1 min *Child:* inject slowly, over 3 minutes	*Adult:* 0.5–2 mg as initial dose; repeat cautiously with 0.5–1.0 mg after 3–4 min until desired effect is reached *Child (6 mo–13 yr):* 0.05–0.1 mg/kg/dose; repeat after 4–5 min until desired effect is reached to maximal total dose of 0.5 mg/kg *Child > 13 yr:* follow adult dosing	2–3 (adult and child)
	IM	*Adult:* 2–5 mg *Child:* 0.1–0.5 mg/kg	*Adult:* 15–20 *Child:* 5
Diazepam (Valium)	IV	*Adult:* 5–10 mg *Child:* 0.04–0.2 mg/kg/dose	5–10 (adult and child)
	IM	*Adult:* same as IV dose *Child:* same as IV dose	30 (adult and child)

IV = intravenous, IM = intramuscular.

For Information Only: Additional Blocks for Procedures on the Upper Extremity

These procedures are technically more difficult and require special equipment. Although discussed for completeness, they are beyond the realm of a health care provider without expertise in delivering anesthesia.

Bier Block

In a Bier block, also called intravenous regional anesthesia, the affected hand or forearm is exsanguinated and an upper arm tourniquet is inflated. The venous circulation of the hand or forearm is then filled with lidocaine via a catheter placed in a hand vein before exsanguination. In this manner, the hand and forearm are anesthetized. The block lasts about 45–60 minutes.

Warning: The tourniquet must work perfectly. If the tourniquet does not hold its pressure, the injected lidocaine may become systemic and cause serious side effects (e.g., seizures, cardiac arrhythmias/arrest). In addition, for a very short procedure (< 15–20 minutes), the lidocaine in the veins will still be at too high a concentration for the tourniquet to be deflated. Usually, the tourniquet can be released safely after 25–30 minutes.

Axillary Block

An axillary block essentially anesthetizes the proximal portions of the nerves that become the median, ulnar, and radial nerves in the forearm and hand. Technically these portions of the nerves are called the cords of the brachial plexus. The axillary block is commonly used to provide anesthesia for hand procedures.

Usually a mixture of lidocaine and bupivacaine is used for infiltration. An axillary block is useful for procedures that take up to $2\frac{1}{2}$ hours.

The landmark for injection of the anesthetic is the axillary artery, which is easy to feel in the inner aspect of the upper arm. However, injecting in the vicinity of the axillary artery is not without risk; possible complications include injury to the artery or accidental intra-arterial injection. A nerve stimulator can be used to help to identify the nerve and thereby lessen these risks. Even so, an axillary block should be done only by health care providers with expertise in delivering anesthesia.

Bibliography

1. Cousing MJ, Bridenbaugh PO: Neural Blockade in Clinical Anesthesia and Management of Pain, 3rd ed. Philadelphia, Lippincott Williams & Wilkins, 1997.
2. Longnecker DE, Morgan GE, Tinker JH: Principles and Practices of Anesthesiology, 2nd ed. St. Louis, Mosby, 1997.

Chapter 4

PROTECTING YOURSELF FROM INFECTIOUS DISEASES

Healthcare providers are at risk for contracting serious infectious diseases. Although the human immunodeficiency virus (HIV) is often the most feared, the hepatitis B virus (HBV) and hepatitis C virus (HCV) are actually much more contagious than HIV, because a smaller inoculum can cause infection.

Healthcare workers who are inexperienced at technical procedures and find themselves having to treat open wounds and perform invasive procedures are especially at risk for two important reasons. First, treatment of an open wound almost always necessitates exposure to blood and body fluids. Blood and body fluids represent the primary mode of transmission of these contagious agents. Second, the treatment of open wounds and the performance of even simple procedures (for example, suturing) involves the use of sharp instruments. Inexperience on the part of the healthcare provider is a major risk factor contributing to an accidental needlestick or other traumatic injury during such procedures.

Scope of the Problem

These statistics are presented not to scare you, but to emphasize that the risk is genuine.

Human Immunodeficiency Virus

World Prevalence: Over 47 million people worldwide have been infected with HIV since the start of the epidemic. In 1998, HIV caused over 2 million deaths. In some countries in Africa, 1 in 4 people is infected with HIV. Ninety-five percent of cases occur in the developing world.

Prevalence in the U.S.   Approximately 1 in 200 people carries HIV.

Hepatitis B Virus

World Prevalence.   There are over 350 million chronic carriers of HBV worldwide. In developing nations, 8–15% of the population are chronic carriers. This percentage drops to less than 5% in developed nations. Five to ten percent of chronically infected people will develop chronic liver disease that may lead to death.

Prevalence in the U.S.   Approximately 1 million people are chronically infected with HBV.

Hepatitis C Virus

World Prevalence.   Three percent of the world's population is infected with HCV. There are more than 170 million chronic carriers of HCV. About 50–70% of infected people will develop chronic liver disease. HCV infection is the leading disease necessitating liver transplantation.

Prevalence in the U.S.   Approximately 4 million people are chronically infected with HCV.

Delta Hepatitis Virus

The delta hepatitis virus (HDV) primarily affects patients infected with HBV. A patient infected with both HBV and HDV has an increased risk for the development of fulminant hepatitis compared with a patient infected with HBV alone (the risk doubles to 20%). About 70–80% of people infected with HBV and HDV develop chronic hepatitis.

Prevalence in the U.S.   Unknown

Simple Precautions that Make a Difference

- **Wash your hands before and after examining every patient.** This is the single most important way to prevent the spread of infectious diseases.

- **Wear gloves.** Gloves should be worn whenever you anticipate contact with mucous membranes, open wounds, or body substances (e.g., urine, feces, blood). Also wear gloves when handling items soiled with blood or body fluids or performing any type of invasive procedure. Do not go from patient to patient wearing the same pair of gloves. Gloves are not a substitute for proper hand washing. After removing your gloves, remember to wash your hands.

- **Double-glove whenever possible during procedures involving sharp instruments.** Double gloves may feel uncomfortable at first, but you will get used to them. Try wearing a glove a half size larger next to your skin, and wear your regular size over the larger glove.

- **Wear goggles.** Eye protection is always advisable during procedures. Get your own pair, and keep them in your pocket. You will be amazed at how much material accumulates on the lenses, even when you are not aware that any material has been sprayed. The goggles used for racket sports are quite comfortable and often very useful. When you wear a mask over your mouth, the goggles may fog up because exhaled air escapes from under the mask around the edges of your nose. To prevent your lenses from fogging, tape the mask to your cheeks and to the bridge of your nose to prevent air escape.

- **Get vaccinated against HBV.** All healthcare providers should be immunized against HBV. The vaccine is 95% effective in preventing infection. The current vaccine is completely artificial, i.e., no human products are part of the vaccine. There is *no* chance of contracting HBV, HCV, or HIV from the vaccine. The vaccine is administered as a series of three intramuscular injections. The second dose is given 1 month after the first injection, and the third dose is given 6 months after the first injection.

- **Observe proper use and disposal of all sharp instruments.** Needles for injection should not be recapped by hand. Accidents often occur during manual recapping. Keep the cap on your tray, and slide the needle back into the cap when you have finished using it. Do not attempt to bend needles or other sharp objects. Use your instruments when placing sutures—*not your fingers!* Suturing is often difficult for the novice, but get in the habit of using only instruments to hold and reposition the needle. With practice, this technique becomes easier. Do not leave needles or other sharp instruments lying around. Always place them in a container marked "sharp instruments" after use.

- **Adequately sterilize all reusable materials.** This practice is vital to protect healthcare providers and their patients from serious infectious diseases. *Never* reuse needles or syringes without properly sterilizing them.

- **Keep all countertops and other surfaces clean.** It is important to regularly clean all surfaces that may have become contaminated by blood or other body fluids. HBV can survive for at least 1 week in dried blood on various surfaces. A disinfectant made of dilute bleach should be used for regular cleaning.

Postexposure Treatment

Exposure to potentially infectious blood or body fluids includes needle-sticks, splashing of fluids in the face or eyes, and contact with body, fluids or blood through an open wound on your skin. Although intact skin is usually a good protective barrier, irritated or chapped skin (for example, from cold weather) can be penetrated by some viruses. If, despite following all of the above recommendations, you are exposed to potentially infectious blood or body fluids, certain steps can be taken to decrease your risk for becoming ill.

- **If you are exposed to HBV and have not been previously vaccinated:** Hepatitis B immunoglobulin (HBIG) should be given (5.0 ml intramuscularly). HBIG is most effective when administered within 24 hours of a needlestick, but some protection is still afforded if it is given in the first few days after exposure. You also should begin the HBV vaccination regimen.

- **If you are exposed to HCV:** Unfortunately, there is no way to prevent infection after HCV exposure. However, close observation is warranted, and at the first sign of hepatitis, interferon therapy should be instituted. Although early interferon therapy, before any signs or symptoms of hepatitis have developed, does not prevent illness, once signs and symptoms become apparent, interferon may prevent serious illness.

- **If you are exposed to HIV:** If you have access to drugs used to treat HIV infection, a short course of medication is often recommended after a significant exposure. Usually, exposure to infected urine does not warrant treatment. Recommendations for treatment usually are related to the patient's HIV titer and to the healthcare worker's degree of exposure. For example, a hollow needlestick from a patient with a high HIV titer definitely warrants postexposure treatment—optimally, a combination of zidovudine, 200 mg 3 times/day; lamivudine, 150 mg 2 times/day, and indinavir, 800 mg 3 times/day. All are given orally.

Bibliography

1. Gilbert DN, Moellering RC, Sande MA (eds): The Sanford Guide to Antimicrobial Therapy, 29th ed. Vermont, Antimicrobial Therapy Inc., 1999, pp 112, 128.
2. www.cdc.gov/epo/mmwr (Postexposure prophylaxis).
3. www.osha.gov (Universal precautions).
4. www.who.int (World Health Organization surveillance statistics).

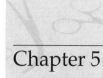

Chapter 5

EVALUATION OF THE ACUTELY INJURED PATIENT

KEY FIGURES:
Emergency cricothyrotomy
Emergency needle thoracostomy

This book primarily describes treatments for stable patients who have a specific injury or problem wound. They have been evaluated previously by a general surgeon, trauma surgeon, or emergency department physician, who has ruled out other, more life-threatening injuries.

Because health care providers cannot know what situation they may face, all of us must be aware of how to evaluate a patient with potentially serious injuries. This chapter provides basic principles for the important, life-saving initial evaluation and treatment of a patient who may have suffered a serious traumatic injury. It is not intended to be a full, detailed description of first-line treatments, but it does provide useful information for all health care providers.

Be sure to get as detailed a history as possible (from the patient, family, or whoever brought the patient to medical attention), but do *not* waste time. Your primary objective is to identify and treat potentially life-threatening injuries.

ABCs of Trauma Care

Following the ABCs (airway, breathing, circulation) and DE (disability and exposure) of trauma care prevents you from getting sidetracked by the patient's obvious injury (arm fracture, for example) and thereby missing a more life-threatening but less obvious injury.

Airway

An open airway (i.e., the path from the nose/mouth to the lungs) is vital for the patient to be able to breathe. You need to determine quickly whether the airway is blocked. Blockage may be due to the tongue, vomit, blood, or foreign bodies.

Signs of Airway Obstruction

In **patients breathing on their own**, signs of airway obstruction include noisy breathing on inspiration and retractions of the supraclavicular space (area above the clavicle) or intercostal space (between the ribs) with attempts at respiration. In **nonbreathing patients**, it may be difficult to diagnose airway obstruction. You must look directly into the mouth and examine for signs of obstruction.

How to Maintain an Open Airway

- Clear out any blood or vomitus in the mouth.
- In an unconscious patient, the tongue may obstruct the airway because of loss of tone in the muscles of the lower jaw (mandible).
- Proper patient positioning often relieves obstruction due to a posteriorly displaced tongue.
- To position the tongue forward, gently lift the chin to bring the mandible forward. Be careful not to extend the cervical spine (because of concerns about possible undiagnosed cervical spine injury).
- An artificial oral or nasal airway tube can be useful, but in a conscious patient it may cause gagging and agitation. Use with caution—such devices are not comfortable.
- Intubation with an endotracheal tube is often the best way to maintain an open airway.
- When intubation is impossible, a surgical airway (cricothyroidotomy or tracheotomy) is required.

Surgical Cricothyroidotomy.   A cricothyroidotomy is done only in emergency situations when no other means is available to maintain an open airway. The following guidelines are helpful:

1. The cricothyroid membrane can be located by running your finger down the center of the neck and feeling the wide thyroid cartilage (Adam's apple). The depression just below the Adam's apple is where you want to place the incision. The rings of the trachea are palpable just below this area.
2. Try to clean the area with Betadine.
3. If you have time, inject the skin with lidocaine and epinephrine to decrease bleeding from the skin edges and to make the procedure a little easier to perform.

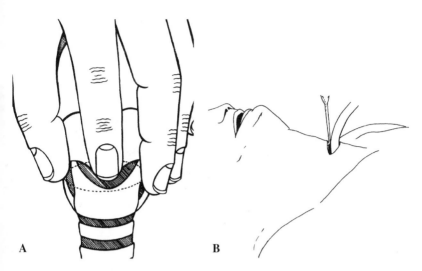

Emergency cricothyroidotomy. *A*, The larynx is stabilized between the left thumb and middle finger. The tip of the index finger is inserted over the cricothyroid membrane. Keep the index finger in this position to identify the position of the cricothyroid membrane as you perform the procedure. *B*, The endotracheal tube in position. (From Simon RR, Brenner BE (eds): Emergency Procedures and Techniques, 3rd ed. Baltimore, Williams & Wilkins, 1994, with permission.)

4. The neck should be in neutral position with the chin held slightly forward.

5. Hold the thyroid cartilage between your thumb and middle finger (actually you are stabilizing the larynx). Use your index finger to help identify the cricothyroid membrane.

6. Using a no. 15 knife blade, make a horizontal incision no more than 2 cm long, just below the Adam's apple. Be sure to stay in the center of the neck. Do *not* make this incision too large, or you may injure a nearby vein, thereby causing significant bleeding and making the procedure very difficult.

7. Staying in the midline, gently push the knife so that it goes through the cricothyroid membrane. Do not push inward too far; use only the knife tip. You do not want to injure the esophagus, which is immediately behind the trachea.

8. Insert the back of the knife handle (not the blade) through the opening that you have just made, and rotate the handle to enlarge the opening.

9. Place the largest possible pediatric endotracheal tube through the opening. Give oxygen and ventilate the patient through this tube.

10. Secure the tube in place with tape or sutures.

Breathing

Breathing relates to getting oxygen to the tissues. All patients with any possibility of having sustained a head injury or with an altered level of consciousness should be given supplemental oxygen, which usually can be administered with a face mask or nasal prongs.

Listen for bilateral breath sounds, demonstrating that both lungs are inflated (see "tension pneumothorax" below). Problems that interfere with oxygen getting to the tissues are often related to significant chest trauma.

Circulation

Circulation pertains to the patient's blood pressure and secure intravenous access. Start an intravenous line with the largest available catheter, and hang a liter of 0.9% saline.

The most common reason for hypotension (low blood pressure) in a trauma patient is blood loss, either external or internal. Control obvious hemorrhage. Be careful of scalp wounds—a lot of blood can be lost from the scalp. A closed fracture of the femur can result in the loss of a liter of blood into the tissues of the thigh, which may not be immediately obvious.

A head injury in and of itself does *not* cause hypotension. Look for another source. In contrast, a spinal cord injury can result in profound hypotension without blood loss (see "Neurogenic shock" below) because of loss of vascular tone.

How to Determine Blood Pressure
Without a Working Blood Pressure Cuff

Feel for palpable pulses at the wrist (radial artery), groin (femoral artery), and neck (carotid artery).

Location of Palpable Pulse	Minimal Approximate Systolic Blood Pressure (mmHg)
Radial artery	80
Femoral artery but not radial artery	70
Carotid artery but not femoral and radial arteries	60

Other Causes of Hypotension/Shock that Can Lead
to Death if not Quickly Diagnosed

Tension pneumothorax occurs when the lung has collapsed and air surrounds the lung. If the air is not removed and the lung reexpanded, build-up of pressure in the chest may cause the lung, great vessels, and even heart to be compressed and pushed to the opposite side. This process impairs blood flow to and from the heart and leads to hypotension.

Cardiac tamponade is a build-up of fluid in the sac around the heart. It can lead to cardiac dysfunction and shock.

Neurogenic shock occurs with an injury that causes paralysis—i.e., a spinal cord injury, *not* a head injury. Because of the loss of nerve input, the blood vessels dilate. Even with minimal blood loss, the patient cannot maintain proper vascular tone, and hypotension develops.

Acute myocardial infarction (heart attack) or any cause of cardiac dysfunction can result in hypotension.

Disability

The following brief exam helps to evaluate patients for the presence of a neurologic deficit:

1. Check the pupils. Are they equal, round, and reactive to light?
2. Is the patient conscious?
3. Can the patient move the fingers and toes?
4. For patients with a suspected head injury, the Glasgow Coma Score (GCS) should be determined. Fifteen, the highest (best) score, indicates that the patient is awake and alert; three, the lowest (worst) score, indicates that the patient is unconscious and unresponsive.

Glasgow Coma Score

Category	Best Response	Points Assigned
Eye opening	None	1
	Opens eyes to painful stimulus	2
	Opens eyes to voice	3
	Opens eyes spontaneously	4
Verbal response	None	1
	Unintelligible sounds	2
	Inappropriate words	3
	Disoriented but converses	4
	Fully oriented and converses appropriately	5
Motor response	None	1
	Decerebrate posturing (abnormal extension)	2
	Decorticate posturing (abnormal flexion)	3
	Moves randomly to painful stimulation	4
	Localizes pain	5
	Obeys commands	6

Add up the points. An uninjured patient who is not intoxicated should score 15 points. A score of 13 points may indicate minor injury; scores of 9–12, moderate injury; and scores < 8, severe injury.

Caution: Do not assume that a low GCS is due to intoxication. A drunk person can definitely have a serious head injury. Do a thorough work-up (usually a computed tomography [CT] scan is required).

Exposure

All clothing should be removed so that the patient is fully exposed. Removal of clothing allows you to examine the patient thoroughly for signs of injury. It may seem silly, but you do not want to be fooled.

Patients usually are lying on their back during the evaluation. To examine the back for evidence of spine injury, log-roll the patient (i.e., roll the patient in one motion, keeping the back straight and preventing any twisting motion of the spine).

Case Study

An 18-year-old man is brought into the hospital after being stabbed in the right upper arm with an icepick. He complains of pain in the arm but otherwise seems to be uninjured. You roll up his sleeve to examine the arm and see entrance and exit sites. Since he has good pulses in the extremities, you think that he is stable. While you are doing some paperwork, he becomes very short of breath and hypotensive. What happened?

If you had removed his shirt, you would have seen that the puncture went through the arm and into the right chest. A pneumothorax developed. Because he was young and healthy, he was able to tolerate it until the pressure built up in the chest cavity. At that point he developed a tension pneumothorax—a true emergency!

Only when the patient is stable from the perspective of the ABCs can you undertake specific evaluation of more obvious injuries.

Needle Thoracostomy

Needle thoracostomy is a life-saving procedure that is easy to do in patients with **tension pneumothorax**. All health care providers should be aware of this technique.

If conscious, the patient with tension pneumothorax is severely short of breath and blood pressure is low. If unconscious, the patient may simply be hypotensive and not breathing well.

If you listen over the chest for breath sounds, you may appreciate a loss of breath sounds on the side of the pneumothorax, but this may be difficult to appreciate in the emergency setting.

Another method is to feel the patient's neck. The trachea shifts **away** from the side with the tension pneumothorax.

If you cannot hear breath sounds in either side of the chest, the trachea is in the midline, and the patient is in shock, treat both sides of the chest. The patient may have bilateral tension pneumothoraces.

Equipment Needed

1. Large catheter for intravenous access (12 or 14 gauge). A large-bore needle can be used if a catheter is not available, but the catheter is safer. The needle can injure an underlying structure more easily.

2. Betadine, if available.

Procedure

1. Apply Betadine to the chest. Simply pour it on—this is an emergency!

2. Place the catheter, with the needle in place, into the affected side of the chest at the second interspace in the midclavicular line (the imaginary line drawn perpendicular to the clavicle at its midpoint).

3. Locate the second interspace.

   • The second interspace is the space between ribs 2 and 3.

   • It can be located by feeling for the spot on the breastbone (sternum) where the manubrium and sternum meet (the point where you can feel an elevation in the bone as you rub your fingers up and down the breastbone).

   • Move your fingers to the right or left chest (depending on where the problem is). You should be at the second interspace when you are at the midclavicular line.

4. The intercostal vessels run just below each rib. To prevent injury to these vessels, the catheter should be inserted into the chest at the second interspace just above the third rib.

5. If you inserted a catheter, remove the needle, but leave the catheter in place. You will hear a big whoosh from the escaping air.

6. Leave the catheter in place until help arrives.

7. If you used a needle, you should hear the air escape as soon as you enter the pleural space. Leave the needle in place until help arrives.

8. The patient requires a chest tube for definitive treatment of the pneumothorax, but you may have just saved the patient's life.

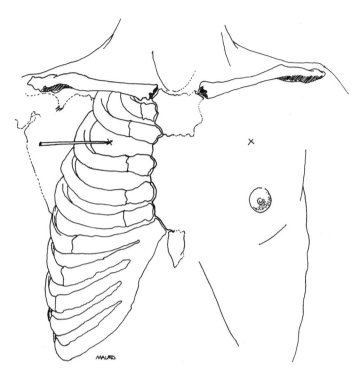

Emergency needle thoracostomy. At the midclavicular line, insert a large (14-gauge) needle or vascular catheter into the chest at the second interspace just above the third rib. You will hear a large rush of air when the needle enters the chest.

Bibliography

1. Creech O, Pearce CW: Stab and gunshot wounds of the chest. Am J Surg 105: 469–483, 1963.
2. Melio FR: Priorities in the multiple trauma patient. Emerg Med Clin North Am 16:29–43, 1998.
3. Simon RR, Brenner BE: Emergency Procedures and Techniques, 3rd ed. Baltimore, Williams & Wilkins, 1994, pp 71–75.
4. Walls RM: Cricothyroidotomy. Emerg Med Clin North Am 6:725–736, 1988.
5. Walls RM: Management of the difficult airway in the trauma patient. Emerg Med Clin North Am 16:45–61, 1998.

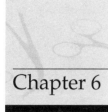

Chapter 6

EVALUATION OF AN ACUTE WOUND

> **KEY FIGURE:**
> Irrigating a wound

This chapter explains the basics for evaluation and treatment of an acute wound. Proper evaluation helps to determine the appropriate next step—formal wound exploration or wound closure.

The **first step** is to control blood loss and evaluate the need for other emergency procedures (see chapter 5, "Evaluation of the Acutely Injured Patient"). The **second step** is to obtain a thorough history about the patient and the events surrounding the injury.

About the Patient

Tetanus Immunization Status

Tetanus is a devastating disease, causing muscle spasms that can lead to muscle rigidity and seizures. Without adequate treatment, one in three adults with tetanus will die. Although immunization has made tetanus uncommon, it always lurks in the background.

If the patient has not had a tetanus booster within 5 years, and the wound is tetanus-prone (see Table 2), a booster should be given. If the wound is not tetanus-prone but the patient has not had a tetanus booster within 10 years, a booster should be given. Patients who have never been immunized need human tetanus immunoglobulin as well as tetanus toxoid followed by completion of the full tetanus toxoid series.

Table 1.   Doses of Antitetanus Drugs

Drug	Number of Doses	Dosage
Tetanus toxoid: booster	1	0.5 ml intramuscularly
Tetanus toxoid: full immuni-zation regimen	3	0.5 ml intramuscularly; repeat in 4 wk and 6–12 mo after second injection
Human tetanus immunoglobulin	1	250 U, deep intramuscular injection

Note: Tetanus toxoid and immunoglobulin must be kept refrigerated at all times during transport from the factory. This requirement may be a problem in remote areas.

Pulsatile Bleeding at Time of Injury

Even if the patient is not bleeding at the time of your examination, the history of bright red, pulsatile bleeding at the time of injury implies an arterial injury. A thorough vascular exam is required, and formal surgical wound exploration is almost always indicated.

Medical Illnesses

Patients with diabetes are more prone to infections and wound-healing problems. Encourage diabetic patients to keep glucose levels well controlled to decrease the risk of complications. Malnourished patients and patients with human immunodeficiency infection (HIV) or a history of cancer also have wound-healing difficulties.

Smoking History

Tobacco smoking dramatically decreases circulation to the skin and slows down the wound-healing process. Medical professionals have a duty to tell all patients not to smoke. But the patient with an open wound should be specifically warned that smoking interferes with and perhaps prevents the healing process. Smoking also increases the risk for wound complications and poor cosmetic outcome.

Events Surrounding the Injury

Timing of the Injury

It is best to close an open wound within 6 hours of injury. Do not close a wound after 6 hours because the risk of infection becomes unacceptably high.

Wounds on the face are exceptions to this rule. The face has an excellent blood supply, which makes infection less likely. In addition, cosmetic concerns are important. It is therefore acceptable to close a wound on the face that is older than 6 hours (perhaps up to 24 hours or at most 48 hours), as long as you can clean it thoroughly.

Nature of the Injury

- A wound caused by a **clean knife** has a low risk of infection.
- A **dirty wound** carries a risk for tentanus. Wood may break off and leave pieces behind, increasing the risk for subsequent infection if the wound is not explored and washed out thoroughly.

- Any wound that may contain a **foreign body** should be explored and the foreign body removed.

- **Animal bites**, especially cat bites, often penetrate more deeply than you think. Bites on the hand should raise concern about involvement of an underlying joint. Oral bacteria may cause severe infections (see chapter 36, "Hand Infections"). Always consider the risk of rabies.

- **Human bites** also are associated with specific oral bacteria that may cause serious infections (see chapter 36, "Hand Infections").

- **If any object penetrated the patient's clothing or shoes** before piercing the skin, the chance for infection is increased because pieces of clothing may become embedded in the underlying tissues. If an object penetrated the patient's tennis shoes, be concerned about a possible pseudomonal infection.

- **Crush injuries** may be associated with greater underlying damage than initially appreciated (see chapter 35, "Crush Injury").

- **Gunshot wounds:** see chapter 37, "Gunshot Wounds."

- **Thermal or electrical injury:** see chapter 20, "Burns."

Concerns about Tetanus

Table 2.   Risks for Tetanus

Wound Characteristics	Tetanus-prone	Not tetanus-prone
Time since injury	> 6 hr	< 6 hr
Depth of injury	> 1 cm	< 1 cm
Mechanism of injury	Crush, burn, gunshot, frostbite, puncture through clothing	Sharp cut (knife, clean glass)
Devitalized tissue	Present in	None present
Contamination (e.g., dirt, saliva, grass)	Yes	No

Concerns about Rabies

Be aware of the risk of rabies in the area where you work. Some countries—England, for example—have no cases of rabies because of tight animal controls. In most other countries, rabies is a real concern.

The primary animals associated with rabies infections include bats, raccoons, skunks, and foxes. Because different areas have a different risk for specific animals, know your area. Dogs and cats also can be infected; be sure to ask if the animal has been vaccinated against rabies. Livestock, rodents (e.g., rats, mice, squirrels), and rabbits are almost never associated with a risk of rabies.

If you have fears that the animal is rabid:

1. Thoroughly clean the wound with soap and water.

2. Administer human rabies immunoglobulin, 20 IU/kg total. If possible, administer one-half of this around the wound, and give the rest in the gluteal area intramuscularly (IM).

3. Administer one of the three types of rabies vaccines currently available: 1.0 ml IM in the deltoid area of adults and older children, outer thigh (*not* gluteal area) in younger children. Repeat on days 3, 7, 14, and 28.

Examination of the Wound

The wound must be cleansed thoroughly to allow full evaluation of the extent of injury.

Cleansing the Wound

Cleansing a wound *hurts*. Often you must start by anesthetizing the area. Infiltrate a local anesthetic around the wound, or administer a nerve block using a few milliliters of lidocaine (see chapter 3, "Local Anesthesia," for a more thorough discussion).

For most simple wounds (i.e., no exposed bone or other vital organ), clean technique is adequate. You can use clean gloves and gauze instead of sterile ones.

The wound needs to be fully washed out to remove all foreign material and decrease bacterial content.

Irrigate the wound with several hundred milliliters of sterile saline until all dirt and foreign material are removed. Then irrigate a bit more (an additional 50–100 ml, depending on the size of the wound).

In patients with a puncture wound, you need to irrigate into the puncture, not just the external opening. You may need to cut into the puncture wound and enlarge it by 1–2 cm to appreciate the full depth of penetration and allow proper cleansing.

Wound Irrigation

Irrigation does *not* mean merely pouring some saline over the wound. You must apply the solution with some force to remove embedded debris and decrease the bacterial count.

The best method is to make an irrigating device out of a syringe (20–50 ml) with a 20-gauge angiocatheter (or whatever you use for intravenous access) or a blunt-tipped needle (a sharp needle can be used, but be careful not to stick yourself). Draw the saline into the syringe and then squirt it out onto the wound. The 20-gauge catheter is best because it delivers the saline at an appropriate pressure to cleanse the wound and costs much less than larger-diameter catheters and needles.

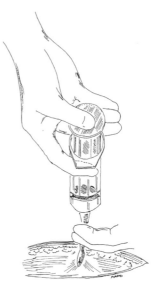

Wound irrigation. Draw saline into a syringe. Place a 20-gauge, blunt-tipped catheter (preferably) or needle on the end of the syringe. Squirt the saline from the syringe onto the wound. Use some force. Repeat until the wound is clean. Usually a few hundred milliliters of irrigation are required.

Removal of Foreign Material, Devitalized Tissue, and Old Blood

Foreign material such as dirt, pieces of wood or grass, and parts of clothing must be removed because they are potential sources of infection.

An exception to this rule is a needle, bullet, or piece of glass deeply embedded in the tissues. In the absence of significant injury to surrounding tissue, these foreign materials usually can be left alone. They often are difficult to locate (even with x-ray guidance), and exploration may cause more local damage. Explain to the patient that the surrounding tissues usually wall off the foreign body. It may then gradually work its way to the skin surface, where it can be easily removed. Warn the patient that the foreign body may cause the area to become infected. If infection develops, localization and removal become much easier because you can follow the pus to the foreign body.

Obviously dead tissue in or around the wound should be removed. Remove any fat that appears to be almost completely detached from the wound, dark purple or black skin, or tissue embedded with debris or foreign material.

Old blood also must be removed. Blood is an excellent media for bacteria proliferation and infection.

If you are unable to remove the objectionable material completely, formal surgical exploration in the operating room with more adequate anesthesia (general and more local) is required.

Evaluation for Injury to Underlying Structures

Vascular Injury

If the injury is near a pulse point (e.g., in the groin near the femoral artery), check to be sure that a pulse is palpable in the nearby vessel—even if there is no active bleeding at the time of examination.

Check also for a palpable pulse in the vessel distal to the injury; for example, check pulses behind the knee or in the foot for a possible femoral artery injury.

Look for pulsatile bright red arterial bleeding or dark red venous oozing.

Ensure that circulation to structures distal to the wound is adequate. Do so by checking capillary refill in the fingers or toes, as appropriate.

Testing Capillary Refill

A well-vascularized finger or toe generally has a pink hue under the nail. If it is blue or very pale, circulation may be impaired. Compare with the uninjured side to determine the patient's baseline status.

If you pinch the tip of the finger or toe, as appropriate, it should blanch (i.e., turn pale.)

Release the pressure. The color should return to normal within 2–3 seconds. A longer period may imply an arterial injury. A shorter period may imply a problem with venous circulation.

An arterial injury usually necessitates urgent surgical exploration in the operating room.

Nerve Injury

If injury occurs along the course of an important nerve, check for sensory and motor function.

A nerve injury in and of itself does not warrant urgent operation at the time of injury. A surgeon should explore the wound thoroughly and repair any injured nerves in the near future. The acute needs are thorough cleansing and loose closure to prevent infection and allow the wound to be fully explored at a later date.

Tendon Injury

If the injury occurs over the course of a tendon, evaluate the action of the affected tendon to ensure that it is appropriate.

A tendon injury in and of itself also does not warrant urgent operation at the time of injury. A surgeon should explore the wound thoroughly and repair any injured tendons in the near future. Again, the acute needs are thorough cleansing and loose closure to prevent infection and allow the wound to be fully explored at a later date.

Fracture or Joint Dislocation

In patients with an obvious bony deformity or a bone that is tender to palpation, get an x-ray to look for fracture or dislocation.

An open wound over a fracture or dislocation classifies it as an "open" or "compound" fracture or dislocation. This distinction is important because an open bone injury is associated with a higher risk of infection than a closed injury. Therefore, patients with an open injury must be placed on antibiotics immediately (a first-generation cephalosporin with or without an aminoglycoside, depending on the amount of bone and soft tissue contamination).

Unless the patient will be treated by an orthopedic surgeon within 24 hours, the wound should be cleansed thoroughly under general or regional anesthesia in the operating room. A finger fracture can be cleansed thoroughly with a digital block for local anesthesia. This procedure can be done in the emergency area or office.

If the wound can be closed, do so loosely. If soft tissue loss is apparent or if the skin is too tight to close primarily, the wound should be packed with sterile gauze moistened with saline or dilute Betadine. Reduce (align) the fracture or dislocation as best as possible, and immobilize the area. The patient should be evaluated by an orthopedic surgeon and possibly a reconstructive plastic surgeon if there is soft tissue loss.

What to Do Next

Active Bleeding

Apply point pressure over the wound. It is not enough to place gauze in the wound and wrap the area with an Ace wrap. You should place a wad of gauze over the injured area and use two fingers to apply point pressure. Push down firmly onto the wound. You may need to hold the pressure for 10–15 minutes before the bleeding will stop. If the bleeding is arterial, exploration is required.

If the patient has an exsanguinating (life-threatening) hemorrhage due to an extremity injury, place a tourniquet or blood pressure cuff proximal (closer to the heart) to the injury. The blood pressure cuff must be inflated to at least 50 mmHg above arterial pressure. *This technique hurts* and places the tissues at risk for ischemic injury. Therefore, the tourniquet should not be left in place for more than 15–20 minutes. If a tourniquet is needed, urgent operative exploration is required.

Foreign Body in the Depths of a Wound

Get an x-ray. Although many materials do not show up on x-rays, you may be able to see air or other indicators that give information about the depth of injury. The x-ray also can tell you whether an underlying joint was violated; air in the joint indicates injury.

Stab Wound over the Chest or Abdomen

You need to be concerned about penetration into the chest or abdominal (sometimes both) cavities. Such injuries should not be closed; they require further examination and evaluation to rule out internal injuries. Call a general surgeon.

* * *

Before further treatment, "paint" (i.e., wipe) the wound and the surrounding tissues with a small amount of Betadine or some other antibacterial agent.

The wound is now ready for one of the following definitive treatments.

Formal Wound Exploration

The patient is taken to the operating room and given general or regional anesthesia so that the wound can be fully cleaned and surgically examined under sterile conditions. Formal wound exploration is indicated in wounds with underlying vascular injuries, open fractures or dislocations, and wounds with extensive contamination, debris, or devitalized tissue.

Wound Closure

The method of closure often depends on the specific characteristics of the wound. Reconstructive plastic surgeons have organized the various techniques for wound closure into a hierarchy, sometimes called the "reconstructive ladder," that ranges from the simplest to the most complex techniques. This hierarchy is set up so that if the first "step" does not work, it will not hinder attempts at the next step on the ladder. The "reconstructive ladder" gives you a logical way to think about how to close an open wound, regardless of its cause. Whether it be an acute, traumatic wound or a wound that resulted from excising a tumor, the same principles apply. A brief overview follows; each step on the ladder is discussed more completely in subsequent chapters.

1. **Secondary closure** (leave the wound open). Sometimes it is best not to close a wound. Treat it with dressings, and allow it to heal on its own (healing by secondary intention). This technique is useful if soft tissue loss is apparent, if the wound cannot be closed without tension, or if you have concerns about infection. Certain wounds, however, require formal closure:

• Wounds with exposed vital structures, such as exposed bone, tendon, or nerve.

• Wounds in areas overlying creases; for example, the front of the elbow (antecubital fossa), back of the knee (popliteal fossa), or armpit. Subsequent scar contracture may severely limit function.

If formal closure is required, one of the following options should be used:

2. **Primary closure**. Skin edges around the wound are sutured together. The wound must be "clean" (i.e., no foreign material, no devitalized tissue, and no active bleeding). Tension in the closed wound should be minimal; therefore, there must be adequate skin to bring together without tension. As described earlier, primary closure is best done within 4–6 hours of injury. Except on the face or over a vital structure, delayed closure results in an unacceptably high infection risk, even with adequate cleansing.

3. **Skin grafting**. When the wound requires closure but cannot be closed primarily, a skin graft is often useful. Skin is taken from one area of the body as a free graft and placed over the wound. There are essentially two types of skin grafts: split thickness and full thickness. Skin grafts will not survive over exposed tendon or bone if the thin connective tissue covering is destroyed by the injury. A flap is required.

4. **Local flaps**. Like skin grafts, local flaps are used when the wound cannot be closed primarily. Flaps are needed for wounds with exposed underlying structures that require more than skin graft coverage. A local flap is created by moving nearby tissue—sometimes skin, sometimes muscle, sometimes both—to the wound for closure.

5. **Distant flaps**. When no useful local tissue is available to close the wound, tissue can be brought from a distant area. Sometimes the tissue is temporarily disconnected from the body; this technique is also called a free flap or a free tissue transfer. Tissue transfers also may be "walked" along the body in stages.

Bibliography

Gross A, et al: The effect of pulsating water jet lavage on experimental contaminated wounds. J Oral Surg 29:187, 1971.

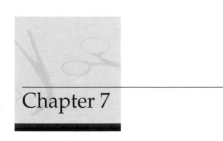

Chapter 7

GUNSHOT WOUNDS

This chapter describes how to treat the external, surface wounds caused by a bullet. The evaluation for underlying injury related to gunshot wounds in an extremity also is discussed. A plastic surgeon is often called to help manage such injuries.

The evaluation of a patient with chest, abdomen, or head/neck gunshot wounds is beyond the scope of this text. However, chapter 5 addresses the initial evaluation of any patient who has sustained a significant traumatic injury.

Initial Treatment of Stable Patients

By definition, a stable patient is awake and alert with stable vital signs. Especially in patients with a gunshot wound, it is preferable that a general surgeon or experienced emergency physician complete a full evaluation before your arrival to ensure that the patient is truly "stable."

Expose the Injured Area

You need to evaluate the injured area thoroughly. All clothing should be removed to ensure that no injury is missed and to allow you to estimate the trajectory (path) of the bullet. This information is important, because knowing the approximate course of the bullet helps you to determine the probability for injury to underlying structures.

Do not probe the wound blindly. Blind probing of the gunshot wound can be dangerous. It may dislodge the clot in an injured blood vessel that has stopped bleeding, thus leading to significant blood loss.

Radiographs

Especially when the gunshot wound is in an extremity, a radiograph is indicated to rule out an underlying fracture and to determine whether the bullet remains in the tissues. It is often helpful to mark the external bullet holes with a small metal object to identify the path of the bullet on the radiograph. Sometimes markers are available in the radiology department for this purpose. Otherwise, a paper clip can be taped to each of the bullet sites.

Neurovascular Exam

When the bullet traverses the path of a major nerve or blood vessel, check for signs of nerve or vascular injury.

- Check the circumference of the injured area. Is it becoming larger (an indication of ongoing bleeding), or is it essentially staying the same size?
- Check for pulses in the vicinity of and distal to the bullet wounds.
- Palpate nearby pulses for a thrill (vibration), and listen with a stethoscope for a bruit. Thrills and bruits may be signs of arterial injury, even if a pulse is palpable.
- Adequate assessment of motor function is often difficult because of pain related to the traumatic injury, but always make the effort. Sensation should not be affected by pain. Test sensation in the extremity distal to the wound to evaluate for nerve injury.

Case Example

A patient arrives with a gunshot wound to the upper thigh. After removing his trousers and undergarments, you note one bullet wound along the inner aspect (medial side) of the thigh, about 15 cm from the pubic symphysis. The thigh is swollen but does not feel very tight. There is no active bleeding from the wound, and the thigh is not increasing in size.

A **radiograph** shows a bullet lodged in the soft tissues of the upper lateral thigh, and small fragments are noted in the soft tissues anterior to the femur. There is no fracture of the bone. This radiograph tells you that the bullet traversed the soft tissues in front of the femur where the femoral artery and femoral nerve travel. You must evaluate the patient for injury to these structures.

Feel the femoral pulse. Does it feel as strong as the opposite, uninjured femoral pulse? Can you feel a thrill with pulsation? Place your stethoscope over the pulse. Can you hear a bruit?

Feel for the distal pulses of the popliteal artery (behind the knee), dorsalis pedis artery (top of the foot), and posterior tibial artery (behind the medial malleolus). The popliteal artery often is difficult to find even in uninjured patients.

Check motor function of the femoral nerve. Can the patient extend the knee? Extension may be difficult because of pain in the thigh. The patient should be able to move his toes and ankle. These functions are under the control of the sciatic nerve, which travels along the posterior aspect of the thigh.

Check sensation. The femoral nerve is responsible for sensation to the anterior and medial aspects of the thigh. Touch the patient with your hand or with the end of a clean needle. Can he feel the touch?

If you identify a problem, further studies (possibly an arteriogram for an injured vessel) or exploration is warranted. The care of this patient then should be **transferred to a specialist**.

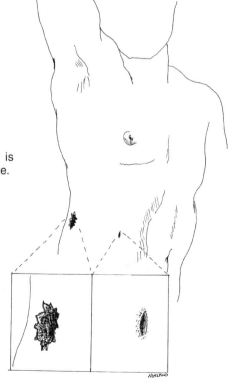

Typically the entrance wound is smaller and tidier than the exit site.

Care of the External Wound

The amount of injury at the entrance and exit (if present) sites is related to the caliber of the bullet, the angle at which the bullet traverses the tissues, the distance from the gun, and even the type of bullet. Usually, there is more damage to the skin at the exit site than at the entrance site (see figure on preceding page).

Excision of the edges of *all* bullet wounds used to be recommended, but now it is not always necessary.

When the bullet wound is relatively clean: Often the entrance wound is very clean, with regular skin edges and no gunpowder imbedded in the surrounding skin.

- Clean the area well with gentle soap and water or an antibacterial scub solution. Then rinse with saline. The wound then may be covered with gauze. If necessary, anesthetize the area with lidocaine before cleansing.
- Such wounds should not be closed primarily (i.e., with sutures).
- Wet-to-dry dressings or antibiotic ointment with dry gauze should be applied 1–2 times/day until the wound has healed.
- Oral antibiotics are not needed.

When the bullet wound has irregular edges embedded with foreign material: Risk for infection is high. Excision of the skin edges is indicated to minimize the risk.

How to Excise the Skin Edges

1. Infiltrate the area around the wound with local anesthetic.
2. Use a scalpel to excise the necrotic skin. Remove only the tissue that is purple or black (i.e., seems dead).
3. If gunpowder is embedded in surrounding skin, which otherwise looks alive, use the flat edge of the scalpel to scrape off the foreign material. Alternatively, use a forceps to grab the debris, and cut it out with the scalpel.
4. Remove any dead fat or subcutaneous tissue visible in the wound.
5. The wound should not be closed primarily. Treat the wound as previously described.

Gunshot Wounds to the Face

Gunshot wounds to the face should be cleansed as described above. Because of the cosmetic concerns, most facial wounds should be loosely closed to reduce the amount of subsequent scarring. Full-thickness wounds (i.e., wounds that communicate with the oral cavity or go down to bone) must be closed in layers. See chapter 16, "Facial Lacerations" for specific details.

Do You Need to Remove the Bullet?

Contrary to television medical shows, the presence of a bullet in the soft tissues, in and of itself, is not an absolute indication for surgery. Operations are required to repair underlying injured structures, not specifically to remove the bullet, unless it is near an important structure and may cause trouble if it migrates.

In certain cases, however, the bullet must be removed. These exceptions are related to the nature of the ammunition. For this reason it is important to have information about the type of gun and bullet that caused the injury.

A **shotgun/buckshot injury** causes a great deal of damage to underlying soft tissue, and numerous pellets and foreign debris are lodged in the tissues. Most importantly, wadding is part of the ammunition and often becomes lodged in the soft tissues along with the pellets. Shotgun/buckshot injuries warrant exploration to remove dead tissue, to remove as many of the pellets as possible, to remove the wadding, and to wash out the wound. If such exploration is not done, the risk for serious infection is high.

It may be tempting to try to remove a single bullet that on radiographs does not seem too deeply embedded in the tissues. If the bullet cannot be easily palpated in the superficial skin, removal is not recommended. Removal is always more difficult than you think, and you risk injury to surrounding structures. It is usually best to leave the bullet alone. Over time, the bullet will either be walled off by the body and stay in place, causing no subsequent problems, or gradually work its way to the surface. Once the bullet can be felt directly under the skin, it can be removed easily with local anesthetic.

Bibliography

1. Fackler ML: Civilian gunshot wounds and ballistics: Dispelling the myths. Emerg Med Clin North Am 16:17–28, 1998.
2. Modrall JG, Weaver Fam Yellin AE: Diagnosis and management of penetrating vascular trauma and the injured extremity. Emerg Med Clin North Am 16:129–144, 1998.

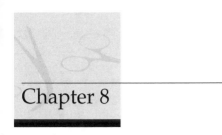

Chapter 8

NUTRITION

Poor nutrition can negate all the benefits of proper wound care or advanced medical interventions. Studies have shown that malnourished patients often require longer hospitalizations, have more postoperative complications, and have delayed wound and fracture healing compared with well-nourished patients.

Usually, patients who do not ingest adequate amounts of calories and protein are also not meeting vitamin and mineral requirements. Malnutrition essentially depletes physiologic reserves and leads to many problems, including impaired wound healing and impaired immune function.

Elective surgery is often contraindicated and therefore not performed in malnourished patients. This illustrates the importance of understanding the basics of nutrition as they affect wound healing.

Types of Malnutrition

Marasmus

Malnutrition due to inadequate caloric intake is called marasmus. The patient has severe physical wasting due to the loss of fat and somatic (skeletal) muscle. This condition is seen not only in the developing world and in times of famine but also in patients with cancer or anorexia. Although the patient is not taking in sufficient calories, he or she is getting sufficient protein. As a result, measured serum protein stores (see below) are adequate.

Kwashiorkor

Patients with kwashiorkor take in sufficient calories but do not meet their protein needs. The typical patient has thin arms and legs with a large protruding belly and peripheral edema (swelling in the soft tissues).

Marasmic Kwashiorkor

Marasmic kwashiorkor is a combination of protein and calorie malnutrition. It is the most common form of malnutrition in the developing world and occurs when a chronically starved patient (e.g., a patient with cancer) suffers an additional stress (e.g., injury, infection).

Assessment of Nutritional Status

Evaluation of protein stores provides a good estimate of nutritional status.

How to Evaluate Protein Stores

The liver produces various proteins, including albumin, prealbumin, and transferrin, that can be measured in the serum. These proteins have been found to correlate well with general nutritional status. Albumin does not correlate with nutritional status as well as prealbumin and transferrin. However, measurement of albumin is useful if the more expensive tests for prealbumin and transferrin are unavailable.

Table 1.   Serum Protein Measurements as a Guide to Nutritional Status

Protein	Normal Value	Moderate Malnutrition	Severe Malnutrition
Albumin (gm/dl)	3.5–5.0	2.1–2.7	< 2.1
Prealbumin (mg/dl)	15–40	5–10	< 5
Transferrin (mg/dl)	200–400	100–150	< 100

How to Estimate Caloric Needs

A patient's daily caloric requirements are affected by a number of factors. Most calories are used to provide the energy for the basic body functions in a resting state, also called the basal metabolic requirements (BMR). These body functions include breathing, maintaining an upright posture, maintaining stable blood pressure, and digestion. The need for additional calories depends on various stresses. Examples of stresses that increase caloric requirement include burns, blunt trauma, fever, infection, surgery, and exercise.

Harris-Benedict Equation

The Harris-Benedict equation is commonly used to estimate the BMR in healthy people. Height (in cm), weight (in kg), and age (in years) are factored into the equation:

BMR for men = 66.47 + [13.75 × weight] + [5.0 × height] – [6.76 × age]

BMR for women = 655.1 + [9.56 × weight] + [1.85 × height] – [4.68 × age]

To determine *total* energy needs, the BMR must be multiplied by factors for activity and stress levels. Activity factors are 1.2 for patients at bedrest and 1.3 for ambulatory patients. Stress factors range from 1.2 for minor surgery or a fracture, to 1.8–2.0 for severe sepsis or severe burns.

Example

A 35-year-old women weighs 60 kg and is 5 feet tall. While working she fell and broke her arm. What are her caloric needs? Because height must by in cm, 5 feet must be converted to 152.4 cm:

$$BMR = 655.1 + [9.56 \times 60] + [1.85 \times 152.4] - [4.68 \times 35]$$

$$BMR = 655.1 + 573.6 + 281.94 - 163.8 = 1346.84 \text{ kcal/day}$$

Total needs = 1346.84 × 1.3 (she is ambulatory) × 1.2 (minor fracture)

Total needs = 2101.07 kcal/day

A Simpler Formula to Estimate Caloric Needs

To get a general estimate of daily caloric requirements, multiply the patient's weight in kg by 25–40, depending on stress level (25 = low stress, 40 = high stress, as in patients with burns or sepsis). For the patient above:

Total needs = 60 × 30 (the fracture adds a little to the stress level) = 1800 kcal/day

Protein

Protein is probably the most important nutrient. It is broken down into individual amino acids, which are important building blocks for bone, muscle, and skin. Thus, adequate protein intake is vital for normal wound healing. Protein is found in food derived from animals and plants. Not all sources of protein contain all of the necessary amino acids required to maintain adequate protein stores; in other words, they are not considered to be "complete" protein sources.

In general, animal sources (e.g., eggs, meat, milk) contain all of the required amino acids. Dried beans, peanuts, and soy-derived foods are the best nonanimal sources of protein. Although protein is present in cereals and grains, they are not complete sources of protein. Corn may be a good source, but often much protein is lost during processing. Fruits and vegetables contain little protein.

Patients who have limited access to animal protein must combine vegetable protein sources carefully to provide complete proteins each day. Sources of vegetable protein include rice and beans, cereal with milk, and noodles with cheese.

How to Estimate Protein Needs

The adult U.S. recommended dietary allowance (RDA) for protein is 0.75 gm/kg of body weight/day, which for an average-sized adult is 45–60 gm/day. Children and infants have higher protein requirements (1–2 gm/kg/day).

Stress, such as infection, burns, or traumatic injury, increases protein breakdown and thus protein requirements. Even under these circumstances, the requirements usually do not increase by more than 50% of the RDA.

During times of stress, precise measurements of nitrogen loss can be determined by collecting the urine produced over a 24-hour period and measuring its urea nitrogen content. Multiply this number by 1.25 to estimate total nitrogen lost. Determine how much nitrogen the patient took in based on diet. If the patient is losing more nitrogen than he or she is taking in, more nitrogen must be ingested to prevent depletion of protein stores.

Important Vitamins and Minerals

The following vitamins and minerals are important for proper wound healing. Because vitamins and minerals cannot be made by the body, they must be ingested. They serve as cofactors in many enzymatic reactions that are necessary for normal physiologic functioning. Although supplements are indicated in patients with deficiencies, little evidence indicates that higher supplemental doses have beneficial effects in patients with adequate vitamin/mineral stores.

Note: These nutrients have other important physiologic effects, but only their effect on wound healing is discussed below. All of the listed minerals (calcium, copper, iron, magnesium, manganese, and zinc) are important in collagen synthesis.

Vitamin A

Because vitamin A is fat-soluble, it can be stored by the body. It is needed for the formation and maintenance of healthy skin and hair. It is a cofactor for collagen synthesis and is also important for normal immune function. Studies have shown that in patients taking chronic, high-dose steroids, Vitamin A is particularly important for proper wound healing. In this specific population, higher daily doses than the RDA may be beneficial for a short period (few weeks). In patients who are not taking steroids and who ingest a healthy diet, extra doses of vitamin A can be harmful.

RDA: 5,000 IU/day.

In patients taking steroids with an open wound: 25,000 IU/day orally; 200,000 IU/8 hr topically.

Sources: liver, egg yolks, fortified milk and cheese, dark green leafy vegetables, deep orange fruits/vegetables, fortified cereals.

Vitamin C (Ascorbic Acid)

Because vitamin C is water-soluble, it is not stored in significant amounts in the body. Patients must take in enough vitamin C on a daily basis to prevent deficiency. It is an important cofactor for collagen synthesis.

RDA: 60 mg/day.

Sources: citrus fruits, potatoes, tomatoes, broccoli, green peppers.

Vitamin E

Vitamin E is needed to maintain proper immune function and proper cell health. In patients with wounds exposed to radiation, vitamin E can counteract the negative effects of radiation on wound healing.

RDA: 30 IU/day.

Sources: vegetable oils, wheat germ, whole grain cereals, dried beans, nuts, green leafy vegetables, eggs, seeds.

Calcium

Calcium is found primarily in bones and teeth. Every day 700 mg of calcium is turned over between plasma and bone.

RDA: 400–1200 mg/day.

Sources: dairy products, green leafy vegetables, dried beans, nuts, whole grains.

Copper

RDA: none at present, but the estimated safe and adequate daily dietary intake (ESADDI) is 1.3–3 mg/day.

Sources: shellfish, dried beans, nuts, organ meats, whole grains, potatoes.

Iron

RDA: men, 10 mg/day; women, 15 mg/day.

Sources: liver, shellfish, meat, poultry, and fish; dried beans and whole grains.

Magnesium

RDA: 250–350 mg/day.

Sources: found widely in vegetables and nuts.

Manganese

ESADDI: 2–5 mg/day.

Sources: whole grains, nuts, dried beans, vegetables, fruits, tea, instant coffee.

Zinc

Zinc is important for wound epithelialization and increases wound strength.

RDA: men, 15 mg/day; women, 12 mg/day.

Sources: meat, fish, poultry, milk products, beans, whole grains, nuts.

Bibliography

1. Mora RJF: Malnutrition: Organic and functional consequences. World J Surg 23: 530–535, 1999.
2. Ruberg RL: Role of nutrition in wound healing. Surg Clin North Am 64:705–714, 1984.
3. Van Way CW: Nutrition Secrets. Philadeplhia, Hanley & Belfus, 1999.

Chapter 9

TAKING CARE OF WOUNDS

KEY FIGURE:
Gauze

Wound care represents a major area of concern for the rural health provider. This chapter discusses the treatment of open wounds, with emphasis on dressing techniques. These techniques can apply to an acute wound allowed to heal on its own (see chapter 10) or to a chronic/longstanding wound.

Definitions

Cellulitis: diffuse infection of the soft tissues.

Clean wound: a wound in the process of healing; usually it has a bed of healthy granulation tissue (see below) without overlying exudate or surrounding cellulitis.

Debridement: the process of removing dead/unhealthy tissue from a wound.

Dirty wounds: wounds covered with exudate or eschar (scab), but not infected.

Exudate: the tan/grayish material that often forms over an open wound. It consists of proteinaceous material from the wound itself. The presence of exudate does not mean that the wound is infected.

Granulation tissue: the red, shiny tissue that forms at the base of an open wound during the healing process. It is composed of inflammatory cells necessary for wound healing, and bacteria. Granulation tissue is highly vascular and bleeds easily. For this reason, a wound covered with granulation tissue frequently bleeds with dressing changes or minor trauma.

Infected wounds: wounds caused by injury with a dirty source (such as a rusted metal object) or associated with dirt/grass contamination.

A chronic wound, covered with necrotic (dead) material and surrounded by cellulitis, also is described as an infected wound.

Supplies

The following supplies are basic for taking care of a wound.

Newly Developed Materials

Currently, in affluent areas of the world, hydrocolloid-type dressings and growth factor formulations aid in the wound-healing process. However, these products are quite expensive and not readily available. As of yet, they do not necessarily yield the superior results that warrant the added expense. For these reasons, hydrocolloid-type dressings and growth factor formulations are not discussed.

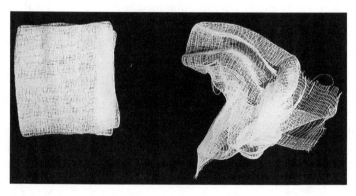

Gauze usually comes folded into a square. For dressings, it is best to open the gauze so that a single layer is in contact with the open wound.

Dressing Materials

The best material to use for dressings is plain cotton gauze. Usually, all that is needed is just enough gauze to cover the wound lightly; multiple layers are unnecessary and wasteful.

There is nothing sterile about your skin or an open wound. Bacteria colonize the surface of both. For this reason, you do not have to use sterile technique to change dressings. Clean technique is usually sufficient.

Sterile Technique vs. Clean Technique

Sterile technique uses instruments and supplies that have been specifically treated so that *no* bacterial or viral particles are present on their surfaces. Examples of sterilized supplies include instruments that have been autoclaved (subjected to high temperatures to kill microorganisms) and gauze and gloves that have been especially prepared at the factory and are individually packaged. Procedures in an operating room are usually done with sterile technique.

Clean technique uses instruments and supplies that are not as thoroughly treated to rid surfaces of all microorganisms. Nonsterile gloves and gauze, which come many in a package, are examples of "clean" supplies. Clean supplies are less expensive than sterile supplies. Hence, appropriate use of clean techniques can save valuable resources.

The occasions when a sterile dressing should be used are noted throughout the text.

Solutions

Various solutions are available for wound care. They are poured onto the gauze, and then the moistened gauze is placed over the wound. They also can be used to cleanse the wound. The following table describes commonly used solutions.

Table 1.   Solutions for Dressings

Solution	Preparation	Usage	Notes
Betadine	Purchased premade in container Best diluted for dressings: 1 part Betadine to at least 3 or 4 parts saline or sterile water	To clean wounds, to use for dressings Especially good for infected wounds	Toxic to healthy tissues; best used in diluted form for few days at time. Then use another solution for dressings. Safe on face and around eyes.
Saline*	To 1 liter of water add 1 tsp salt Boil solution for at least 60 sec Cool before use Essentially equivalent to and cheaper than prepackaged liter of saline solution	To clean wounds, to use for dressings	Safe anywhere on body
Sterile water*	Boil 1 liter of water for at least 60 sec Cool before use	To clean wounds	Safe anywhere on body
Dakin's solution*	To 1 liter of saline solution add 1–2 tsp (5–10 cc) liquid bleach Some pharmacies keep Dakin's solution in stock When available, best diluted: 1 part Dakin's to 3–4 parts saline or sterile water	To use for dressings	Better antibacterial agent than saline Do not use around eyes

* Keep the solution in a sealed container; refrigerate if possible. Solutions stay fresh for several days.

Useful Antibiotic Ointments

Some wounds (e.g., burn) are best treated with antibiotic ointments. The antibiotic is absorbed into the tissues of the wound to prevent infection. The ointment keeps the wound moist and helps to decrease the pain caused by a wound that has become too dry.

Table 2.   Examples of Antibiotic Ointments and Their Uses

Ointment	Indication	Comments
Silver sulfadiazine (Silvadene)	Burns	Do not use around eyes
Bacitracin	Open wounds, face burns	Do not use around eyes*
Triple antibiotic	Open wounds, face burns	Do not use around eyes

* Use only a topical antibiotic ointment specifically labeled for ophthalmologic use around the eyes. Bacitracin has an ophthalmologic formulation, as do garamycin and erythromycin ointments.

Types of Dressing Techniques

The following dressing techniques are easy to do and require the least amount of materials. Unless otherwise noted, clean technique is sufficient. Pain medication is sometimes needed to make the dressing change process more tolerable for the patient. Usually, an oral agent can be used; it is best to administer it 30 minutes before the dressing change.

Note: At least once a day, usually at the time of a dressing change, the wound should be cleaned with gentle soap and water or washed with saline.

Wet-to-Dry

Indication

The objective of the wet-to-dry dressing technique is to clean a wound or to prevent build-up of exudate. It is called a "wet-to-dry" dressing because you place a moist dressing on the wound and allow it to dry. When the dressing is removed, it takes with it the exudate, debris, and nonviable tissue that have become stuck to the gauze. Wet-to-dry dressings are indicated for wounds that are dirty or infected.

Technique

Moisten a gauze dressing with solution, and squeeze out the excess fluid. The gauze should be damp, not soaking wet. Completely open the gauze (it usually comes folded), and place it on the wound. You do *not* need many layers. Then cover with a thin layer of dry gauze.

When changing the dressing, pour a few milliliters of saline (or water) on the bottom layer of gauze if it has completely dried out. This techique prevents the removal of healthy new tissue from the surface of the wound. Remove the dressing gently to avoid causing pain.

How Often?

Optimally, a wet-to-dry dressing should be changed 3–4 times/day, depending on how much debridement is needed. The dressing should be changed more frequently for a dirty wound than for a clean wound. However, depending on the availability of dressing material and personnel, the dressings may be changed less often. Gradually the wound will become cleaner and heal.

Wet-to-Wet

Indication

A wet-to-wet dressing does not debride the wound, which remains as it is. The dressing remains wet so that when the gauze is removed, the top layers of the healing wound are not removed with it. This dressing should be used on clean, granulating wounds with no overlying exudate in need of removal.

Technique

Moisten the gauze dressing with solution. It should not be soaking wet, but it should be a little wetter than damp. Unfold the gauze, place it over the wound, and then cover with dry gauze. The dressing should still be wet or damp when it is changed. If the bottom layer of gauze has dried out, saturate the gauze with saline or water before removal.

How Often?

The wet-to-wet dressing should be changed at least twice a day to prevent drying.

Antibiotic Ointment

Indication

Antiobiotic ointment may be used as an alternative to wet-to-wet dressings for a clean wound that is healing well and has no need for debridement.

Technique

Coat the wound with a small amount of ointment. A thick layer of antibiotic ointment over the wound offers no advantage and wastes supplies. Cover with a dry gauze if the wound is large or if it is in an area that will be covered with bedclothing or rubbed by clothing. Otherwise the wound can be left open to air with the antibiotic ointment alone.

How Often?

Remove the old ointment with gentle soap and water or saline, and reapply the ointment once or twice a day.

When to Use Which Dressing

- For wounds that are infected or covered with exudate, use a wet-to-dry dressing.

- For uninfected wounds that are in the process of healing and have no need of debridement, use a wet-to-wet dressing or antibiotic ointment. You may use a wet-to-dry dressing, but it may cause more pain than the other two options.

Bibliography

1. Ladin DA: Understanding dressings. Clin Plast Surg 25:433–441, 1998.
2. Steed D: Modifying the wound healing response with exogenous growth factors. Clin Plast Surg 25:397–405, 1998.

Chapter 10

SECONDARY WOUND CLOSURE

KEY FIGURE:
Dead space under skin closure

Secondary wound closure is also referred to as closure by secondary intention. The skin edges of the wound are not sutured together; the wound is left "open." Dressings are applied regularly to keep the wound clean, and the wound gradually closes and heals on its own. Secondary wound closure requires little technical expertise. It is the simplest and, therefore, lowest rung on the "reconstructive ladder." This chapter discusses the important background knowledge you must have when deciding to allow secondary wound closure.

Caveats

Although it is often true that the easiest treatment is the one to choose, you must be aware of what secondary wound closure involves from the patient's perspective.

Extended Healing Period

It may take several weeks to even months for the wound to heal using dressings alone. This extended healing period can cause considerable hardship for the patient. From a financial standpoint, the patient may not be able to return to work with the open wound. In addition, dressing supplies, no matter how simple you make them, can get expensive.

Wound Location

The location of the wound may make it impossible for the patient to change the dressings. For example, the patient will require outside assistance to care for a wound on the back or the buttocks. It also may be difficult to keep the dressings in place during treatment of a facial wound.

Pain

The sensation associated with an open wound can range from somewhat bothersome to quite painful. Dressing changes are often painful as well. Some pain medications are addictive when given for the long period required for a large wound to heal.

Scarring

Wounds that are allowed to heal secondarily tend to have **larger and more noticeable** scars than the scars that results from primary closure. Secondary healing also has a greater tendency for hypertrophic scar/keloid formation, which can be bothersome and unsightly.

Scar tightness and contracture can be especially problematic in areas such as the upper cheek, where a tight scar can pull down and distort the lower eyelid, or in the arm pit (axilla), where scar problems can lead to limited shoulder mobility and function.

A wound that heals secondarily has a **less stable** scar—that is, the scar is more easily injured than the scar from a wound with primary closure. Over the years less stable scars may be chronically injured. They may reheal only to be reinjured again and again. This cycle can be quite troublesome and also is associated with a risk for the development of an aggressive skin cancer.

Acceptable Settings for Secondary Closure

Wounds that will heal with an acceptable scar if the skin edges are not sutured together can be allowed to heal secondarily. Examples include:

- **Relatively small wounds.** Wounds smaller than $1\frac{1}{2}$ cm often heal quite well by secondary intention. Even wounds with a diameter of 3–4 cm or larger, with no exposed tendons, bones, or other important structures, can be allowed to heal secondarily when lack of surgical expertise allows no other option. Be sure to keep in mind the above caveats when wounds > 2 cm are allowed to close by secondary intention.

- **Second-degree burns.** Second-degree burns are often allowed to heal with local wound care alone. See chapter 20, "Burns," for a more thorough discussion.

Secondary Closure as the Treatment of Choice

Some wounds should *not* be closed with sutures. Instead, they should be left open and treated with dressing changes until they heal. Examples include:

- **Wounds that come to your attention more than 6 hours after occurrence.** With the exception of facial wounds, you should not use primary repair for a wound that is more than 6 hours old. The risk of infection is greatly increased after this amount of time has lapsed.

- **Highly contaminated wounds.** A dirty wound should not be closed because of concerns about wound infection. Examples of dirty wounds include human bites on the hand or wounds deeply embedded with dirt or grass.

- **Wounds with dead space under the skin closure.** Sometimes empty space rather than subcutaneous tissue is seen beneath the repaired skin when you try to bring the skin edges together. This "dead" space occurs due to loss of subcutaneous tissue or swelling of the skin around the wound. If such wounds are closed primarily, the risk for blood collecting under the skin closure is high, increasing the likelihood of infection and problems with wound healing.

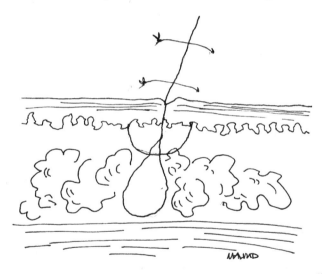

After the skin is sutured together, the underlying tissues are not well approximated. This dead space promotes hematoma (a collection of old blood) formation and infection.

- **Wounds with too much swelling or skin loss.** Excessive swelling or skin loss makes the skin closure very tight. A tight skin closure decreases blood circulation to the skin edges, thereby causing the tissues to become ischemic (low supply of oxygen and nutrients). If the tightness does not soon resolve, the skin may die. Skin death results in a wound that is larger than the initial wound and even more problematic to close.

Contraindications to Secondary Closure

Certain wounds should not be allowed to heal by secondary intention. These are wounds that are associated with exposure of an important underlying structure or are located in areas where a tight scar will be particularly problematic. Such wounds should be closed primarily. If primary closure is not possible, one of the other options from the reconstructive ladder must be chosen (see following chapters).

Exposure of a Vital Structure

Sometimes wounds occur over important structures such as fracture sites, tendons, or prosthetic devices (e.g., artificial joints). If these structures are not covered by healthy soft tissue, there is an almost 100% risk for the structure to become infected or die.

To avoid permanent disability, a wound that results in exposure of an important structure should optimally be closed quickly (within days) with healthy tissue.

Areas Where a Tight Scar is Undesirable

Wounds over Creases

Secondary closure is not useful on wounds that are larger than 3–4 cm and located over creases (e.g., front of the elbow [antecubital fossa], armpit [axilla]). The scar that results from secondary closure will cause tightness across the crease and may result in significant limitation of movement. If splints and movement exercises are used diligently (see chapter 15, "Scar Formation"), this problem may be avoided. But even with the best of care, limitation of movement often results.

Face Wounds Near the Lower Eyelid

In many areas of the face, a wound can be allowed to heal secondarily without significant cosmetic ill effects. However, wounds on the cheek near the lower eyelid may pull the eyelid downward if allowed to heal secondarily. The result not only is cosmetically unacceptable but also may expose the eye to injury.

Guidelines for Use of Secondary Closure

If you decide to treat a wound by secondary intention, the wound must be evaluated thoroughly and cleaned rigorously. The appropriate dressing regimen must then be implemented. See chapter 9, "Taking Care of Wounds," for specific dressing recommendations.

Unless the wound involves a human or a deep animal bite, antibiotics (oral or intravenous) are not required. However, you should see the patient within a few days to ensure that no signs of infection are present and that the wound is being cared for properly.

Signs of Infection

Signs of wound infection include redness, warmth, swelling, and tenderness in the tissues around the wound. Drainage of pus from the wound is also a sign of infection.

Gray exudate on top of the wound does *not* mean that the wound is infected. It is often just proteinaceous debris from the wound itself. A green, somewhat sweet-smelling, creamy material is a sign of colonization by *Pseudomonas* bacteria. Without signs of surrounding soft tissue infection, antibiotics are not required. However, you should treat the wound with wet-to-dry dressing changes, preferably with Dakin's solution, and increase the number of changes each day.

Change in Dressing Regimen

Do *not* be afraid to change dressing regimens. You may start with a dressing regimen of antibiotic ointment covered with dry gauze. After a few days, a lot of exudate covers the wound. At this point you should change to a wet-to-dry dressing and observe how the wound progresses. Once the wound has improved in appearance, you can go back to the antibiotic ointment or continue with the wet-to-dry dressings.

Duration of Wound Dressing

The dressings should be continued until the wound heals. Often during the course of secondary healing, the wound develops a dry eschar (scab). The patient can cover the area with dry gauze or even leave it uncovered. As the wound heals, the eschar gradually falls off.

If the wound is near a crease, encourage the patient to exercise the area to prevent formation of a tight scar. Splints also may be useful. See chapter 15, "Scar Formation," for more details.

Bibliography

1. Goldwyn RM, Rueckert F: The value of healing by secondary intention for sizable defects of the face. Arch Surg 112:285, 1977.
2. Montandon D, D'Andiron G, Gabbiani G: The mechanism of wound contraction and epithelialization. Clin Plast Surg 4:325, 1977.

Chapter 11

PRIMARY WOUND CLOSURE

> **KEY FIGURE:**
> Everting skin edges

In primary wound closure, the skin edges of the wound are sutured to-gether to close the defect. Whenever possible and practical, primary closure is the best way to close an acute open wound.

Advantages of Primary Wound Closure

- Primary wound closure simplifies wound care for the patient, who simply needs to keep the suture line clean and dry. Secondary wound closure requires several dressing changes per day.

- A wound closed primarily heals much more quickly and with less pain than a wound allowed to heal with dressings alone.

- Primary closure involves fewer problems with abnormal scarring and has a better cosmetic outcome.

- All vital, underlying structures are covered.

Contraindications to Primary Wound Closure

Concern about wound infection is the main reason not to close a wound primarily. If infection develops, the resultant deformity may be worse than that caused by the initial injury alone. The following cir-cumstances are associated with an unacceptably high risk of infection:

- An acute wound > 6 hours old (with the exception of facial wounds)

- Foreign debris in the wound that cannot be completely removed (e.g., a wound with a lot of embedded dirt that you cannot clean completely)

- Active oozing of blood from the wound

- Dead space under the skin closure

- Too much tension on the wound

Before Primary Closure

Clean Wound

The wound must first be evaluated thoroughly for injury to underlying structures to rule out the need for urgent exploration in the operating room. (See chapter 6, "Evaluation of an Acute Wound," for specific details.)

The wound must then be cleansed.

Evaluating and cleansing a wound can hurt; remember pain control.

Anesthetize the Area Before Suturing

If local anesthetic was administered for wound cleansing, check to ensure that the anesthesia is still effective.

Pinch the tissues with your forceps, or gently touch the skin edges with a needle. If the patient feels *sharp* pain, more anesthetic is required.

Pressure sensation is not dulled by local anesthetics. With adequate anesthesia, the patient may still feel a sensation of pressure when you pinch the tissues with the forceps, but it should not hurt.

Agents

Injectable lidocaine (lignocaine) or bupivacaine should be used. For wounds of the face or scalp, the addition of epinephrine decreases bleeding caused by the placement of sutures. The effects of lidocaine last approximately 1 hour; the effects of bupivacaine last 2–4 hours.

Administration

1. Inject the anesthetic with as small a needle as possible. A 25–gauge needle is acceptable, but use the smallest needle that you have. The larger the number, the smaller the needle: a 25-gauge needle is much smaller than an 18-gauge needle.

2. Inject slowly. It is acceptable to inject into the wound after it has been cleaned. If the tissues are dirty, however, inject into the skin surrounding the wound to prevent foreign material from being pushed into the uninjured surrounding tissues.

3. Inject enough anesthetic to make the tissues swell just a little.

4. If the injury is in an area where a nerve block can be done (e.g., on the finger), do a nerve block. It provides better anesthesia.

5. Allow 5–10 minutes for the anesthetic to take effect.
   See chapter 3, "Local Anesthetics," for more details.

How to Suture the Wound

Most wounds can be closed by suturing the skin edges together. Chapter 1, "Suturing: The Basics," contains a detailed description of the various suturing techniques, but some reminders are included below.

Suture Size

On the Face

Small sutures such as 5-0 or 6-0 should be used to repair facial lacerations. Smaller sutures decrease scarring, which is a major concern with facial wounds. Again, the bigger the number, the smaller the suture. (See chapter 16, "Facial Lacerations," for more details.)

All Other Sites

Usually, in areas where cosmetic concerns are less important, 3-0 or 4-0 sutures are best because of their larger size and increased strength.

Absorbable vs. Nonabsorbable Sutures

For most skin suturing, nonabsorbable sutures are best because they are associated with less noticeable scarring. Exceptions include patients who cannot return for suture removal, children (because of the difficulty in removing sutures from a frightened, crying child), and some facial lacerations.

Suture Placement

When you suture a wound, it is important to evert the skin edges—that is, the underlying dermis from both sides of the wound should touch (see figure at top of following page). If the edges are inverted (i.e., the epidermis turns in and touches the epidermis of the other side), the wound will not heal as quickly or as well as you would like.

Choose the suture technique (simple vs. mattress sutures) that allows the best dermis-to-dermis closure for optimal wound healing.

For most areas of the body except the face, the sutures should be placed 3–4 mm from the skin edge and 5–10 mm apart. There is no need to drive yourself crazy by placing too many sutures.

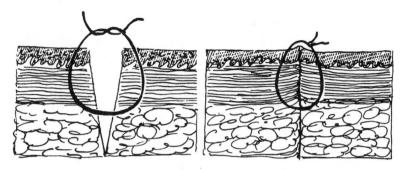

For optimal healing, sutures should be placed so that the skin edges are everted, allowing the dermis on both sides of the wound to be well approximated. (From McCarthy JG (ed): Plastic Surgery. Philadelphia, W.B. Saunders, 1990, with permission.)

Interrupted vs. Continuous Closure

In an interrupted closure, you tie the suture once it has passed through each side of the wound. In a continuous closure, you place the sutures one right after the other without tying each suture individually.

In a relatively simple laceration with smooth edges that line up easily, it makes no difference which method you choose. On the average, a continuous closure is faster to perform, but you should choose the method with which you are most comfortable.

In a laceration with irregular edges, an interrupted closure is preferred because it allows better alignment of the tissues.

If you have any concern that the wound may become infected, it is better to do an interrupted closure. If an area of the wound begins to look inflamed, the sutures in that area can be removed and the other sutures left in place. By removing a few sutures and placing the patient on oral antibiotics, you may be able to treat the infection adequately without having to reopen the entire wound. This approach results in a smaller scar and a happier patient.

Closure in Layers vs. Simple Skin Closure

Although most wounds require only skin closure, sometimes it is necessary to close the wound in layers. The layers may involve muscle, fascia (the layer of connective tissue that overlies the muscle and is actually quite strong), or dermis, depending on the particular wound.

If the muscle or fascia is widely separated, a few absorbable sutures can be placed in a figure-of-eight fashion to bring the tissues together.

If the wound is widely separated or the closure will be under some tension, a few buried dermal sutures are useful. Such sutures are placed in the skin layer just below the epidermis and should be made of an absorbable material.

Aftercare

1. After suturing the wound closed, apply a small amount of antibiotic ointment over the suture line and cover the area with a dry gauze.

2. After 24 hours, remove the original dressing.

3. The patient can wash the area with gentle soap and water the day after the repair. A shower is fine, but if the patient wants to take a bath, the injured area should not be allowed to soak in the water for more than a few minutes.

4. A small amount of antibiotic ointment can be applied daily for the first few days; then leave the area open to air.

5. If the injured area is on the hand, foot, or calf, have the patient elevate the affected extremity. Elevation decreases swelling in the injured area and thereby improves healing.

Suture Removal

Sutures should be removed according to the following guidelines:

• Face: 5–7 days

• Hand: 10–14 days

• Elsewhere: 7–10 days

To decrease scarring, skin sutures are removed while the scar tissue is still relatively weak compared with the final scar strength (which is not attained for several months). To help maintain the wound closure, it is useful to place Steristrips (if available) across the scar once the sutures have been removed. These strips fall off on their own, and the patient can wash the area, even with the strips in place.

What to Do if the Suture Line Becomes Red

If the suture puncture sites start to become red and irritated-looking but the surrounding skin area is not tender or red, simply remove the sutures. No antibiotics should be needed. This reaction probably represents nothing more than inflammation and irritation from the sutures. As a precaution, you should check the patient within 24–48 hours to be sure.

If the area around the sutures becomes red, tender, and swollen, an infection probably has developed. Remove a few sutures, and open the wound. Try to express any underlying fluid or pus, and clean the area with saline or other antibacterial solution. If you cannot fully drain the underlying fluid or fully cleanse the area by taking out a few sutures, all of the sutures should be removed, the wound opened, and the area treated with wet-dry dressings. Oral antibiotics are also needed.

Delayed Primary Closure

Delayed primary closure is a compromise between primary repair and allowing an acute wound to heal secondarily. This option may be considered for a wound with characteristics that require secondary closure (e.g., a wound over 6 hours old) even though primary closure is preferable (e.g., a large wound or a wound near a skin crease).

In delayed primary closure, you initially treat the wound with wet-to-dry dressing changes for a few (2–3) days with the hope of being able to suture the wound closed within 3–4 days.

During the few days of dressing changes, the reasons for not closing the wound initially may resolve. The dressings should clean the wound, the tissue swelling caused by the trauma may subside, and all bleeding may be fully controlled. If the wound shows no signs of infection and can be closed without tension, it may be possible to close the wound primarily within a few days.

Delayed primary closure is a relatively simple technique and avoids having to choose a more complex method for wound closure.

Bibliography

Millard DR: Principlization of Plastic Surgery. Boston, Little, Brown, 1986.

Chapter 12

SKIN GRAFTS

A skin graft involves taking a piece of skin from an uninjured area of the body (called the donor site) and using it to provide coverage for an open wound. When primary closure is impossible because of soft tissue loss and closure by secondary intention is contraindicated, a skin graft is the next rung on the reconstructive ladder. It is not a technically difficult procedure but does require some surgical skills. For a successful result, you need a thorough understanding of how skin grafts heal and how to perform the procedure.

Background information

Anatomy of Skin

The thickness of human skin is quite variable. The eyelids have the thinnest skin (0.5 mm), and the thickest skin is found on the soles of the feet (> 5.0 mm).

Epidermis

The epidermis is the top portion of the skin. The outer layers of the epidermis are formed by essentially dead, nonreplicating cells. The innermost layer contains the cells capable of replication, which are responsible for wound healing and skin pigmentation.

Dermis

Immediately below the epidermis is the dermis. It is made primarily of collagen and is much thicker than the epidermal layer. The dermal-epidermal junction is irregular and has the appearance of ridges. This anatomic arrangement accounts for the skin's strength and prevents injury from normal shear forces. Nerve endings, hair follicles, and sweat glands are located in the dermis. *All skin grafts must include at least a portion of the dermal layer for survival.*

Subcutaneous Tissue

The subcutaneous fatty tissue below the dermis provides padding for the skin. The base of many hair follicles and sweat glands, as well as many important nerves for pressure sensation, reside in the subcutaneous tissue. Because of these important skin components, I include the subcutaneous tissue as a layer of the skin. However, it is not included in a skin graft. Fat attached to the graft interferes with transport of nutrients to the important upper skin layers. Therefore, no fat should be included in the skin graft.

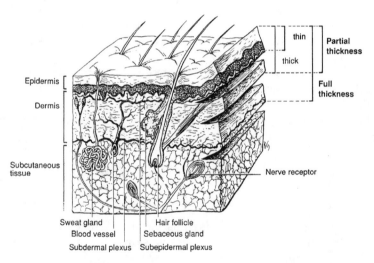

Cross-section of human skin showing the epidermis and dermis (derived from two different germ layers). The relative thickness of skin grafts is shown. The thicker the graft, the more characteristics of normal skin it will provide. (From Cohen M (ed): Mastery of Plastic and Reconstructive Surgery. Boston, Little, Brown, 1994, with permission.)

How a Skin Graft Survives

When the skin graft is harvested from the donor site, it is completely separated from its blood supply. In its new position covering the open wound, the graft initially survives by diffusion of nutrients from the wound bed into the graft. Diffusion of nutrients keeps the skin graft alive for, at most, 3–5 days. During this period, blood vessels begin to grow from the wound bed into the graft. By the time the graft is no longer able to survive by diffusion of nutrients alone, this vascular network has formed and becomes the primary mechanism for providing nutrients to the graft.

In the first several weeks after the procedure, the skin graft looks quite red and irregular compared with normal surrounding skin. Reassure the patient that the appearance will improve dramatically over the next several months, but the skin-grafted area will never look completely normal. It can take at least 1 year to see the final appearance of the graft. See chapter 15, "Scar Formation," for more details

When is a Wound Ready for Grafting?

A wound will accept a skin graft when there is no overlying dead tissue and the wound is clean, beefy red (from granulation tissue), and without surrounding infection. Skin grafts heal well over muscle. Therefore, if muscle is exposed in the wound, skin can be grafted at any time, as long as the wound is otherwise clean.

Table 1. Compensating for Factors that Interfere with Graft Survival

Factor	Compensation
Dirty wound (e.g., surrounding infection, necrotic tissue over wound)	Debride the wound and treat it with wet-to-dry dressings until the wound looks clean. Use antibiotics to clear signs of surrounding infection. The skin graft can be done once the wound has improved in appearance and there are no signs of surrounding infection.
Fat in base of wound	Fat has a poor blood supply and may not be able to support the graft. Treat the wound with wet-to-dry dressings until granulation tissue* begins to appear. Then do the skin graft.
Shear forces between graft and base of wound	Movement of the graft over the wound interferes with vascular ingrowth. The graft must be kept well secured to the wound by the dressing. If the graft is on an extremity, consider using a splint for immobilization of the limb.
Blood or serum collection under graft	Fluid collection under the graft prevents the ingrowth of blood vessels necessary for graft survival. Fluid collection can be prevented by cutting holes in the graft and keeping the graft well secured to the wound. If the graft is on the leg, the patient should be kept on bedrest, with the leg elevated at all times for at least the first 4–5 days.

* Granulation tissue is the beefy red tissue that develops as a wound heals. It has an excellent blood supply but also contains bacteria in its crevices.

Contraindications to Wound Closure with a Skin Graft

A wound that has exposed tendon or bone can be successfully covered with a skin graft only if the thin layer of tissue connecting the tendon or bone (paratenon or periosteum, respectively) is intact. These connective tissues contain the vascular structures necessary for skin graft survival. If the paratenon or periosteum is absent, the graft will not survive. Under these circumstances, some type of flap is needed for wound closure.

Split-thickness Skin Graft

A split-thickness skin graft (STSG) is composed of the top layers of skin (the epidermis and part of the dermis). The graft is placed over an open wound to provide coverage and promote healing. The STSG donor site is essentially a second-degree burn because only part of the dermis is included in the graft. The donor site will heal on its own because some dermal elements remain.

Indications

An STSG is indicated in most wounds that cannot be closed primarily and when closure by secondary intention is contraindicated. It is also indicated for a relatively large wound (> 5–6 cm in diameter) that would take many weeks to heal secondarily. A skin graft provides more stable coverage for large wounds than the scar that results from secondary closure. A large wound also heals more quickly with a skin graft than with dressing changes alone. The wound must be clean. All necrotic tissue must be removed before skin grafting, and there should be no signs of infection in the surrounding tissues.

Anesthesia of the Donor Site

Because of the relatively large size of the graft to be taken, the patient usually requires either general or spinal anesthesia for adequate pain control. However, if the required graft is no more than several centimeters in diameter, the donor site can be anesthetized by local infiltration of tissues with lidocaine or bupivacaine.

Preparation of the Donor Site

The most common donor site is the anterior or lateral aspect of the thigh. If the wound to be covered is on the back, try to take the graft from the lateral thigh, but the posterior thigh is also acceptable. Use of the posterior thigh as a donor site is a bit more painful and difficult for the patient to care for postoperatively.

Any betadine or other antibacterial solution used to prepare the donor site should be washed off with saline. Then the donor site should be dried. Apply a sterile lubricant (e.g., mineral oil, K-Y jelly) to the donor site and to the instrument you will be using to harvest the graft.

Procedure for Taking the Graft

A thin layer of skin (epidermis with some underlying dermis) is taken with a dermatome or a Humby knife (sometimes called a Watson knife). A dermatome is powered by air or electricity, but it is not available in all hospitals, especially in rural settings. Remember: you are *not* taking full-thickness skin; some dermis must be left at the donor site.

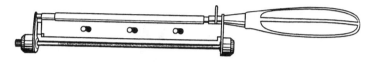

Skin-graft (Humby) knife. (From Padgett Instruments, Inc., with permission.)

Both the Humby knife and dermatome have settings that can be adjusted to set the thickness of the graft. Place the settings at 0.011–0.015 inch (0.25–0.4 mm). Unfortunately, these settings are often unreliable. Another technique to ensure proper thickness of the graft is to adjust the opening of the blade so that you can snuggly fit the beveled edge of a no. 10 blade into the opening.

Caution: Always check the knife settings just before you take the graft. This safety check prevents the accidental taking of too thick or too thin a graft.

An assistant should help to spread and flatten out the donor site by placing tension on the skin with gauze or tongue depressors.

If you have a dermatome:

1. Turn on the power while the dermatome is in the air before it comes into contact with the skin.

2. Hold the dermatome at a 45° angle with the skin and hold it firmly against the skin.

3. Slowly move down the donor site until you have taken the properly sized graft.

4. At this point do *not* turn off the power. Remove the dermatome from the skin with the power on so that the graft is completely freed from the donor site.

5. The entire movement is evocative of landing an airplane and taking off again right away.

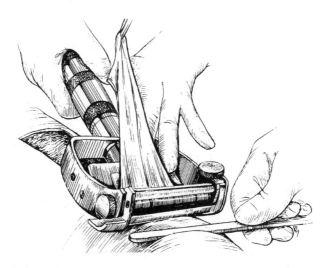

Harvesting a split-thickness skin graft with a power-driven dermatome. (From Cohen M (ed): Mastery of Plastic and Reconstructive Surgery. Boston, Little, Brown, 1994, with permission.)

If you have a Humby knife:

1. Hold it with the sharp edge at about a 45° angle with the skin.

2. With a back-and-forth motion run the knife over the tight skin.

3. When you have taken a large enough graft, continue the back-and-forth motion, and twist your wrist into supination to remove the knife from the skin. Another option is to stop the knife movement and then use a scalpel to cut the skin graft from the donor site at the

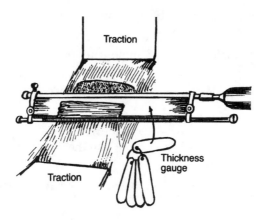

Harvesting a split-thickness graft with the Humby knife. (From McCarthy JG (ed): Plastic Surgery. Philadelphia, W.B. Saunders, 1990, with permission.)

blade edge. You may need to open the knife fully to remove the skin from the instrument.

Preparation of the Skin Graft

It is best to cut multiple slices in the graft to prevent blood and serum from accumulating under the graft. The cuts also help to expand the graft, allowing you to take a graft that is slightly smaller than the open wound. Use the tip of a knife or a small scissors to create the cuts in the graft. Some operating rooms have special equipment, called meshers, for this purpose. The mesher is a hand-cranked instrument that creates pie-cuts in the skin.

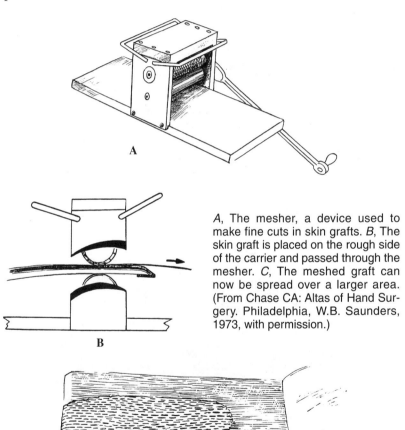

A, The mesher, a device used to make fine cuts in skin grafts. B, The skin graft is placed on the rough side of the carrier and passed through the mesher. C, The meshed graft can now be spread over a larger area. (From Chase CA: Altas of Hand Surgery. Philadelphia, W.B. Saunders, 1973, with permission.)

How to Use the Mesher

1. Place the skin on a plastic carrier. Carriers are available in different sizes, but the best size to use is 1.5:1 (i.e., the graft is expanded 1.5 times).

2. Spread out the skin graft *on the rough side* of the carrier. If you put it on the smooth side, you will get spaghetti when you place the graft through the mesher. It does not matter which side of the skin faces upward on the carrier, but the dermis side is the more shiny side.

3. Pass the carrier with the skin graft through the mesher, taking care that the graft stays on the carrier and is not pulled into the blades of the mesher.

Placement of the Graft onto the Recipient Site

1. Be sure that the wound is clean. Remove any small areas that appear unhealthy.

2. To decrease the amount of contamination in the top layers of the healing wound, scrape the wound with the edge of a knife. Do not push the knife edge into the wound; instead, scrape it over the wound. Rinse the wound with saline.

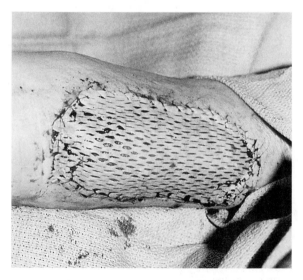

Wound covered with a split-thickness skin graft. The graft has been meshed 1.5:1.

3. Scraping the wound will make it bleed, but the bleeding is easily controlled by placing gauze over the wound and applying gentle pressure for a few minutes. Remember: hemostasis is important.

4. Place the skin graft over the wound with the **dermis side** (the shinier side) **down**, next to the raw surface of the wound.

5. Suture the graft in place with absorbable sutures. Leave a long tail on a few of these sutures so that they can be used to hold the dressing in place (see below).

6. Alternatively, the skin graft can be stapled in place, but the staples must be removed. Removal can be painful.

Application of Wound Dressing

1. A layer of nonstick material, such as antibiotic-impregnated gauze, should be placed directly over the graft. If you do not have this type of gauze, apply a layer of antibiotic ointment over the graft.

2. Moisten a sterile gauze with mineral oil (if available) or saline.

3. Fluff the gauze and place it over the nonstick layer; then cover the area with dry gauze.

4. Try to keep the dressing as secure as possible, either by wrapping with gauze or by tying the dressing in place.

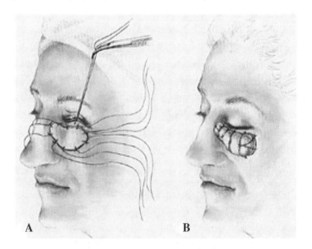

Tying the dressing in place. In suturing the skin graft to the wound edges, leave the ends of each suture long *(A)*. Then use the long ends to secure the dressing in place *(B)*. This technique immobilizes the dressing and underlying graft. (From Edgerton M: The Art of Surgical Technique. Baltimore, Williams & Wilkins, 1988, with permission.)

Removal of Wound Dressing

- The dressing should be kept in place for 3–5 days. Check the dressing each day. If it develops an odor or has a lot of drainage, remove the dressing sooner.

- Be careful not to lift the graft from the wound with the dressing change. Wet the dressing with saline (mixed with a little hydrogen peroxide, if available) to prevent the dressing from sticking.

Aftercare

- Gently apply antibiotic ointment, or use a wet-to-wet saline dressing once or twice a day for the next few days. The area can be cleansed very gently with saline at each dressing change.

- After 10–14 days, once the wound looks like it is healing (i.e., the graft is pink and well-adherent to the wound), the dressings can be left off. A gentle moisturizer should be applied daily.

- The skin graft site should be kept out of the sun as much as possible. Sunscreens can be used once the graft has fully healed.

- Vigorously counsel the patient not to smoke during the healing period. Smoking probably will cause the skin graft to die.

Care of the Donor Site

- At the time of surgery, the donor site should be covered with a layer of antibiotic gauze. A thick layer of gauze should be placed on top.

- After 24 hours, remove the outer gauze dressing—not the antibiotic layer—and leave the entire area open to air. The layer of antibiotic gauze will dry out over the next 24–48 hours and gradually peel off as the underlying wound heals.

- An alternative treatment is to treat the donor site like a burn: apply antibiotic ointment twice a day until the wound has healed.

- Apply moisturizer regularly to the donor site once it has healed.

- The donor site also should be kept out of the sun. Sunscreens can be used once the wound has fully healed.

Full-thickness Skin Graft

A full thickness skin graft (FTSG) includes the epidermis and entire dermis but no subcutaneous fat. Because the entire thickness of skin is taken, the graft donor site must be closed primarily.

Indications

FTSGs are rarely done, because the wound must be *very* clean for the graft to survive. Most often they are used for a small wound, usually one created surgically (such as a wound on the face created by excision of a malignant skin lesion).

The other common use is for open wounds on the palmar surface of the hands and fingers. These areas may scar too tightly if the thinner STSG is used.

Preparation of the Donor Site

The best donor site is usually just above the inguinal crease on the lower abdomen. If the graft is needed to cover a facial wound, extra skin of a reasonable color match often can be taken from the supraclavicular area in the neck or from behind the ear.

An ellipse is drawn at the donor site. Make sure that it is large enough to cover the defect but not too large to close the donor site.

You can tell how large a graft you can take by seeing how much skin you can pinch or pull up at the donor site. At the inguinal area, you can flex the patient's hip to decrease tension on the closure. After a few days the patient will be able to extend the hip fully. This approach causes no long-term problems.

Anesthesia of the Donor Site

Because you are taking a relatively small graft, the FTSG can be harvested with a local anesthetic. Lidocaine and marcaine work equally well.

Procedure for Taking the Graft

1. The ellipse of skin is excised with the full layer of dermis. To facilitate the procedure, take the graft with some underlying fat attached.

2. You must remove the attached fat, which will interfere with graft survival.

How to Defat the Graft

1. The skin graft should be placed under tension. Place clamps on the ends of the graft, lay the graft over your hand, and let the clamps hang freely.

2. Use scissors to remove the fat on the dermis. Place the scissors flush with the skin, and cut away the fat. Do not worry if you take a little dermis or cut into small areas of the epidermis.

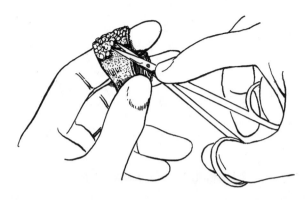

Defatting the undersurface of a full-thickness skin graft with a pair of scissors. (From McCarthy JG (ed): Plastic Surgery. Philadelphia, W.B. Saunders, 1990, with permission.)

Placement of the Graft onto the Recipient Site

1. The recipient site must be *very* clean.

2. If you are using the FTSG for a wound on the palmar surface of the hand, decrease the amount of contamination in the top layers of the healing wound by scraping the wound with the edge of a knife. Do not push the knife edge into the wound; simply scrape it over the wound and then rinse with saline.

3. Scraping makes the wound bleed, but the bleeding is easily controlled by placing gauze over the wound and applying gentle pressure for a few minutes. Remember: hemostasis is important.

4. A few small slits can be cut in the graft to prevent fluid from accumulating under the graft. In general, the graft is placed as an intact sheet. Do *not* mesh a FTSG.

5. The graft is placed over the wound, dermis side down, and sutured in place with absorbable sutures. Leave a long tail on a few of these sutures so that they can be used to hold the dressing in place.

Application of Wound Dressing

1. A layer of nonstick, antibiotic-impregnated gauze should be placed directly over the graft. Alternatively, place a thin layer of antibiotic ointment over the graft.

2. Moisten sterile gauze with mineral oil (if available) or saline.

3. Fluff the gauze and place it over the nonstick layer and cover with dry gauze.

4. Keep the dressing as secure as possible, either by wrapping with gauze or by tying the dressing in place.

Removal of Wound Dressing

The dressing should be kept in place for 3–5 days. Check the dressing each day. If the wound develops an odor or has a lot of drainage, remove the dressing sooner.

Be careful not to lift the graft off of the wound with dressing changes. If necessary, wet the dressing with saline (mixed with a little hydrogen peroxide if available) to prevent it from sticking.

Aftercare

Apply antibiotic ointment, or use a wet-to-wet saline dressing once or twice a day for the next few days.

Cleanse the area gently with saline at each dressing change.

The epidermis (very top layer) may become black and peel off. Do not be overly concerned. As long as the underlying dermis is attached and vascularized, the graft should heal.

After 7–10 days, once the graft looks like it is healing (i.e., it is pink and well-adherent), the dressings can be left off. A gentle moisturizer should be applied.

The skin graft site should be kept out of the sun as much as possible. A gentle sunscreen should be used.

Vigorously counsel the patient not to smoke during the healing period. Smoking probably will cause the skin graft to die.

Care of the Donor Site

The donor site should be closed primarily and covered with antibiotic ointment and dry gauze. The dressing can be removed after 24 hours.

Apply a small amount of antibiotic ointment and dry gauze for 2–3 days. Then the area can be left open.

Clean daily with gentle soap and water.

Remove the sutures after 7–10 days.

Bibliography

Reus WF, Mathes SJ: Wound closure. In Jurkeiwicz MJ, Krizek TJ, Mathes SJ, Ariyan S (eds): Plastic Surgery: Principles and Practice. St. Louis, Mosby, 1990, pp 20–22.

Chapter 13

LOCAL FLAPS

KEY FIGURES:
Axial flap noting pedicle
Random flap noting
   pedicle and 3:1 ratio
Rhomboid flap
Rotation flap
V-Y advancement flap

Definitions

A **flap** is a piece of tissue with a blood supply that can be used to cover an open wound. A flap can be created from skin with its underlying subcutaneous tissue, fascia, or muscle, either individually or in some combination. Depending on the reconstructive requirements, even bone can be included in a flap.

A **local flap** implies that the tissue is adjacent to the open wound in need of coverage, whereas in a **distant flap**, the tissue is brought from an area away from the open wound.

Local flap coverage of a wound is the next higher rung up the reconstructive ladder after a skin graft. Examples of wounds that require flap coverage include wounds with exposed bone, tendon, or other vital structure and large wounds over a flexion crease, for which a split-thickness skin graft or secondary closure would result in tight scarring.

Donor site: where the flap originates.

Recipient site: the open wound/soft tissue defect in need of coverage.

Pedicle: the blood supply of the flap (i.e., its arterial inflow and venous outflow). The pedicle varies from a wide bridge of tissue (skin, subcutaneous tissue, muscle, or some combination) to an isolated artery and vein.

Most local flaps can be classified as either (1) **skin flaps**, which are skin and subcutaneous tissue with or without the underlying fascia, or (2) **muscle flaps**, which are created from a muscle with or without the attached overlying skin.

Skin Flaps

A portion of skin and subcutaneous tissue and, when possible, the underlying fascia (the thin layer of connective tissue overlying muscle that has an excellent vascular supply) is moved to fill the defect. This movement of tissue results in a new defect at the donor site. Often the donor site can be closed primarily, but sometimes a skin graft is needed.

Classification

Skin flaps are classified as either **axial** or **random**. The classification is based on the blood supply.

Axial Flaps

The circulation of an axial flap is supplied by specific, identifiable blood vessels. Careful anatomic study has identified several donor sites with a single artery and vein responsible for circulation to a particular area of skin. Examples include the volar forearm skin supplied by the radial artery and skin on the back supplied by the circumflex scapular artery (a branch of the thoracodorsal artery).

Circulation based on specific vessels results in a highly reliable blood supply and a reliable flap. You can be confident that unless there is an injury to the vessels, the majority of the flap tissue should survive in its new position.

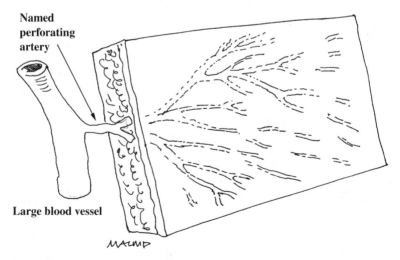

Axial flap. Note that the blood supply comes from an identifiable vessel. As a result, the pedicle can be quite thin, which makes transferring the flap to its new site an easier task.

An axial flap can be completely detached from all surrounding tissue as long as it remains connected to its supplying blood vessels. These vessels serve as the pedicle. The thin pedicle allows axial flaps to be easily positioned to fill the wound defect (unlike the random flap [see below]).

The difficulty with an axial flap is locating the blood vessels. You must be very careful not to injure the vessels when creating the flap. The necessary technical expertise is beyond the realm of most providers without reconstructive surgical training. Thus, no specific axial skin flaps are discussed in this chapter.

Random Flaps

Circulation to a random flap is provided in a diffuse fashion through tiny vascular connections from the pedicle into the flap. The pedicle must be bulky to increase the number of vascular connections. The more vascular connections, the better the circulation to the flap. The better the circulation to the flap, the better its survival.

In general, a random flap does not have as reliable a blood supply as an axial flap. Nonetheless, the relative ease of creating random flaps makes them useful almost anywhere on the body. The circulation and thus the reliability of the flap can be increased by "delaying" the flap before final transfer.

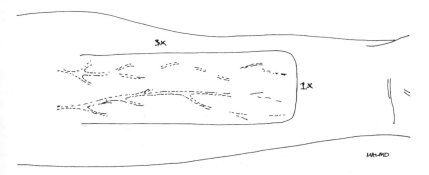

Random skin flap. The blood supply comes diffusely from the remaining skin attachment, which serves as the pedicle. For optimal circulation and flap survival, the flap should be designed so that the length is no more than three times the width.

Delay Procedure

Before the flap is created, the tissue gets its blood supply via all of the surrounding skin and underlying tissue attachments. When the flap is created, the circulation to the flap comes only from the pedicle.

The purpose of the delay procedure is to enable the pedicle to assume its role as the main source of circulation before the flap is moved to its new position. This goal is obtained by making some of the incisions needed to create the flap but not separating the flap from the underlying tissues. The flap is not moved to its new position; instead, the skin edges are sutured together loosely.

The total blood supplied to the flap initially decreases when the incisions are made. This decrease promotes opening of new vascular channels between the pedicle and flap. Thus, more blood will flow into the flap through the pedicle than if the delay procedure had not been done.

Delaying the flap before final transfer allows more confidence in the viability of the flap. Wait about 7–10 days after the delay procedure before moving the flap to the recipient site.

Techniques for Creating Random Local Flaps

When creating a random local skin flap, you take advantage of the relatively loose, excess skin in the vicinity of the skin defect. Random flaps require less technical expertise than axial flaps. Because they can be quite useful for covering an open wound, several types of random flaps are discussed in detail below.

General Information

Random flap procedures often can be done under local anesthesia if the area (flap plus defect) is not too large (< 8–10 cm). For larger areas, general anesthesia probably will be required.

Be sure to clean the wound thoroughly before creating and placing the flap. Use a scrub brush or the flat part of a scalpel to scrape away the top layer of granulation tissue from the wound. Then wash with saline. The wound probably will bleed, but gentle pressure should control the bleeding.

Hint: Outline the flap before making any incisions. A water-based magic marker allows you to make corrections to your design before making any incisions. Incorrect marks can be removed by wiping with alcohol.

The part of the flap at highest risk for poor circulation is the tip of the flap (the tissue farthest from the pedicle). Unfortunately, the tip of the flap is usually the most important part of the flap because it is the part that provides coverage for the open wound.

To optimize circulation and reliability of a random flap, plastic surgeons heed the 3:1 rule. The flap should not be longer than 3 times its width. Delaying the flap is also useful.

Unfortunately, the thickness of the pedicle can make it difficult to move the flap to its new position. *Minimal tension should be applied to the flap when it is sutured into place.* Tension on the flap decreases circulation and can lead to tissue necrosis (death). You can tell that too much tension has been applied if portions of the flap look pale once it is in its new position.

If the donor site cannot be closed primarily without placing tension on the flap, avoid primary closure. A skin graft can be used to cover the donor site defect—or, if the defect is just a few cm, it can be allowed to heal secondarily.

For coverage of a wound > 7–8 cm, it is useful to place a drain under the flap to prevent collection of fluid, which will interfere with healing. The drain can be a suction drain, if available, or a passive drain (e.g., Penrose drain). A piece of sterile glove can substitute for a Penrose drain. The drain usually can be removed after 48 hours.

Rhomboid Flaps

Indications

Rhomboid flaps are useful for wounds up to 4 or 5 cm in diameter on the face, trunk, or extremity. They are especially useful when there is not enough laxity in the surrounding tissues to create one of the other flaps discussed below.

Procedure

1. Measure the diameter of the defect.
2. Determine the site of greatest surrounding skin laxity (pinch the tissues to see where it is easiest to pull up on the skin). Draw a line from the wound edge into this tissue. This line, which represents the first incision, should be approximately 75% of the wound diameter.
3. Draw another line at a 60° angle to this extension, parallel to the edge of the defect. This line should be the same length as the line in step 2. These lines outline your flap.
4. Be careful not to make the pedicle of the flap too narrow.
5. Make the incisions along the lines placed in steps 2 and 3. Incise the skin and subcutaneous tissue of the flap down to, but not including, the underlying muscle.
6. Use a knife to lift the flap off the underlying muscle, trying to keep the fascia attached to the flap to enhance circulation. You should also separate the pedicle and some of the tissues around the wound

defect from the underlying muscle. This technique is called **undermining**. Undermining allows more mobility in the flap and surrounding tissues, which in turn facilitates wound and donor site closure.

7. The flap now should be ready to be moved into the wound, and the donor site should be closed primarily.

8. Loosely suture the flap in place, taking care to avoid tension on the pedicle. Place a few dermal sutures, and then do an interrupted skin closure. Be sure that the skin closure is not tight. It is better to have small gaps in the skin closure (which will heal) than to make a tight closure and lose part of the flap.

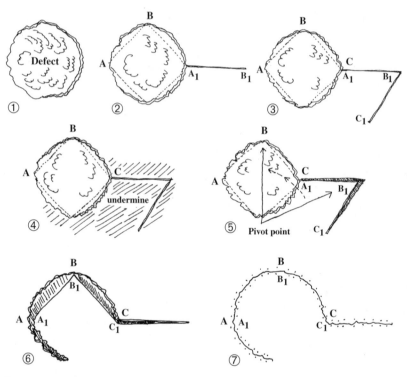

Rhomboid flap. *1:* Open wound in need of coverage. *2:* Draw a circle or rhomboid around the defect and, at the area of maximal skin laxity, a line 75% of the wound diameter. *3:* Draw another line of the same length at a 60° angle to the first line, taking care not to narrow the base of the flap. *4, 5, and 6:* Incise the lines. Undermine the area widely to allow transfer of the flap to the desired position and primary closure of the defect. *7:* Final appearance of closed wound.

Rotation Flaps

Indication

Commonly used for coverage of sacral pressure sores. This type of flap can cover wounds of various sizes.

Procedure

1. Draw the flap before making any incisions so that you can make corrections.

2. Determine the site of greatest laxity in the surrounding tissues.

3. Make the flap larger than you think you need.

4. Extend the wound in a curved fashion until you think the flap can be moved into the defect. Be sure that the flap has a wide base (at least 8–10 cm).

5. Separate the flap from the underlying tissue attachments, and undermine the flap pedicle and surrounding skin edges.

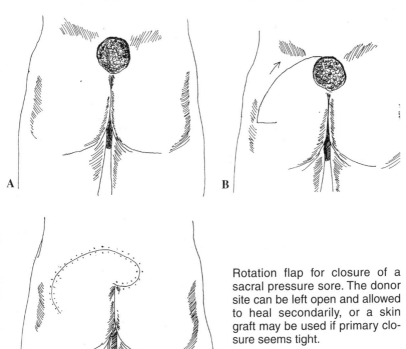

Rotation flap for closure of a sacral pressure sore. The donor site can be left open and allowed to heal secondarily, or a skin graft may be used if primary closure seems tight.

6. If necessary, a small back cut can be made at the lateral edge of the base of the flap to help it turn onto the wound. Do not narrow the base by more than 1–2 cm.

7. Loosely suture the flap in place, avoiding tension on the pedicle. Place a few dermal sutures, and then do an interrupted skin closure. Be sure that the skin closure is not tight. It is better to have small gaps in the skin closure (which will heal) than do a tight closure and lose part of the flap.

8. Sometimes the donor site may need to be closed with a split-thickness skin graft or allowed to heal secondarily.

V-Y Advancement Flaps

Indications

V-Y advancement flaps are useful for covering ischial pressure sores and other wounds with very lax surrounding tissues. They may be used for both large (> 7–8 cm) and small wounds. V-Y advancement flaps are slightly different from those described above. The pedicle is not a bridge of surrounding skin and subcutaneous tissue; it is the deep tissue underlying the flap.

Procedure

1. Determine the site where the laxity of the surrounding skin is greatest.

2. Draw the flap before making any incisions so that you can make corrections.

3. Mark the V with the widest area at the edge of the wound, tapering gradually to a point.

4. Incise the skin edges through the subcutaneous tissue down to, but not into, the underlying muscle. The flap remains attached to the deep tissues.

5. The flap then should be advanced into the wound defect.

6. Close the defect primarily at the narrow point of the V. This step creates the Y limb.

7. Suture the flap loosely, under no tension. Place a few dermal sutures, and then close the skin with interrupted sutures. Do not make the skin closure too tight. It is better to have small gaps in the skin closure (which will heal) than do a tight closure and lose part of the flap.

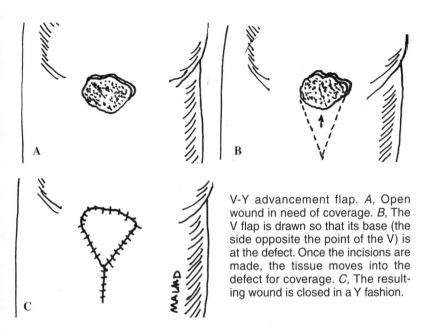

V-Y advancement flap. *A*, Open wound in need of coverage. *B*, The V flap is drawn so that its base (the side opposite the point of the V) is at the defect. Once the incisions are made, the tissue moves into the defect for coverage. *C*, The resulting wound is closed in a Y fashion.

General Postoperative Care

Cleanse the suture lines with gentle soap and water and apply antibiotic ointment 1–2 times per day.

Remove the sutures within 7–10 days.

TROUBLE-SHOOTING

What to Do if the Flap Becomes Swollen and Bluish Within Hours after the Operation

A swollen, bluish flap indicates a problem with circulation into or out of the flap. Usually it is a venous (i.e., outflow) problem.

Make sure that the patient is positioned properly and that nothing is compressing or pulling on the pedicle. Loosen surrounding dressings and tape. Sometimes it is helpful to remove a few stitches to ensure that the flap is not under too much tension.

Be sure that no fluid has collected under the flap. Any collection of fluid requires drainage. Place a clamp between some of the sutures, and spread the skin edges. This technique helps to drain the fluid.

Ensure adequate pain control. Pain stimulates the sympathetic nervous system, which decreases blood flow through the pedicle.

What to Do If Part of the Flap Dies

A few days after the procedure, you may notice that a part of the flap has become purplish. A purple color indicates inadequate circulation to that part of the flap, and the tissue may eventually die.

If there is no evidence of infection, you may simply leave the flap alone. With time, this tissue will demarcate and die and then separate—or you may have to cut off the dead tissue. While this process is occurring, the underlying tissues will heal.

Muscle Flaps

Muscle flaps involve moving a local muscle to cover a defect. A muscle flap is often done to cover an exposed bone or fracture, usually in the calf. The muscle is freed from the surrounding tissues but left attached to its blood supply. A muscle flap is an axial flap.

Compared with skin flaps, muscle flaps bring in a robust, new circulation to the injured site and thus enhance wound healing. The use of muscle flaps to cover exposed fractures has markedly decreased the morbidity associated with open (compound) fractures.

For rural practitioners without access to a specialist, the muscle flaps of greatest utility involve primarily the lower extremity (see chapter 21, "Fractures of the Tibia and Fibula").

Bibliography

1. Dhar SC, Taylor GI: The delay phenomenon: The story unfolds. Plast Reconstr Surg 104:2079–2091, 1999.
2. Taylor GI, Corlett RJ, Caddy CM, Zelt RG: An anatomic review of the delay phenomenon. II: Clinical applications. Plast Reconstr Surg 89:408–418, 1992.

Chapter 14

DISTANT FLAPS

A distant flap involves moving tissue (skin, fascia, muscle, bone, or some combination) from one part of the body, where it is dispensable, to another part, where it is needed. A distant flap is required when there is no healthy soft tissue adjacent to an open wound with which to provide adequate coverage.

These complex procedures are at the highest rung of the reconstructive ladder. Therefore, a distant flap is the treatment of choice when other, simpler procedures are *not* applicable.

Types of Distant Flaps

Distant flaps are divided into two categories: attached and free.

An **attached distant flap** implies that the area with the open wound initially is attached to the flap at the distant donor site. For example, the patient may have an open wound on the hand that requires soft tissue coverage. The donor site for the distant flap may be the chest (see chest flap below). Thus, the patient's hand initially is attached to the chest.

The blood supply to the flap initially comes from its pedicle (the bridge of tissue connecting the flap to its donor site). Gradually, over a few weeks, the flap develops in-growth of vessels from the recipient site (the wound). These new vessels bring blood to the flap, and the flap gradually becomes less dependent on the donor site circulation for survival. After a few weeks, the flap can be separated from its donor site and survive in the new area.

Patient inconvenience is a major drawback to attached flaps. Also, attached flaps are usually random flaps (see chapter 13, "Local Flaps"); therefore, they are not always completely reliable.

Free flaps, which are axial flaps, were developed to circumvent the problems inherent in attached distant flaps. Tissue supplied by a named vascular pedicle is detached completely from the donor site. The flap is then transferred to the open wound. With the aid of a microscope or other form of magnification, the flap's blood vessels (often just a few millimeters in diameter) are painstakingly connected to blood vessels at the recipient site. As you can imagine, a free flap is a technically difficult procedure and requires special equipment not readily available in many rural areas.

In contrast, attached distant flaps do not require such highly skilled specialists, but they do require basic surgical skills. Attached flaps often are quite useful when specialty care is unavailable. For example, an attached flap can make the difference between a healed functional hand and a severely damaged dysfunctional hand in a rural patient who has sustained severe soft tissue injury. This chapter focuses primarily on attached distant flaps.

Attached Distant Flaps

The procedure for creating and placing attached distant flaps follows many of the same rules that apply to local flaps. You should review chapter 13, "Local Flaps," for important background information.

Remember the 3:1 rule: for optimal circulation the flap length should be no more than 3 times the flap width. A delay procedure should be done if a larger flap is required.

As always, be sure that the wound is thoroughly cleansed before attaching the flap. All necrotic tissue must be removed. For a wound on the hand, it is best to debride the wound using a tourniquet. This technique allows you to remove the dead tissue carefully and avoid injury to important nearby structures. Be sure to remove the tourniquet and stop all bleeding before suturing the flap to the defect.

If the wound is covered by necrotic tissue, debride the wound a day or two before flap closure. If the wound is clean and granulating, use a scrub brush or the flat part of a scalpel blade to remove the top layer of granulation tissue before covering the wound with the flap.

Chest Flap

Indications

An open wound on the hand or forearm with exposed tendons/bones.

Anesthesia

A chest flap can be done under general anesthesia. However, local anesthesia for the donor site and a block for the recipient site is sometimes preferable. Local anesthesia and recipient site block ensure that the patient will not accidentally pull the flap attachments apart when awakening from general anesthesia.

Procedure

1. Ask the awake patient to position the injured hand over the chest in the most comfortable position. Stay away from breast tissue.

2. Mark this area. The flap should be drawn in such a way that the hand can be comfortably attached to the chest, but you must make sure that the pedicle does not become kinked. Usually the flap is drawn so that the pedicle is based inferiorly, but it can be designed with almost any orientation. Be sure that no scars from previous injuries are located within the flap or pedicle.

3. Design the flap so that it is slightly larger than the defect.

4. Make the incision through skin and subcutaneous tissue and into the underlying fascia (the thin layer of connective tissue over the muscle). Do not incise the muscle. The fascia contributes to the blood supply of the flap; therefore, it is important to keep it attached to the flap whenever possible.

5. Elevate the flap off the deep underlying tissues.

6. Loosely stitch the three free sides of the flap in place. Use a few dermal sutures, and then close the skin with interrupted, simple sutures. The closure does not have to be perfect. If the flap is stitched too tightly, it may compromise circulation and result in partial flap loss.

7. If possible, the donor site on the chest should be closed primarily, but usually a split-thickness skin graft is needed. Alternatively, if the wound is just a few cm in diameter, the donor site may be allowed to heal secondarily.

8. Antibiotic ointment and saline-moistened gauze dressings should be placed on the exposed undersurface of the flap. Apply antibiotic ointment around the edges of the flap.

Postoperative Care

Donor site: Dressings should be changed daily as appropriate, depending on how you decide to treat the donor site. For example, use wet-dry dressings if the wound is allowed to close secondarily, antibiotic ointment with dry gauze if it is closed primarily.

Flap: Keep the recipient site and flap uncovered so that the patient and caregivers can be sure that the flap pedicle has not kinked. Any signs of venous congestion (the flap becomes purplish and swollen, with fast capillary refill) necessitates repositioning of the recipient site.

While the patient is in bed, it often helps to place a pillow under the elbow to help support the forearm and wrist. Change the dressings daily, and clean the suture lines with saline or gentle soap/water. The patient can get out of bed after surgery but must take care not to pull on the flap.

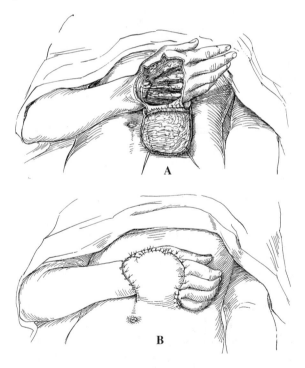

Chest flap. *A,* Open wound on the dorsum of the hand. *B,* An inferiorly based chest flap is created to cover the defect. A split-thickness skin graft is used to close the chest skin defect. (From Chase RA: Atlas of Hand Surgery. Philadelphia, W.B. Saunders, 1973, with permission.)

Cross Arm Flap

Indications

A cross arm flap is a good choice to cover a relatively small (maximal diameter of 2–4 cm) open wound on the hand or fingers. Usually such wounds are associated with an exposed tendon or bone.

A cross arm flap is useful when positioning makes the chest flap too uncomfortable for the patient. It is also the flap of choice if the patient prefers not to have scars on the chest or if no donor sites are available on the chest.

The inner aspect of the upper arm is the donor site.

Anesthesia

A cross arm flap can be done under general anesthesia, but local anesthesia with a nerve block is preferable. Local anesthesia and nerve block ensure that the patient will not accidentally pull apart the flap attachments on awakening from general anesthesia.

Procedure

1. Before surgery, ask the patient to hold the injured hand so that the wound is next to the inner aspect of the opposite upper arm.

2. The flap should be designed so that the hand can be comfortably attached to the inner arm, making sure that the attached part of the flap does not become kinked. Pick a position that allows some gentle shoulder motion to prevent shoulder stiffness.

3. Mark this area.

4. Draw the flap so that it is slightly larger than the defect. Stay away from any scars.

5. Make the incision through the skin and subcutaneous tissue; do *not* include muscle.

6. Elevate the flap off the underlying tissues.

7. Loosely stitch the three free sides of the flap in place. Use a few dermal sutures, and then close the skin with interrupted, simple sutures. The closure does not have to be perfect.

8. If possible, loosely close the donor site primarily. Alternatively, a wound no larger than a few centimeters may be allowed to close secondarily.

9. Antibiotic ointment covered with saline-moistened gauze dressings should be placed on the free undersurface of the flap. Antibiotic ointment should be placed around the edges of the flap.

Postoperative Care

Donor site: Dressings should be changed daily as appropriate, depending on how you decide to treat the donor site.

Flap: Keep the recipient site and flap uncovered so that the patient and caregivers can be sure that the flap has not kinked. Any signs of venous congestion (the flap becomes purplish and swollen, with fast capillary refill) necessitates repositioning of the hand.

While the patient is in bed, it often helps to place a pillow under the elbow to help support the forearm and wrist. Change the dressings daily and clean the suture lines with saline or gentle soap and water. The patient can get out of bed after surgery but must take care not to pull on the flap.

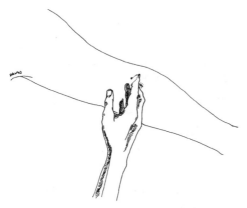

The cross arm flap is useful for smaller defects, especially those involving the fingers.

Cross Leg Flap

Indications

The most common indication for a cross leg flap is an open wound with an exposed fracture or exposed tendons of the lower third of the calf or foot. The lower calf or foot is sewn to the calf of the opposite leg for 3–4 weeks. Keeping the legs in this position can result in marked leg and hip stiffness. Therefore, a cross leg flap is best used in children or young adults; it is not recommended in patients older than 35 years.

Anesthesia

Either general or spinal anesthesia is required for cross leg flaps.

Procedure

1. Before administration of anesthesia, determine the best position for the patient's legs so that a flap of tissue taken from the noninjured posteromedial calf will lie easily over the defect with the least discomfort.

2. Draw the flap on the posteromedial side of the calf, overlying the gastrocnemius muscle. The flap should be slightly larger than the wound defect.

3. The flap should be designed so that it is superiorly based.

4. Incise the skin, subcutaneous tissue, and fascia overlying the gastrocnemius muscle. Elevate the flap along the plane between the fascia and underlying muscle. The fascia must stay attached to the flap.

5. Move the flap over to the open wound.

6. Loosely stitch the three free sides of the flap in place. Place a few dermal sutures, and then close the skin with interrupted sutures. The closure does not have to be perfect.

7. The donor site should be covered with a split-thickness skin graft.

8. Place antibiotic ointment and saline-moistened gauze along the free undersurface of the flap. Apply antibiotic ointment around all suture lines.

9. The patient's legs must be immobilized together to prevent accidentally separating the legs and tearing the suture line. This is best achieved with plaster. Use a lot of padding under the plaster.

10. Cut out a window in the plaster and padding over the flap so that the flap can be observed and cleansed daily.

Postoperative Care

Donor site: Treat as you would the site of a split-thickness skin graft.

Flap: Keep the recipient site and flap uncovered so that the patient and caregivers can be sure that the flap has not kinked. Any signs of venous congestion (the flap becomes purplish and swollen, with fast capillary refill) necessitates repositioning of the legs.

In adults, plaster immobilization often can be removed after 4–5 days. Then a splint or gauze wrap can be created to keep the legs in the proper position.

Children must be fully immobilized in plaster until the flap is divided. You may need to change the plaster in the operating room under anesthesia.

Change the dressings daily and clean the suture lines with saline or gentle soap and water. Be careful not to pull on the flap.

Division of Distant Flaps

Gradually the flap will experience an in-growth of circulation from its new site. After no less than 2 weeks, you can start to divide the pedicle, using local anesthesia such as lidocaine or bupivacaine. Do not add epinephrine to the anesthetic solution.

Cut approximately one-fourth of the way across the pedicle, and loosely stitch down the free edge to the recipient wound. A week later continue another fourth of the way across the pedicle of the flap. At 4 weeks you should be able to divide the flap completely.

Alternatively, you may divide the flap completely in one stage 4 weeks after the initial procedure. Gradual division, however, gives the flap time to adjust to less input from the pedicle.

Suture the flap loosely to the skin edges of the recipient site. Small areas of skin separation will heal; all areas along the edge of the wound do not have to be closed completely.

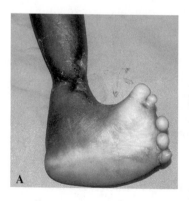
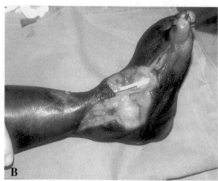

Cross leg flap. *A,* Child with a congenital deformity that caused the foot to grow in an inverted position. Several previous operations failed to correct the problem. Definitive treatment required excision of the tight scar and repositioning of the foot. *B,* This procedure resulted in an open wound with exposed tendons in need of soft tissue coverage. *(Figure continued on following page.)*

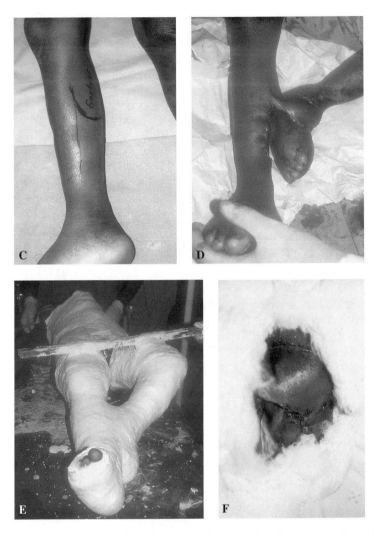

Cross leg flap *(continued)*. *C*, Design of the cross leg flap. *D*, The flap after being sewn in place. *E*, The legs immobilized together in plaster. *F*, A window cut in the plaster to allow dressing changes and observation of the flap.

Groin Flap

The groin flap is an axial flap, whereas the previously discussed distant flaps are random flaps. The groin flap is more reliable but also more technically difficult. Thus, only providers with advanced surgical skills should attempt this procedure. Because the groin flap may be used to save a hand with a large soft tissue defect but otherwise intact tendons and nerves, it is described in detail below.

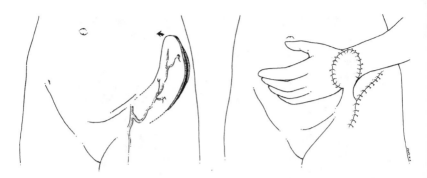

Design of groin flap. In contrast to the previously mentioned distant flaps, the groin flap is an axial flap, and its blood supply is by way of an identifiable vessel. It is a highly reliable flap for coverage of hand wounds. (From Cohen M (ed): Mastery of Plastic and Reconstructive Surgery. Boston, Little, Brown, 1994, p 59, with permission.)

Indications

The indication for a groin flap is an open wound on the hand or fingers in which the tendons or bones are exposed. It is also possible to take a piece of iliac bone with the flap, if needed, to reconstruct a bony defect in the hand.

Anesthesia

The groin flap is usually done under general anesthesia. However, it is possible to perform the procedure using spinal anesthesia with a wrist block.

Design

Landmarks

- Anterosuperior iliac spine (ASIS)
- Pubic tubercle
- Course of the inguinal ligament
- Femoral artery

The artery that nourishes the flap comes off the femoral artery within two finger widths below the point where the femoral artery meets the inguinal ligament. This artery travels in the direction of the axis of the flap toward the ASIS.

Medial flap border	The course of the femoral artery
Upper flap border	Two fingerwidths above the inguinal ligament parallel to the artery nourishing the flap
Lower flap border	Two fingerwidths below the take-off of the nourishing artery from the femoral artery; again, it runs parallel to the direction of the femoral artery
Lateral flap border	Lateral to the ASIS, as determined by the size of the wound. Once the flap is lateral to the ASIS, keep the length-to-width ratio at 1:1.

Always draw the flap first. The portion of the flap overlying and lateral to the ASIS is used to cover the open wound. Most of the medial portion of this flap is tubed and serves as the pedicle (see below).

Dissection

1. Proceed from lateral to medial.

2. Start by incising the lateral half of the upper and lower markings and the lateral border of the flap.

3. Elevate the skin and subcutaneous tissue off the underlying fascia. Dissect medially until you reach the lateral aspect of the sartorius muscle; look for the muscle fibers traveling in an inferomedial direction from the ASIS to the medial knee.

4. At the lateral border of the sartorius muscle, make an up-and-down incision into the fascia.

5. Keeping the fascia attached to the skin and subcutaneous tissue of the flap, continue the dissection until enough of the flap is raised to allow inset of the flap over the wound.

6. If a branch of the blood vessel runs deep to the fascia, ligate it to prevent accidental injury.

7. Take care to avoid injury to the lateral femoral cutaneous nerve when you incise the sartorius fascia.

Inset of the Flap

1. The pedicle of the flap (approximately the medial half of the flap) is sutured loosely to itself to make a tube. Simple, interrupted skin sutures are adequate. The tube allows the patient to move the shoulder without risking injury to the flap or hand attachment. It also increases postoperative comfort and makes dressing care easier.

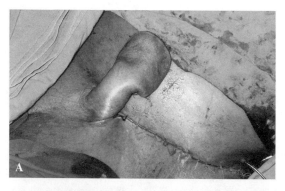

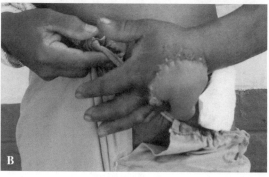

Groin flap. *A,* Elevation of the groin flap; the medial portion is sewn together to form a tube. The donor site has been closed primarily. *B,* The patient with the hand attached to the flap.

2. Manipulate the hand/forearm into pronation or supination to determine the appropriate hand position for suturing the flap to the wound.

3. The lateral portion of the flap should be loosely sutured to the edges of the wound.

4. If the portion of the flap used to cover the wound seems too bulky, you can thin it by removing some of the subcutaneous tissue. Do not be too aggressive. The flap can be thinned at a later date once it has been divided from the donor site. Better a bulky flap than a dead one.

5. *Do not thin the flap medially, where you are making it into a tube.* You may injure the blood supply to the flap.

Donor Site

The donor site should be closed primarily. You may need to flex the patient's hips to bring the wound edges together. The patient should remain flexed for a few days after surgery. Then you may allow the patient to straighten the leg gradually over a few days.

Place a Penrose drain or a strip of sterile glove to prevent fluid from accumulating under the suture line. The drain can be removed on the day after surgery.

Postoperative Care

Apply antibiotic ointment along the suture lines and saline-moistened gauze along the undersurface of the flap between the part of the flap that is tubed and the patient's hand. Change the dressing daily.

You may want to wrap the patient's arm to the chest for the first day to prevent too much arm movement. Once the patient is fully awake, this precaution is usually unnecessary.

Watch for signs of venous congestion. Check the flap regularly to ensure that the pedicle is not twisted or kinked.

Division of the Flap

1. Gradually the flap will develop an in-growth of circulation from its new site.

2. After no less than 3 weeks, you may start to divide the pedicle. Cut one-fourth of the way across the pedicle, and loosely stitch down the edge to the recipient site. Local anesthetic without epinephrine should be used.

3. One week later, divide another small portion of the pedicle.

4. At 5 weeks you should be able to divide the flap completely from its pedicle. Gradual division is best; do not completely separate the flap at one time. However, if gradual division is not possible, it should be safe to divide the flap all at once at 5 weeks.

5. Suture the flap very loosely. Small areas of skin separation will heal; so do not worry that all skin edges have to be completely closed.

What to Do if Part of the Flap Dies

If a portion of the flap becomes ischemic and dies, the wound often heals with local care. See chapter 13, "Local Flaps," for further details.

Free Flap

A free flap involves complete detachment of a piece of tissue (skin, fascia, muscle, bone, or some combination) with its blood supply (artery and vein). The tissue is transferred to the wound in need of coverage. The blood vessels of the flap are then reattached to an artery and vein near the wound.

To reconnect the blood vessels requires magnification capabilities (4 × glasses at least or a microscope), tiny suture material (8-0, 9-0 nylon), and delicate instruments. The procedure takes several hours and is most efficiently done with two teams of surgeons (one working to find the vessels at the wound site, one working to dissect the flap).

In experienced hands, a free flap can achieve remarkable results. Examples include reconstruction of the tongue or jaw after ablative on-cologic surgery, breast reconstruction after mastectomy, or coverage of a badly fractured ankle with soft tissue loss. Obviously, these proce-dures can be done only by highly experienced reconstructive surgeons with extensive microvascular training and expertise.

The following photographs show a patient with a squamous cell car-cinoma of the lateral aspect of the tongue. Because of the extent of the tumor, almost one-half of the tongue and floor of the mouth needed

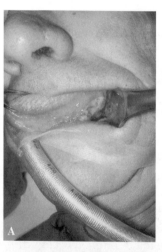

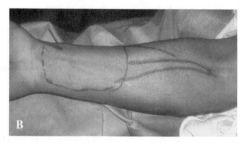

Free flap reconstruction. *A*, Squamous cell cancer of the lateral tongue. *B*, Design of the radial forearm flap. *C*, Blood vessels from the flap are reattached to blood vessels in the neck. *D*, Final result 1 year postoperatively.

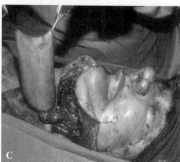

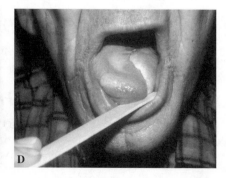

to be resected. The reconstruction was done with a free flap taken from the volar surface of the forearm and based on the radial artery (called a radial forearm flap).

The reconstructed tongue is almost normal in size. Thus the patient was able to eat and speak normally. The flap also tolerated postoperative radiation treatment without complication. These results would be hard to attain with any other reconstructive technique.

Bibliography

1. Chase RA: Atlas of Hand Surgery. Philadelphia, W.B. Saunders, 1973, pp 120–127.
2. Chuang DCC, Colony LH, Chen HC, Wei FC: Groin flap design and versatility. Plast Reconstr Surg 84:100–107, 1989.
3. Daniel RK, Taylor GI: Distant transfer of an island flap by microvascular anastomoses. Plast Reconstr Surg 52:111–117, 1973.
4. Puckett CL, Reinisch JF: Gastrocnemius musculocutaneous cross-leg flap. In Strauch D, Vasconez LO, Hall-Findlay EJ (eds): Grabb's Encyclopedia of Flaps. Boston, Little, Brown, 1990, pp 1703–1705.
5. Strauch B, Yu HL (eds): Atlas of Microvascular Surgery. New York, Thieme Medical Publishers, 1993.

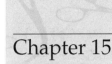

Chapter 15

SCAR FORMATION

KEY FIGURES:
Hypertrophic scar
Buried dermal suture

This chapter gives background information about the scarring process. Treatment options for problematic scars are also discussed.

Normal Course of Scar Maturation

Strength

Scar tissue is never as strong as normal, uninjured skin. For the first 3–4 weeks after injury, the wound can easily be reopened by minimal trauma. By 6 weeks, the scar has attained approximately 50% of its final strength. During the next 12 months, the scar gradually increases its ability to withstand injury, but it never attains normal strength.

Appearance

The period of maximal collagen production (the primary component of skin and scar tissue) is the first 4–6 weeks after a wound has closed. During this period the scar may appear red and be slightly firm and raised.

Over the next several months, changes in the rate of collagen production and degradation occur. Normal healing results in normal types and amounts of collagen in the area. On the surface, normal healing is illustrated by the fading of redness and softening of the scar.

I usually tell patients that it will take at least 1 year for the scar to achieve its final appearance. Scars in children may continue to change and improve for several years.

Abnormal Scarring

For various reasons, such as genetics, nature of initial injury, or bad luck, some scars become exceptionally red, thick, and tight. Such scars can be problematic on the hand or other flexor surfaces, because they may lead to limitation of movement and loss of function.

Hypertrophic scars are a bit thicker and redder than the fine scar that usually results after primary healing. At the extreme, scars may become **keloids**—that is, they may enlarge beyond their initial area. Keloids can become large and unsightly. They also can cause annoying symptoms, such as itching and pain.

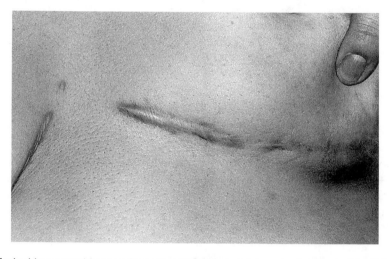

Typical hypertrophic scar. Note that the scar is thick and raised but still within the confines of a normal scar.

In addition, the scar may be **unstable**. An unstable scar is easily reinjured with minimal trauma; it heals but is easily injured again. This cycle can go on for years and ultimately result in the development of an aggressive form of skin cancer.

Abnormal scarring is usually the result of abnormal collagen production and degradation. Although we do not know the exact cause of these abnormal processes, the manner in which a wound is closed may play a role. In addition, there are interventions that can improve an abnormal scar.

Method of Wound Closure

Primary Wound Closure

Usually, the best (i.e., least noticeable) scar results when a wound is closed by suturing the skin edges together. Usually the sutures are removed before the 14th day after repair. As explained above, at this point the scar is not very strong; in fact, it has < 15% of its final strength. Normal everyday movements will pull on the scar and may result in widening of the scar.

For this reason, most plastic surgeons place buried dermal sutures as well as the usual skin sutures when they close a wound (see figure below). Buried dermal sutures are not difficult to place, but this extra step is time-consuming. The dermal sutures add strength to the repair site during the weeks to months required for their absorption. The anticipated result is less widening and an improved appearance of the scar.

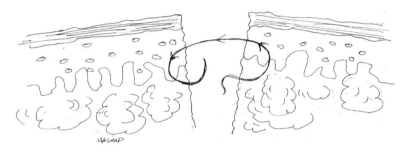

Buried dermal sutures are used to hold together the skin edges and thereby decrease tension on the external sutures. In theory, placement of a few buried dermal sutures decreases the risk for hypertrophic scarring and keloid formation.

When dermal sutures are not used, be sure that the skin sutures provide good dermis-to-dermis approximation. It also is important to remove the sutures at the appropriate time (see chapter 1, "Suturing: The Basics"). Sutures that are left in place too long cause an inflammatory response that worsens scar appearance.

If Steristrips are available, put them across the suture line when the sutures are removed. This simple step gives the scar a bit of extra strength during the period when it is vulnerable to injury.

Secondary Wound Closure

Wounds that are allowed to heal secondarily often have larger, more noticeable scars than ones closed primarily. Secondary wound closure also is associated with a higher incidence of hypertrophic scarring and keloid formation.

How the Patient Can Help

Once the sutures have been removed and the wound looks well healed, **rubbing or gently massaging the scar** with a mild moisturizing cream (e.g., Vaseline, aloe, cocoa butter) a few times each day promotes softening and lightening of scar tissue, especially on the face and hands. A cream with vitamin E may be helpful. Patients should not spend a large sum of money on fancy creams because no conclusive evidence indicates that expensive formulations improve the scar's final appearance. Gentle massage should be continued for at least 4–6 weeks.

Patients should stay out of the sun as much as possible, and always **use a sunscreen** (SPF > 20). Scars exposed to the sun (especially if sunburn dvelops) not only stay red longer but also may not fade as much as normally expected.

All patients should **maintain good nutrition**, and diabetics should maintain good glucose control.

Providers must counsel patients aggressively about the **ill effects of tobacco products** on wound healing. Some of the components in cigarettes cause a decrease in blood circulation to the skin, which results in poor wound healing and may even lead to tissue loss. Dramatic adverse reactions due to the effects of smoking have been reported.

Interventions for Problematic Scars

Scars that are Too Tight

These treatments can be tried individually or in some combination.

Gentle Massage

Instruct the patient in the massage techniques described above.

Silicone Gel Sheets

Once the sutures have been removed and the wound looks well healed, you can cover the wound with silicone gel sheets. Although it is not entirely understood how they work, silicone gel sheets can be quite effective. They can be obtained from pharmacies but usually require a prescription (although this policy is changing in the United States).

How to use the silicone gel sheet

1. Cut a piece large enough to cover the scar completely.

2. The sheet should be left in place as long as tolerated—even all day. The longer it is in place, the better.

3. The patient should remove the sheet to wash. Deodorant soaps should not be used to cleanse the area; they may cause a rash. One piece of gel sheet can be used repeatedly.

4. Sheets should be used for at least 2–3 months to make an appreciable difference.

Splinting

The purpose of splinting is to prevent loss of function and restriction of movement from a tight scar. Especially on the hand and in a crease, splinting can be quite useful. The splint should be molded so that it stretches the tight scar.

Case example: If a tight scar across the front of elbow prevents the patient from fully extending the forearm, the following steps may help:

• Make a splint that holds the elbow in as much extension as tolerated. Gradually the scar will become less tight because of the remodeling due to splinting and scar massage (remember, you can add other "scar is too tight" treatments). With time the patient will be able to extend the elbow more fully.

• The splint can be made out of simple plaster of Paris (see chapter 28, "Hand Splinting and General Aftercare").

• If the splint interferes with the patient's ability to work, encourage the patient to wear it at night.

• New splints should be made as the patient can more fully extend at the elbow.

• This process may take many months, but is worth the effort to improve function.

Pressure Garments

Pressure garments, measured and fitted to the individual patient, can be worn under everyday clothing. They are designed to apply continuous pressure over the area of concern. Theoretically, the pressure causes the underlying scar to become ischemic and thus leads to remodeling.

Pressure garments should be worn 18–24 hours/day for a minimum of 4–6 months. Medical supply stores and pharmacies can order pressure garments, which are expensive. Prescriptions usually are required.

Scars that are Too Red

Reassurance and Reminders

Reassure the patient that scars will fade on their own, but the process takes time. Remind the patient to avoid sun exposure whenever possible and to use sunscreen when exposure cannot be avoided. Ultraviolet light injures normal skin as well as scars. A sunburned scar may not fade as well as normally expected.

Make-up

Once the sutures have been removed and the wound looks well healed, the patient can apply gentle make-up until the scar fades on its own. It is best to use make-up with a sunscreen to prevent sun injury. Make-up alone does not protect the tissues from the ill effects of the sun.

Keloids and Hypertrophic Scars

Try the treatments described under "Scars that are Too Tight." Massage, silicone gel sheets, splinting, and pressure garments may help. In addition, the treatments listed below may be useful. Each can be tried individually, but often they work better in combination with another method. For example, inject the keloid with steroids and use a pressure garment daily. Or excise the keloid, close the wound meticulously, and then use silicone gel sheeting after the sutures have been removed.

Steroid Injection

Inject triamcinolone acetonide into the dermis of the keloid—approximately 1 mg for every 1–2 cm of scar. It is best to use a tuberculin syringe because you are working with small amounts of medication. Be sure to check the mg/ml of the solution (different bottles may have different drug concentrations). The total amount of injected triamcinolone should not exceed 30 mg.

Caution: Steroid injection hurts. You can add 0.5–1.0 ml of lidocaine to the steroid solution.

It takes several weeks to see any noticeable change in the scar. Steroid injection can be repeated after 4–6 weeks, but I do not recommend injecting the same area more than 2 or 3 times. The response to steroid injection is quite variable. The reported percentages of patients obtaining some improvement (not necessarily resolution of the scar) after steroid use range from 50% to 100%.

The patient should be warned of the risks associated with the injection of steroids. Infection may develop at the injection site, and the injected area may become lighter in color than the surrounding skin. Be especially careful in treating diabetic patients. Steroids may cause an elevation of blood glucose level.

Pressure Earrings

Some patients develop keloids after ear piercing. Earrings designed to apply pressure to the earlobe are commercially available. They work best on small keloids (< 1 cm). Pressure earrings are especially useful when combined with excision of the keloid. Once the excision sutures have been removed, the patient should wear the earring for at least 2 or 3 months (longer is better). This approach may prevent recurrence of the keloid.

Excision

Caution: Excision of a keloid often results in formation of another keloid. The recurrence rate after excision ranges from 45% to 100%.

At times, however, it is worthwhile to excise the bothersome keloid. For example, patients with a keloid associated with ear piercing may have a successful outcome if, as previously described, after excision they wear a compression earring regularly. Another example when excision may be successful is if the initial injury was not closed with sutures (i.e., it was allowed to heal secondarily). In this case, excision of the keloid followed by primary skin closure may be helpful. Even under these more favorable circumstances, you must warn patients that the keloid may recur.

If you excise the keloid, a close dermal approximation of the skin edges is especially important. Close approximation requires placement of buried dermal sutures prior to skin closure. Therefore, excision of a keloid and primary closure should be undertaken only by clinicians with excellent suturing skills.

Radiation Therapy

If radiation therapy facilities are available, low-dose therapy helps to prevent the development of a keloid. Usually it is performed only on patients known to develop severe keloids who are scheduled for surgical procedures. The radiation is administered as early as the first postoperative day.

As with other treatment methods, the success rate is variable, ranging from 10% to 94% in different studies.

Unstable Scars

When larger wounds or wounds over creases are allowed to heal secondarily, the scar may be easily injured and reopen. Although usually it heals with local wound care measures, this cycle often repeats itself again and again. Excision of the entire scar may be indicated. The resultant skin defect requires closure with a more durable skin graft or flap (see chapters 12, 13, and 14 on "Skin Grafts," "Local Flaps," and "Distant Flaps" for details about these techniques).

Bibliography

Niessen FB, Spauwen PHM, Schalkwijk J, Kon M: On the nature of hypertrophic scars and keloids: A review. Plast Reconstr Surg 104:1435–1458, 1999.

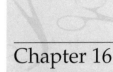

Chapter 16

FACIAL LACERATIONS

The face has several unique properties that dictate the choice of treatment after injury. This chapter describes basic principles for the treatment of facial wounds as well as treatment recommendations for injuries involving specific areas of the face.

Unique Properties of Facial Lacerations

Cosmetic Concerns

Although most people do not want an unsightly scar anywhere on the body, they are especially concerned about scars on their face. Thus, primary closure, which usually results in the least noticeable scar, is the preferred treatment for most facial lacerations. Fortunately, because of the laxity of facial skin, most wounds can be repaired primarily unless they have significant tissue loss or tissue swelling.

Better Blood Supply and Circulation

The skin of the face has a more abundant blood supply compared with other areas of the body. As a result, lacerations on the face can be closed more than 6 hours after injury (the usual time limit for closure of an acute laceration) without a high risk for subsequent wound infection. As long as the wound can be cleansed thoroughly, facial lacerations often can be closed even the day after injury.

Because of the better blood supply, a wound that is closed primarily can tolerate more tension on the suture line than is usually allowed. But do *not* take this principle to an extreme. If there is significant blanching of the skin with the closure, you may not want to close the wound completely. In this instance, merely place a few sutures to close the wound partially and thus decrease the size of the scar.

Initial Care

The initial care of a facial wound is the same as the care applied to any wound. As explained in chapter 6, "Evaluation of an Acute Wound," the wound needs to be cleansed fully and examined thoroughly. All foreign material, blood, and necrotic tissue should be removed. Debridement of skin edges should be kept to a minimum, unless the tissue is obviously dead. Because of the excellent blood supply of the face, tissue that seems ischemic often survives.

Paint the injured area with an antibacterial solution before closing the wound. Be careful: some solutions can cause injury to the eyes. Ten percent povidone iodine solution is commonly available and will not injure the eyes. It also can be used safely on oral mucosa.

Anesthesia

A more thorough description of the administration of local anesthetics is found in chapter 3, "Local Anesthesia." Below is a brief overview.

Agents

Lidocaine with epinephrine is the best choice of anesthetic with one exception: when a flap is raised by the injury. In this case, it is best to use plain lidocaine in order not to diminish circulation to the flap.

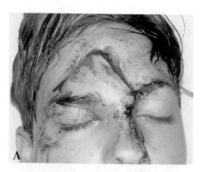

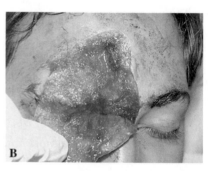

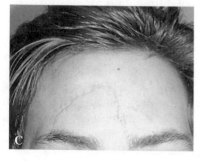

Tissue flap in patient who fell through a glass window. *A,* Irregular forehead laceration. *B,* The skin is separated from the deep tissue layers of the forehead, creating a skin flap with marginal blood supply. Do *not* add epinephrine to the anesthetic solution; it will decrease circulation to the flap and may cause the tissue to die. *C,* One month after repair. All of the skin has survived and is healing without complication.

Bupivacaine is also acceptable. Add bicarbonate to decrease the pain of injection.

Administration of Local Anesthetic

For **smaller lacerations** (a few centimeters or less), it is often easiest to inject the anesthetic along the wound edges.

For **larger lacerations** or lacerations around the edge of the lip (where local injection can distort landmarks), a nerve block is usually more effective.

Nerve Blocks on the Face

Mental nerve block: lower lip, skin below the lip.

Infraorbital nerve block: upper lip, lateral nose, lower eyelid, medial cheek.

Supraorbital/supratrochlear nerve block: forehead.

Suture Choice

Nylon is the suture material of choice to close a skin wound on the face.

Chromic or other absorbable material should be used for mucosal lacerations.

If you believe that the patient will not return for suture removal or if the patient is a child in whom suture removal is likely to be quite difficult, chromic (absorbable material of choice) sutures can be used on facial skin.

The appropriate size of the suture is discussed in the sections describing specific injuries.

Suture Placement

Sutures on the face should be placed a little closer together than usually recommended because of cosmetic concerns. The sutures should be placed 1–2 mm from the skin edge and 3 mm apart to achieve better tissue approximation. Exceptions are noted in specific descriptions below.

If you have access to magnifying glasses, use them. They help to achieve better tissue alignment because the magnification allows more accurate placement of the sutures.

Most facial lacerations can be closed in one layer. Exceptions will be noted.

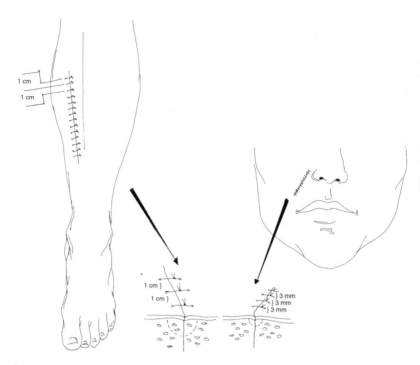

Suture bites: face vs. rest of the body. Sutures placed on the face should be approximately 1–2 mm from the skin edge and approximately 3 mm apart. This technique requires the use of small suture material.

Continuous vs. Interrupted Closure

A laceration in which skin edges can be aligned easily and without tension can be closed with either technique.

Irregular lacerations or lacerations in which you are concerned about the potential for infection should be closed in an interrupted fashion for the following reasons:

1. If, a few days after wound closure, a localized area starts to look infected, you can treat the infection without having to open the entire wound. Just remove a few sutures in the area that looks red, open the skin, and wash the wound with saline. This will allow the wound to drain and may allow the infection to resolve while keeping the resultant scar relatively small. The patient also should be given antibiotics.

2. If the wound had been closed by placing the sutures in a continuous fashion, partial removal of the suture is not possible. If the wound looks infected, the entire suture will need to be removed and thus the entire wound will reopen. This results in a much larger scar.

Suture Removal

Sutures should be removed after 5–7 days to minimize scarring.

Postrepair Instructions

1. After the wound edges are sutured together, apply a small amount of antibiotic ointment over the suture line. Cover with a dry gauze. The dressing can be removed on the following day.

2. The area should be cleansed once or twice daily with gentle soap and water. The patient can shower and wash the face as usual on the day after the repair.

3. After cleansing, a small amount of antibiotic ointment or a petrolatum type ointment should be applied over the suture line. If the patient desires, dry gauze can be used to cover the area, although it usually is not necessary unless the patient is in a dirty environment.

4. Facial injuries cause the tissues to swell. Be sure to warn your patient that the face will be swollen for several days after injury. To minimize swelling, instruct the patient to keep the head elevated at all times. When reclining, an extra pillow (or folded sheet) should be placed under the head.

5. The patient also should avoid bending and heavy lifting for several days after the injury because such activities promote facial swelling.

Specific Wounds

Lip Lacerations

The **vermilion border** is the edge of the lip where the red part of the lip ends and the white skin begins. It is vital to realign the vermilion border meticulously to prevent a noticeable notched irregularity.

The red part of the lip is the **mucosal surface**, which can be divided into two parts. The part of the lip that you see when the lips are barely separated is called the **dry mucosa** because it feels dry to touch. The mucosal surface that lies against the teeth and appears and feels wet is called the **wet mucosa**. These distinctions are important. Try to align the border between these two surfaces to prevent a relatively subtle, but noticeable irregularity.

To make it easier to see the various "borders," it is best to use a nerve block for repair of lip lacerations. If you are unable to do this, inject the local anesthetic a few millimeters away from the wound edge and wait longer than usual (5–10 min) for the swelling from the injection to resolve.

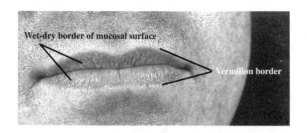

Important anatomic landmarks of the lip.

Mucosal Lacerations

- The key to successful repair is to realign the wet-dry mucosal border, as explained above.
- Place the first stitch at the border between the wet and dry surfaces.
- Use absorbable sutures, 4-0, and try to sew the wet mucosa to wet mucosa and the dry mucosa to dry mucosa.
- It is important to evert the edges; use mattress sutures if necessary.
- Tie at least 4 or 5 knots in the sutures to prevent the sutures from coming undone because the patient unconsciously pulls at them with the tongue.

Partial-thickness Lacerations that Cross the Vermilion Border

- The key to successful repair is to approximate the vermilion border as well as possible.
- Align the red/white margin first. Place the initial suture just above the vermilion border in the white upper lip skin. Use a 5-0 or 6-0 suture.
- If the stitch does not seem to be well-placed, remove it and try again.
- Place the remaining sutures in the lip skin (5-0 or 6-0) and lip mucosa (4-0 or 5-0). Be sure to evert the skin edges.

Full-thickness Lacerations

In full-thickness lip lacerations, the outer skin, lip muscle, and mucosa have all been cut. Full-thickness lip lacerations often look scary. Because muscle retracts when cut, the lip wound looks larger and more complex than it is. Most of these wounds can be repaired easily. Primary repair is possible even if approximately one-fourth of the upper or lower lip is lost. Repair includes the following steps:

1. It often helps to place a gauze pad between the gums and lip to collect blood or other fluids.

2. **If bleeding is significant:** injection of lidocaine with epinephrine usually controls bleeding from the lip surface. However, if the bleeding is coming from a cut artery, you may need to place a stitch in the artery. Use a 4-0 absorbable suture, and place a simple or figure-of-eight suture at the site of bleeding. When you tie the suture, the bleeding should stop.

3. **Repair the mucosa:** repair the inner aspect of the lip first, as described above under "Mucosal Lacerations." Use an absorbable 4-0 suture, and try to evert the edges.

4. **Irrigate the wound** with saline again after the mucosa is closed to cleanse the wound.

5. **Repair the muscle:** use an absorbable suture, 3-0 or 4-0, and place one or two figure-of-eight sutures in the muscle. If you look carefully at the wound edges, the muscle and musosa have a different appearance and texture. Take care not to catch any mucosa in the stitches; if you do, you will cause a pucker in the mucosa.

6. **Repair the skin:** as well as possible, align the vermilion border as described above. Remember to tie 4 or 5 knots in the lip sutures, which often come undone because the patient unconsciously pulls at them.

Intraoral Mucosal Lacerations

Lacerations may occur inside the mouth. When they occur along the inside of the cheek, you must be careful to *avoid injury to the opening of the parotid duct* (through which the secretions of the parotid gland enter the mouth) during the repair. The opening of the duct into the mouth is a small, raised mound of mucosa inside the cheek across from the upper second molar. You do not want to accidentally place a suture across this structure.

• Use absorbable sutures, 4-0 or 3-0.

• Do *not* take big bites of tissue. Go about 2–3 mm from the edge of the wound and include only the mucosa in your suture. Do *not* include muscle or other underlying tissues.

• Be sure to evert the edges.

• You do *not* need to place the sutures close together. Usually only a few are needed (0.5–0.7 cm apart) to approximate the edges.

Tongue Lacerations

- Use lidocaine with epinephrine to control bleeding.

- Because the tongue is a muscle, the edges retract when it is cut, making the wound appear more complicated than it is.

- If you can, place an absorbable 3-0 suture in a figure-of-eight fashion in the inner muscle. If you cannot place this stitch, take deeper than usual bites when repairing the tongue edges. Use 3-0 or 4-0 absorbable sutures.

- Take larger bites, 4–5 mm from the edge, and include the underlying muscle to control bleeding.

Full-thickness Cheek Lacerations

A full-thickness cheek laceration implies that the cheek skin, underlying subcutaneous tissue/muscle, and intraoral mucosa have been injured. Such wounds must be repaired in layers.

Intraoral Mucosa

- The intraoral mucosa should be repaired first, using the previously described technique.

- When the mucosa is closed, it separates the oral cavity from the outer wound.

- To decrease contamination by oral flora, the wound again should be irrigated with saline once the opening into the mouth is repaired. Paint the area with an antibacterial solution.

Skin and Subcutaneous Tissue/Muscle

- Skin and subcutaneous layers often can be brought together simply by repairing the skin. Use 5-0 nylon sutures for skin closure.

- If bringing the skin edges together does not allow the subcutaneous tissue to fill in the wound, place one or two (depending on the size of the wound) 4-0 absorbable simple sutures to approximate the muscle or subcutaneous tissue.

- Do not place too many sutures, or you risk injury to the facial nerve or other deep structures.

Full-thickness Nasal Lacerations

A full-thickness nasal laceration includes injury to the external skin, cartilage, and nasal mucosa.

Skin

- It is best to use plain lidocaine on the skin of the nose.

- Small, 5-0 nonabsorbable sutures are preferable, placed a few millimeters from the edges.

- Try to align the alar rim (the edge of the nostril) as well as possible to prevent notching. This goal is often problematic if the laceration completely tears the alar rim.

Cartilage

The cartilage usually is brought to an acceptable position when the skin laceration is repaired. Placement of sutures directly in the cartilage is not usually recommended.

Nasal Mucosa

- Primary repair of nasal mucosa can be challenging because you are working in a small, dark space; nevertheless, it is important to try. If the nasal mucosa is not properly repaired, the result may be a tight scar inside the nose, which can obstruct nasal breathing.

- To control bleeding from the mucosa, use lidocaine with epinephrine for local anesthesia.

- Use small, absorbable 5-0 chromic sutures. You do not need many.

- Once the repair is complete, loosely pack the affected nostril with gauze coated with antibiotic ointment. Leave the gauze in place for a few days to encourage healing with less scar contracture. The patient should take an oral antibiotic (e.g., cephalosporin) as long as the packing is in place.

Eyelid Lacerations

Caution is mandatory when an antibiotic ointment is used around the eye. Use only an ophthalmic ointment because regular antibiotic ointment can cause conjunctivitis.

Eyelid Skin Alone

The eyelid skin should be repaired loosely with simple sutures. Use 5-0 or 6-0 sutures, absorbable or nonabsorbable. If you use nonabsorbable sutures, remove them in 3–4 days.

Full-thickness Injuries

In full-thickness eyelid lacerations, skin, muscle, usually tarsal plate, and underlying conjunctiva are cut. The conjunctiva does not usually need to be closed as a separate layer. It will heal if the overlying tissues are well aligned. Use the following procedure:

1. Start by placing a small suture (5-0 or 6-0 is best) to reapproximate the gray line (where the eyelid meets the conjunctiva, i.e., the lash margin).

2. Keep the knot away from the eyeball because irritation or potentially an ulceration may result if the knot rubs on the conjunctiva or cornea.

3. Use absorbable 5-0 sutures to reapproximate the tarsal plate and orbicularis muscle in one layer.

4. Close the skin as described above.

Tearduct Injuries

An injury to the tearduct should be considered in full-thickness eyelid lacerations within 6–8 mm of the medial canthus (where the upper and lower eyelids meet near the side of the nose). If tearduct probes and stents are available, the duct should be probed and possibly stented. Probing a tearduct is quite difficult and requires special technical expertise and training. Do *not* attempt to probe a tearduct if you have not done it before.

Injuries with Tissue Loss

Primary closure of the eyelid can be done even with up to 25% full-thickness tissue loss. More than 25% full-thickness tissue loss requires more complicated flaps.

Partial-thickness loss (i.e., skin loss with underlying muscle and conjunctiva intact or repairable) can be covered with a full-thickness skin graft. In the medial canthal area, a defect smaller than 1 cm often can be allowed to heal by secondary intention.

The full-thickness skin graft can be taken from the other upper eyelid, if the patient has redundant upper eyelid skin. See more details in chapter 12, "Skin Grafts."

Eyebrow Lacerations

A laceration that involves the eyebrow should be reapproximated to recreate the natural curve of the eyebrow as well as possible. Leave the suture ends long so that you can easily distinguish them from the eyebrow hairs.

One caveat: do *not* shave the eyebrow. The hair may not grow back normally.

Full-thickness Forehead Lacerations

A full-thickness forehead laceration involves skin and underlying muscle. The bone of the skull is usually exposed. Such wounds must be repaired in layers to prevent a significant contour irregularity.

Frontal Sinus Fractures

The paired frontal sinuses are found at the center of the forehead, just above the bridge of the nose. If you can see a fracture of the anterior wall of the frontal sinus, the patient must have a computed tomography (CT) scan of the head to evaluate injury to the posterior wall of the frontal sinus and brain. If such injuries are present, a neurosurgeon is needed.

If the anterior wall is depressed, try to bring the bones outward to the appropriate position before closing the wound. Optimally, the bones should be immobilized with tiny plates and screws. This procedure requires a specialist and may be done at a later date. The following sections describe only soft tissue repair.

Frontalis Muscle with Overlying Fascia

The muscle and fascia should be brought together with a few simple or figure-of-eight, 3-0 or 4-0 absorbable sutures.

Skin

Repair the skin with 5-0 simple sutures.

Full-thickness Scalp Lacerations

Full-thickness scalp lacerations can be quite serious. Because of the abundant blood supply to the scalp, patients can lose a significant, even life-threatening amount of blood. It is acceptable to shave the surrounding hair to allow thorough examination of the wound. The hair will grow back.

Layers of the Scalp

Classically, the scalp is described as having five layers. From outside to inside, they can be remembered with the mnemonic **SCALP**:

S = **S**kin

C = sub**C**utaneous tissue

A = galea **A**poneurosis (essentially the muscle layer)

L = Loose connective tissue

P = **P**eriosteum (also called pericranium), which overlies the bone

For practical purposes, in patients with a full-thickness scalp laceration (i.e., all layers of the scalp are divided and the skull is exposed), you must close the galea and the skin.

Closing the galea layer often controls the brisk bleeding associated with scalp wounds. If a wound infection develops at the site of injury, closure of the galea layer also prevents the infection from spreading under the entire scalp. Once infection reaches the loose connective tissue plain (deep to the galea), it can spread widely. Closure of the galea prevents this potentially serious complication.

How to Control Bleeding as Well as Close the Wound

1. Lidocaine with epinephrine should be used whenever possible for local anesthesia.

2. Suture together the galea layer with 3-0 or 4-0 Vicryl or chromic sutures. They can be placed in a simple fashion or in a figure-of-eight fashion.

3. Close the skin with a continuous locking suture of 3-0 nylon or Vicryl. The skin stapler (if available) is a useful, fast technique for scalp closure.

Full-thickness External Ear Lacerations

Posterior Side of the Ear

Use 4-0 or 5-0 absorbable sutures. It is best to place them in an interrupted fashion.

Cartilage

1. If the cartilage is highly irregular, gently trim the edges to smooth it out.

2. Be sure to cleanse the wound meticulously when the cartilage is involved. All foreign material must be removed. If dirt is embedded in the cartilage, the cartilage should be trimmed to remove the dirt particles.

3. No sutures need to be placed in the cartilage. When placing sutures in the skin, try to include the perichondrium (the thin layer of loose tissue overlying the cartilage). In this way, the cartilage edges are brought together as the skin is repaired.

Anterior Side of the Ear

Use 4-0 or 5-0 nonabsorbable sutures placed in an interrupted fashion. Absorbable sutures also may be used.

How to Prevent Hematoma Formation

A particularly concerning complication associated with ear lacerations is the development of a hematoma. If blood collects and pressure builds up between the skin and cartilage, the result may be a noticeable ear deformity, so-called cauliflower ear. A properly placed dressing helps to prevent this complication. You should see the patient on the next day, if possible, to check for a hematoma.

Dressing

1. Add antibiotic ointment to a piece of gauze, and place it over the repair site. Gently press it onto the external ear to conform to the shape of the ear.

2. Open and fluff up several dry gauze pads, and place them around the ear, filling the contours of the ear with gauze. Make sure to place some gauze behind the ear as well.

3. Gently wrap the head and ear with gauze wrap and a light Ace wrap. Do not make the wrap tight. Try to leave it in place for 24–48 hours.

What to Do if a Hematoma Develops

If the patient returns (usually within the first few days after injury) with pain and swelling of the ear, a hematoma may be present. The ear looks purplish, and the swelling demonstrates some "give" when you push on it. Blood may ooze out of the suture line, and the ear may be slightly warm. If a hematoma develops, follow the procedure outlined below:

1. The sutures should be removed and the blood drained.

2. The wound should be thoroughly washed and then closed loosely.

3. Use fewer sutures than you used the first time.

4. Apply a dressing similar to the original one.

5. An oral antibiotic, taken for 24 hours, may be a useful precaution.

Summary of the Optimal Suture Material for Specific Facial Wounds

Site of Injury	Optimal Suture Size*	Optimal Suture Material (Good Alternate Choice)
Cheek, forehead, or nose skin	5-0,6-0	Nylon, Prolene[†] (chromic for children or patients who cannot return for suture removal)
Ear skin	4-0	Nylon (chromic)
External tongue mucosa	4-0	Chromic (Vicryl/Dexon)[‡]
Eyelid skin	5-0, 6-0	Nylon (chromic)
Frontalis (forehead) muscle	3-0, 4-0	Polydioxanone (Vicryl/Dexon, chromic)
Galea (scalp)	3-0, 4-0	Polydioxanone (Vicryl/Dexon, chromic)
Lip or intraoral mucosa	4-0	Chromic (Vicryl/Dexon)
Lip muscle	4-0	Vicryl/Dexon (chromic, polydioxanone)
Lip skin	5-0, 6-0	Nylon (chromic)
Nasal mucosa	5-0	Chromic
Scalp skin	3-0, 4-0	Nylon (staples, chromic)
Subcutaneous tissue	4-0, 5-0	Vicryl/Dexon (chromic)
Tongue muscle	3-0	Vicryl/Dexon (chromic, polydioxanone)

* If you have a choice, these sizes are recommended.
[†] Prolene can be substituted whenever nylon is recommended.
[‡] Vicryl is a polyglactic acid; Dexon is a polyglycolic acid. They are essentially interchangeable.

Facial Lacerations with Soft Tissue Loss

If the laceration is relatively small (< 1 cm), it often may be left alone and allowed to heal secondarily, especially if it is located in the medial canthal area, the skin around the upper and lower lip, or the lateral aspects of the bridge of the nose.

Larger wounds (even a few cm in size) involving the lateral cheek area (in front of the ear but not near the lower eyelid) and the forehead also may be allowed to heal secondarily with good results.

Be careful around the cheek near the lower eyelid. Allowing a skin defect to heal secondarily in this area may result in a pulling down of the lower eyelid (called an ectropion). This serious complication may result in injury to the cornea. To prevent an ectropion, a full-thickness skin graft or local flap should be used for soft tissue loss near the lower eyelid.

A local flap or full-thickness skin graft also may be required for other larger face wounds or wounds involving the nasal tip. See chapter 12, "Skin Grafts," and chapter 13, "Local Flaps," for details. Significant soft tissue loss of the lip or eyelid (> 25%) requires the help of a specialist.

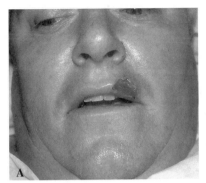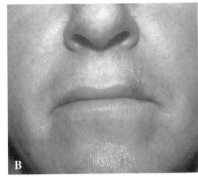

Soft tissue loss. *A*, Dog bite to the upper lip resulting in soft tissue loss. The wound was allowed to heal secondarily. *B*, One year after injury. the lip has a nice contour with minimal scarring.

Bibliography

Goldwyn RM, Rueckert F: The value of healing by secondary intention for sizable defects of the face. Arch Surg 112: 285, 1977.

Chapter 17

PRESSURE SORES

Pressure sores are chronic wounds caused by prolonged pressure applied to a specific area of the body. The involved tissue usually overlies a bony prominence. When a pressure sore develops because the patient is in the recumbent position for long periods, it is called a **decubitus ulcer.**

Pressure sores are often large wounds and may seem difficult to manage. However, by combining the wound care knowledge from previous chapters with the information given here, you will find these wounds more manageable. Often they can be treated successfully with debridement of necrotic (dead) tissue and local wound care measures alone. The result is a healed wound.

Only in specific instances is a flap indicated for the treatment of a pressure sore.

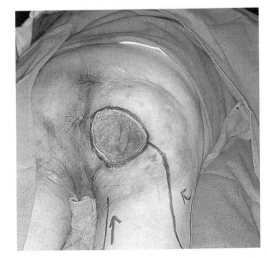

Large ischial pressure sore. (Photo courtesy of Jeffrey Antimarino, M.D.)

Causes of Pressure Sores

The basic problem that leads to the development of a pressure sore is application of elevated pressure to soft tissue for too long a time. The pressure causes direct injury to the tissues. Unrelieved pressure elevation for as little as 2 hours can cause permanent tissue injury and subsequent tissue death.

People at Risk

Communication between the central nervous system and the body (via the peripheral nervous system) allows detection of elevated pressure at the tissue level. Feedback mechanisms result in the diminution of pressure so that tissue injury does not occur. People who are ambulatory and without neurologic abnormalities make regular, subtle position changes without conscious effort because of these feedback mechanisms. Thus, under normal circumstances, people do not develop a pressure sore when they sleep in a recumbent position for several hours.

Any condition that prevents these subtle position changes or interferes with the communication between the central nervous system and peripheral nervous system places the person at risk for the development of a pressure sore.

Patient Populations at High Risk

- **Paraplegic or quadriplegic patients**, who usually are wheelchair-dependent or bedridden and need help in changing positions. They also may lack the ability to sense an elevation in tissue pressure when they remain in the same position for too long a time.

- **Patients with decreased sensation due to neurologic disorders.** For example, children with meningomyelocele have diminished sensation below the spinal cord abnormality. Thus, the central nervous system cannot monitor the pressure in the insensate areas.

- **Patients with impaired mental capacity.** Patients with severe dementia or patients who have suffered debilitating head injuries are often bedridden and move very little when left alone.

- **Seriously ill patients in an intensive care unit.** Patients who have sustained serious burns or multiple fractures are particularly at risk. They are often in considerable pain, which may be exacerbated by movement. Thus they tend to stay in one position unless assisted by a caregiver. In addition, pain medications keep them drowsy, which also inhibits movement.

Additional Risk Factors

- **Malnutrition** makes the tissues more prone to injury. It also delays wound healing.

- **Incontinence** can cause the skin in the buttocks and perineal area to be chronically moist. The tissues become macerated and more susceptible to breakdown with minimal trauma. In addition, contamination of an open wound with urine and feces interferes with wound healing.

- **Tobacco use.** The nicotine in tobacco decreases circulation to tissues, thus exacerbating the lack of circulation caused by the effects of pressure on the tissues. Tobacco use also contributes to poor wound healing.

Table 1.   Areas Prone to the Development of Pressure Sores

Area of Body	Underlying Bony Prominence	Comments
Base of buttocks	Ischium	Tends to occur in patients confined to wheelchair and in seated position for much of the time
Upper outer thigh	Greater trochanter	Tends to occur in patients who spend prolonged periods in bed
Heel of foot	Calcaneus	May occur in both of above patient populations
Back of head	Occiput of skull	Tends to occur in patients who spend prolonged periods in bed
Lower back	Sacrum	Tends to occur in patients who spend prolonged periods in bed

Prevention

For patients at high risk for developing a pressure sore, prevention is the key. To avoid the development of pressure sores in bedridden patients, encourage the patients (and their caregivers) to change positions regularly (*at least* every 2 hours). Paraplegic patients who spend prolonged periods in a wheelchair should lift themselves off their buttocks for just a few seconds every 15 minutes.

Cushioning of pressure points is also important. For example, place pillows or cushions between the patient's knees and ankles to prevent pressure in these areas. Have the patient sit on a pillow as well. Special pressure-dissipating cushions can be fitted to the patient's wheelchair.

Cessation of smoking and maintenance of adequate nutrition are vital for prevention. Proper hygiene of the buttocks and perineum is also important.

Pressure Sore Staging System

A staging scale is important for documentation and communication. Recognition of a pressure sore in its early stages allows aggressive intervention, which may prevent the development of a large, full-thickness wound.

The staging system is based on skin appearance. However, the skin is much more resistant to the effects of pressure than the underlying fat and muscle. Thus by the time you see significant changes in the skin, damage has already occured in the underlying soft tissue fat and muscle. You must institute treatment measures quickly.

Stage I   Redness of intact skin that does not blanch (when you press on the area the redness does not go away). Earliest stage, before start of skin breakdown.

Stage II   Partial-thickness skin loss involving the epidermis and dermis. The ulcer is superficial and may look like a blister or shallow crater.

Stage III   Full-thickness skin loss involving the underlying subcutaneous fat but not the muscle.

Stage IV   Full-thickness skin loss with extensive destruction, tissue necrosis, or damage in muscle, bone, or supporting structures (e.g., tendon, joint capsule).

From U.S. Department of Health and Human Services: Pressure Ulcers in Adults: Prediction and Prevention. Clinical Practice Guideline No. 3, Publication 97-0047, 1992.

Treatment

All Patients in the Process of Developing a Pressure Sore

1. Reinforce the necessity of regular position changes to patient and caregivers.

2. Institute measures to relieve the pressure in the at-risk area. Pillows, foam mattresses, and foam splints are useful.

3. Proper nutrition is a must. High-protein drinks and puddings are useful. Supplemental vitamins and minerals also should be given (especially vitamin C and zinc).

4. Patients should remain active. They should *not* be placed on bed rest or kept from their usual activities.

5. The patient should refrain from using tobacco products.

6. The wound should be kept free from urine or fecal contamination. Temporary use of a Foley catheter (or intermittent catheterization)

should be considered. A diverting colostomy should be considered if persistent fecal contamination is a problem.

Stage I or II Pressure Sore

1. Keep the affected tissue clean and the surrounding area dry.

2. Apply antibiotic ointment (e.g., Bacitracin, silver sulfadiazine) daily to areas that have blistered.

3. DuoDERM (also called Granuflex or Varihesive) is a useful dressing alternative for the treatment of a relatively superficial pressure sore. Cut it to the proper size (a little larger than the wound), and place it directly over the injured tissue. You may need to put tape around the edges to keep it in place. DuoDERM promotes healing by providing a moist environment for the injured tissue. This dressing often may be left in place for up to 7 days, which makes it convenient for patients and caregivers.

Stage III or IV Pressure Sore

If the wound is covered with a dry, dark, leathery eschar (scab): If the wound has no surrounding cellulitis and no drainage, *leave it alone.* This dry eschar is easy to care for. Clean the area with saline or povidone-iodine solution daily. You may cover the wound with dry gauze if the patient desires. The underlying tissues will gradually heal, and the eschar will separate and detach. The eschar should be removed if signs of infection (e.g., redness, warmth, fever) are present.

If the wound has a red, granulating base but is covered with areas of gray exudate: Apply wet-dry saline dressing changes at least twice daily, if possible. Once the wound is clean, you may change to wet-wet dressings, an antibiotic ointment with dry gauze dressings, or other topical material.

If the wound contains foul-smelling, necrotic tissue: Surgical debridement (described below) is necessary to remove large amounts of dead tissue. Follow with wet-dry dressings, using saline or preferably Dakin's solution to clean the wound and promote healing.

If the wound is surrounded by cellulitis: Red, warm, and indurated skin around the pressure sore indicates an infection in the soft tissues (cellulitis). Treat the patient with a course of antibiotics. Ordinarily, a pressure sore without signs of surrounding tissue infection does not require antibiotics. Use antibiotics only if the wound is infected.

With the above treatments, most pressure sores heal on their own. The key is to institute treatment early, before the wound gets out of control. Serial debridement of necrotic tissue and the above treatments promote gradual healing even of a large pressure sore. Although it may take weeks to months for the wound to close completely, this is the optimal course of treatment for a pressure sore. On rare occasions, local flaps can be used to obtain wound closure (see descriptions below).

Surgical Intervention

Surgical intervention is required when the wound has so much dead tissue that formal debridement is needed to clean the wound. Occasionally, the wound can be closed with a local flap.

Debridement

Debridement of small, necrotic areas can be performed at the bedside. But for large or deep wounds, it is better to do the debridement in the controlled environment of the operating room.

The patient will lose blood when large amounts of dead tissue are cut away. Be sure to check the patient's hemoglobin/hematocrit before debriding a large pressure sore. A transfusion may be required.

Often the patient has no feeling in the area of the pressure sore. Sedation (to allay fears and increase comfort on the operating table) may be all that is needed.

Using a scalpel (or a scissors) and forceps, cut away all dead tissue.

If the tissue bleeds, it is probably healthy; if it does not bleed, it is probably dead.

Dead bone or tendon in the wound must be removed. Place a clamp on the tendon, and put the tendon under tension (i.e., pull on the clamp). Then cut off all of the exposed tendon. Bone can be removed with a bone rongeur or an osteotome. Remove the outer layers of the exposed bone until you reach bleeding bone.

Clean the wound with saline mixed with a small amount of povidone-iodine solution if available, and pack the wound with a gauze dressing. Leave the dressing in place for 24 hours. Then remove the packing, and start regular wet-dry dressings.

Debridement may be repeated (serial debridement) if, because of concerns about blood loss, all necrotic tissue cannot be removed at one time.

Local Flaps

Closing a pressure sore with a local flap is an advanced treatment that requires surgical expertise. A local flap is not indicated for all pressure sores. Most heal with local care. Unless you are particular about whom you operate on, the risk for recurrence of the pressure sore is quite high (often over 50%).

If you perform a flap on a patient who is not a good surgical candidate (e.g., a patient who is malnourished, actively smoking, or noncompliant with position changes), he or she may end up not only with a recurrent pressure sore but also with a poorly healing donor site.

Indications

Specific reason for development of the pressure sore. For example, a paraplegic patient who has had no previous pressure sores (despite being in a wheelchair for 10 years) but develops one when he or she is hospitalized for pneumonia and unable to change positions.

Excellent nutritional status. Albumin > 3.5 gm/dl, prealbumin > 20 mg/dl, transferrin > 250 mg/dl (2.5 gm/L). If the patient is malnourished, the flap will not heal and surgery is pointless. There is also a high risk that the donor site will heal poorly.

The patient must not smoke.

Highly motivated patients who want to be at home. Some patients live alone or have little home support. They may be unable to go home because of concerns about wound care. If patients in this situation meet the nutritional requirements and show that they are motivated enough to change positions regularly, local flap closure may be indicated.

Preoperative Considerations

Before flap closure, the pressure sore must be debrided thoroughly. It is often useful to debride the wound surgically a day or so before the planned flap. All necrotic tissue and dead bone must be removed.

Caution: Debridement of pressure sores and flap closure can lead to significant blood loss. The patient's hematocrit must be above 27 (hemoglobin at least 8–9), and blood must be available for the operating room.

A closed suction drain should be available to place under the flap to prevent fluid accumulation postoperatively. If a closed suction drain is not available, a passive drain (Penrose drain or a piece of sterile glove) should be placed under the flap. See chapter 13, "Local Flaps," for additional information.

Sacral Pressure Sores

Buttocks Rotation Flap

1. Draw the flap before making any incisions. This step allows you to make corrections.

2. Design the flap larger than you think you will need to ensure a tension-free closure.

3. Design the flap so that it extends in a curvilinear fashion superiorly (a few cm) and laterally from the wound. It should have a wide base (at least 8–10 cm).

4. Separate the flap from the underlying tissues and transfer it into the wound. Undermine the surrounding skin edges as needed to allow the flap to be sutured in place without tension.

5. If necessary, a small back cut can be made at the lateral edge of the base of the flap to help it turn into the wound. Do not narrow the base more by more than 1–2 cm.

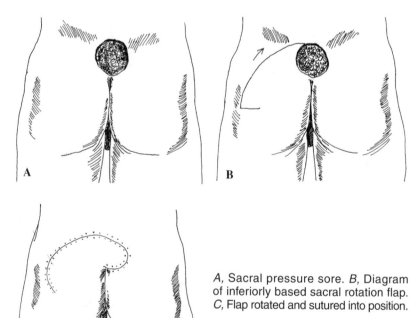

A, Sacral pressure sore. *B,* Diagram of inferiorly based sacral rotation flap. *C,* Flap rotated and sutured into position.

6. Suture the flap in place over a drain. Place a few dermal sutures, and then do an interrupted skin closure. The skin closure should not be tight. It is better to have little gaps in the closure, which will heal, than to do a tight closure and lose part of the flap.

Trochanteric Pressure Sores

Tensor Fascia Lata Flap

The tensor fascia lata (TFL) flap is the most commonly used flap for closure of a trochanteric pressure sore. The TFL flap is adjacent to the wound and runs anterior to it, along the lateral aspect of the thigh. The widest donor defect that can be closed primarily is approximately 6 cm. Pinch the thigh tissues to see how much skin you should be able to remove while still being able to close the donor site primarily. The flap is composed of the skin and fascial extension from the TFL muscle.

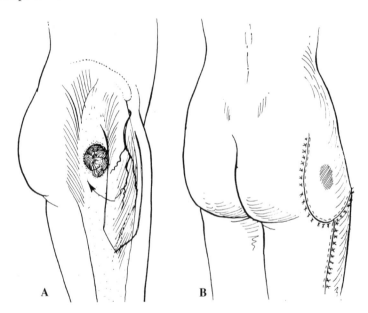

A tensor fascia lata flap is the best choice for coverage of a trochanteric pressure sore. A, Outline of tensor fascia lata musculocutaneous flap. B, Tensor fascia lata flap used to reconstruct trochanteric pressure sore. (From Jurkiewicz MJ, et al (eds): Plastic Surgery: Principles and Practice. St. Louis, Mosby, 1990, with permission.)

1. Draw the flap before making any incisions. This step allows you to make corrections.

2. The anterior border of the flap is a line drawn from the anterior superior iliac spine to the lateral margin of the kneecap.

3. The posterior border is about 5 cm posterior to the anterior border.

4. The flap can extend inferiorly to within 10 cm of the kneecap.

5. The skin is incised, and the incision is taken down through the subcutaneous tissue to the underlying thick TFL fascia. The fascia stays attached to the flap.

6. Elevate the flap off the underlying tissues. You will see an obvious separation between the undersurface of the TFL fascia and the deeper tissues. It is useful to place a stitch in the distalmost part of the flap to connect the fascia to the skin so that you do not accidentally separate the skin/subcutaneous tissue from the TFL fascia during dissection.

7. The flap is moved into the wound defect and loosely sutured in position. Place a few dermal sutures, and then do an interrupted skin closure. The skin closure should not be tight. It is better to have little gaps in the closure, which will heal, than to do a tight closure and lose part of the flap.

8. The donor site is closed primarily with dermal sutures and interrupted skin sutures. A suction drain or a passive drain should be placed under the skin closure at the donor site as well as the site of the pressure sore.

Ischial Pressure Sores

Posterior Thigh Flap

The posterior thigh flap is a V-Y advancement flap. It is quite useful for covering large ischial pressure sores (8–10 cm diameter). The pedicle of this flap is not a bridge of surrounding skin or subcutaneous tissue. The deep tissues underlying the flap supply the circulation.

1. Draw the flap before making any incisions. This step allows you to make corrections.

2. Mark the V with the widest area at the lower edge of the pressure sore, tapering gradually to a point. The V should go at least half way down the back of the thigh.

3. Incise the skin edges going through the subcutaneous tissue down to (but not into) the underlying muscle.

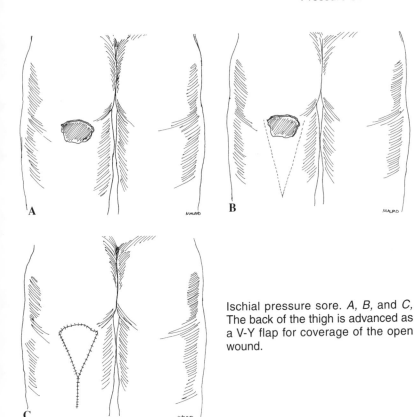

Ischial pressure sore. *A*, *B*, and *C*, The back of the thigh is advanced as a V-Y flap for coverage of the open wound.

4. You should be able to advance the flap superiorly into the wound defect. Place a drain at the base of the wound.

5. Close the narrow part of the V flap defect primarily. This step creates the Y limb.

6. Suture the flap loosely, under no tension. Place a few dermal sutures, and then do an interrupted skin closure. The skin closure should not be tight. It is better to have little gaps in the closure, which will heal, than to do a tight closure and lose part of the flap.

General Postoperative Care for the Above Procedures

1. Cleanse and apply antibiotic ointment to the suture lines daily.

2. If a suction drain was used, it should stay in place until the drainage is < 50 ml in 24 hours. Try to keep it in place at least 1 week. If you do not have a suction drain, remove the passive drain after 3–4 days.

3. In general, the patient should apply no pressure to the surgical site until the suture line has healed (usually 2–3 weeks). The patient then should be allowed to place weight over the area for limited periods (10–15 minutes 3 or 4 times daily). If the suture line stays intact (i.e., it does not start to separate), gradually decrease the restrictions on positioning.

4. Leave the skin sutures in place for at least 14 days unless there are signs of irritation from the sutures.

Bibliography

1. Cervo FA, Cruz AC, Posillico JA: Pressure ulcers: Analysis of guidelines for treatment and management. Geriatrics 55(3):55–60, 2000.
2. Disa JJ, Carlton JM, Goldberg NH: Efficacy of operative cure in pressure sore patients. Plast Reconstr Surg 89:272–278, 1992.
3. Hopkins A, Gooch S, Danks F: A programme for pressure sore prevention and management. J Wound Care 7:37–40, 1998.

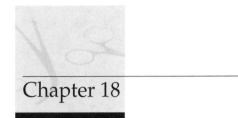

Chapter 18

CHRONIC WOUNDS

KEY FIGURES:
Open wound   Wound covered with skin graft

Chronic wounds are open wounds that for some reason simply will not heal. They may be present for months or even years. Often, especially in rural settings, the wounds have not received adequate care. The most important component of the overall treatment plan must be to identify and treat the underlying cause that interferes with normal wound healing.

Begin by taking a thorough history to find out about the patient's medical status as well as information about the events that contributed to the development of the wound. Next, thoroughly examine the wound. From this information, the underlying cause for the nonhealing wound usually can be identified.

Once the cause is identified and properly treated, the basic principle of chronic wound treatment is essentially the same as those of secondary wound healing: regular dressing changes. For large wounds, a skin graft or flap may be required for final closure.

This chapter discusses the most common underlying causes (with treatments) for a nonhealing wound. In addition, a few specific, problematic chronic wounds are described.

Common Causes and Treatments

Neglected Wound/Poor Wound Care

Especially in the rural setting, many chronic wounds do not heal simply because of inadequate wound care. Without proper care, the wound becomes covered with dead (necrotic) tissue. To achieve wound closure, all necrotic tissue must be removed (debrided), either with wet-to-dry dressings or with surgical debridement.

Surgical Debridement

When a wound is covered with black, dead tissue or thick gray/green exudate, dressings alone may be inadequate. Surgical removal of a significant amount of necrotic tissue may allow successful wound closure with wet-to-dry dressings.

Using a forceps, pick up an edge of the dead tissue and cut it off the wound with a scalpel or scissors. This procedure usually is not painful because the tissue that you are cutting into is already dead. If it hurts, you are near healthy tissue.

Bleeding tissue is a good sign and indicates that you are in an area of healthy tissue. Dead tissue does not bleed.

This procedure can be repeated as often as necessary. You do not have to remove all necrotic tissue with one procedure.

Once the necrotic tissue has been removed, regular dressing changes should be started. Wet-to-dry dressings are the most appropriate choice. Dressings should be changed at least 2 times daily and optimally 3 or 4 times (in areas where dressing supplies are plentiful) until the wound heals. See chapter 9, "Taking Care of Wounds," for a detailed description of dressing options.

Foreign Material in the Depths of the Wound

A foreign body in the depths of a wound may prevent healing. Foreign material such as glass, wood, or metal fragments can cause an inflammatory reaction in the tissues that will not resolve until the foreign material is removed.

The history often provides information that leads you to suspect that foreign materials may be the problem. An x-ray may be useful, but many foreign objects do not show up on x-rays.

Often foreign material is removed with overlying dead tissue during surgical debridement, allowing the wound to heal with dressing changes.

Infection

If signs of surrounding soft tissue infection (redness, warmth, pain, swelling) are present, oral or intravenous antibiotics should be given. The presence of an open wound, in and of itself, does not necessitate oral or intravenous antibiotic administration.

Infection of the underlying bone (**chronic osteomyelitis**) may cause a chronic nonhealing wound. An x-ray may show irregularity in the periosteum (the thin layer of connective tissue around the bone), and signs of bone destruction may be seen.

Infection of the bone often requires at least 6 weeks of antibiotics. In addition, orthopedic and reconstructive surgical expertise is usually required for successful treatment because bone debridement and coverage with a muscle flap may be required for control and resolution of the infection—especially when an infection develops after an open fracture.

Tobacco

Tobacco use interferes with wound healing through a combination of two mechanisms:

1. The vasoconstrictive effects of nicotine decrease local blood circulation to the skin. Thus, less blood and oxygen (and other factors that promote healing) reach the wound.

2. The carbon monoxide present in tobacco smoke further decreases oxygen delivery to the tissues because carbon monoxide decreases the ability of hemoglobin to release oxygen to the tissues.

All patients should be counseled not to smoke, especially patients with open wounds. When the patient stops smoking, the improvement in the wound may be dramatic.

Cancer

In a long-standing wound that looks clean but still will not heal, the wound may be harboring an underlying cancer. Often such wounds look a little different from the usual chronic wound. The tissues around the wound edges may be raised and highly irregular, and irregular red patches may be seen in the surrounding skin.

The concern about an underlying cancer is especially applicable in chronic wounds in elderly patients and on sun-exposed areas of the body.

We tend to expect basal cell or squamous cell skin cancers to be relatively small (< 2–3 cm), but, if left untreated, they can grow to be quite large. Cancer of the breast and soft tissue sarcomas can erode through the skin to create a chronic open wound. Usually, these two types of cancer are associated with a large soft tissue mass underlying the wound.

For such wounds to heal, the entire lesion—i.e., the entire area involved with cancer—must be excised. If the wound is small (< 1–2 cm), immediate excision is indicated. In larger wounds, an incisional biopsy should be done to get a preliminary diagnosis, which helps to plan the definitive resection. See chapter 22, "Skin Cancer," for details.

Malnutrition

For a wound to heal, the patient's nutritional status must be sound. An adequate diet supplying the proper amount of calories and protein on a daily basis is very important. The importance of nutritional factors in wound healing is illustrated by the fact that elective surgery often is contraindicated in patients without adequate protein stores.

How to Assess Nutritional Status

The liver produces various proteins that have been found to correlate well with nutritional status. Examples include albumin, prealbumin, and transferrin. Although albumin does not correlate with nutritional status as well as the other two, measurement of serum albumin is helpful if the more expensive tests for prealbumin and transferrin are unavailable.

Protein	Normal Value
Albumin	3.5–5.0 gm/dl
Prealbumin	10–40 mg/dl
Transferrin	200–400 mg/dl

Vitamin C, vitamin A, iron, and zinc are also important nutrients for proper wound healing. In malnourished patients, vitamin/mineral supplements may be beneficial. In adequately nourished patients, however, extra doses of these nutrients are not necessarily useful.

As stated below in the discussion of radiation, vitamin E may be useful in a wound exposed to radiation. However, high doses of vitamin E interfere with normal wound healing in patients without a deficiency.

Although nutritional supplements may be required in severely malnourished patients, nutritional counseling may be all that is needed for most patients. Nutritional supplements, such as high protein/calorie drinks/puddings, are often quite expensive and unnecessary. See chapter 8, "Nutrition," for more detailed information.

Diabetes

An elevated blood glucose level decreases the body's natural ability to heal wounds. For this reason, patients with diabetes must watch their diet and regularly check glucose levels. High glucose levels should be treated with the appropriate medications (insulin or an oral agent) to maintain the best possible blood glucose control.

Medications

Ask all patients about use of prescription and over-the-counter medications. Several classes of medications interfere with wound healing:

Steroids

Steroids significantly interfere with normal wound healing. Vitamin A may counteract the effects of steroids and promote healing. Try giving vitamin A orally (25,000 IU/day) or topically (200,000 IU/8 hours) for 1–2 weeks, and see if the wound begins to heal.

Nonsteroidal Anti-inflammatory Drugs (NSAIDs)

NSAIDs (e.g., aspirin, ibuprofen) interfere with wound healing by decreasing collagen production. The precise mechanism is not fully understood. If the patient has a chronic wound and is taking NSAIDs, see if switching to another type of medication (e.g., acetaminophen) results in improved wound healing.

Radiation Injury

The patient may give a history of previous radiation therapy to the area around the wound. Radiation damages the ability of the tissues to promote new blood vessel growth as well as interferes with cellular functions necessary for wound healing. These effects are not reversible once the radiation exposure has been completed and in fact may worsen with time. Because of these effects, a seemingly minor injury in an area that previously received radiation may result in a chronic, open wound.

Vitamin E has been shown to improve wound strength in areas exposed to radiation. It may be useful to try a short course (1–2 weeks) of oral vitamin E supplementation (100–400 IU/day) to see whether the status of the wound improves.

Often the entire wound may need to be excised to remove the damaged, radiated tissue. Especially if no reconstructive specialists are available, try local wound care for a few weeks after excision to see whether the wound begins to heal. If this treatment is unsuccessful, a split-thickness skin graft or, more likely, a flap may be required for wound closure.

Specific Problematic Wounds

Leg Ulcers

Leg ulcers usually are caused by problems in either the arterial circulation or the venous circulation (or sometimes a combination of the two).

Arterial Insufficiency

Leg ulcers due to blockages in the arterial circulation tend to develop over the medial aspect of the ankle. Compare the temperature of the patient's feet: is one foot cooler than the other? Coolness is a sign of inadequate arterial blood flow.

Check for the presence of palpable pulses in the foot and ankle. If you cannot feel the dorsalis pedis artery (on the top of the foot) or the posterior tibial artery (behind the medial malleolus), the patient probably has a problem in the arterial circulation. Even if you cannot feel a pulse in the foot vessels, blood flow to the foot may be sufficient to allow a properly treated wound to heal. Absence of a pulse, however, does indicate that the vessels are significantly diseased.

There are many high-tech ways to examine the patency of the blood vessels of the legs. Some are invasive (e.g., arteriogram, in which dye is injected into the vessels and x-rays are taken), and some are not (e.g., Doppler studies using sound waves to examine the vessels). A simple test to measure blood flow to the foot is as follows:

1. Measure the systolic blood pressure in the foot and divide this number by the systolic blood pressure in the arm (at the brachial artery, the usual place to check blood pressure).

2. The result is the **ankle/brachial index** (ABI), which compares blood flow to the ankle with blood flow through the upper extremity. Because the upper extremity is rarely affected by vascular disease, the ABI allows you to determine the degree of diminution of blood flow to the foot.

3. An ABI > 0.5 indicates that sufficient blood reaches the foot to allow wound healing.

4. An ABI < 0.4 indicates poor blood flow to the foot. Healing probably will not occur unless a vascular bypass is done to bring more blood into the lower extremity.

Venous Insufficiency

Ulcers due to problems with the venous circulation tend to be on the lateral side of the ankle or lower calf. Arterial pulses are usually normal. Such ulcers can become quite large (10–15-cm wounds are common).

The foot, ankle, or calf around the wound is often chronically swollen, and obvious skin changes are present. Skin changes include woody induration (the skin feels very hard) and brawny discoloration. Enlarged varicose veins are usually present.

Combination Arterial and Venous Insufficiency

Unfortunately, many patients with leg ulcers do not have purely arterial or purely venous problems. Often the disease involves both arteries and veins.

Treatment

Leg ulcers are often quite difficult to treat. Although we try to avoid amputation, sometimes it is the only successful treatment option.

If the cause is inadequate arterial circulation:

1. If the ABI is > 0.5, the wound has a high likelihood of healing with proper local care (dressings) or a skin graft.

2. If the ABI is < 0.4, the chance of healing without vascular bypass to bring more blood to the area is low.

3. If no one with vascular surgical expertise is available, it is worth trying local wound care to see if the wound improves. If this attempt is unsuccessful, amputation may be the only way to obtain a closed wound.

If the cause is venous insufficiency:

An important component of treatment is to decrease the swelling in the foot or calf:

1. The patient should elevate the affected leg as much as possible. In bed the foot should be propped on a pillow. When the patient is seated, the foot should be propped on a stool so that it does not dangle dependently.

2. The patient also should wrap the leg with Ace wraps or wear support stockings to improve blood flow through the veins and out the lower leg. This strategy also helps to decrease leg swelling.

3. The Ace wraps should start at the toes and gradually go up to the calf. Be sure that the wrap is not too tight. It should be tighter at the toe than at the ankle and tighter at the ankle than at the calf. If the Ace wrap is not properly applied (i.e., if it is tighter at the ankle than the foot), it will cause constriction at the ankle and worsen the swelling in the foot.

4. In patients with arterial and venous problems, take care that the Ace wraps and support stockings do not impede arterial circulation.

Venous ulcers are notoriously difficult to treat. In some patients, especially those treated before the tissues of the leg become hard and woody, control of swelling and proper wound care allow venous ulcers to heal. For large venous ulcers, a split-thickness skin graft may be indicated, but there is a high chance that the graft will not work.

If the problem is a combination of arterial and venous insufficiency:

Each problem must be addressed separately. However, if the arterial inflow is poor, no matter how aggressively the venous problems are treated, wound healing will not occur.

Pressure Sores

A pressure sore is a chronic wound caused by prolonged application of pressure to an area of soft tissue. Usually these wounds develop over, a bony prominence. (See chapter 17, "Pressure Sores," for detailed information.)

Overview of Treating Chronic Open Wounds

The key strategies to promote healing of a chronic open wound can be summarized as follows:

- Remove all dead tissues overlying the wound with either dressings or surgical debridement.

- Remove any foreign material from the wound.

- Treat with oral or intravenous antibiotics if signs of underlying or surrounding infection are present. The presence of an open wound in and of itself does not necessitate antibiotic administration.

- Identify other underlying causes that may prevent wound healing. Provide appropriate treatment.

- Because good nutrition is essential for wound healing, be sure that the patient gets enough calories and protein. A multivitamin may be helpful, but encourage the patient to eat a nutritious diet.

- Stop smoking.

- Adequate local wound care is essential. Dressings should be changed at least twice daily (3–4 times is optimal for a dirtier wound), and the wound should be cleansed with gentle soap and water or saline with each dressing change. Wet-to-dry dressings are often the method of choice. Wet-to-wet dressings or antibiotic ointment can be used once the wound is clean.

It may take weeks or even months for a wound to heal in this manner, but you should see gradual improvement. It is a good idea to measure the dimensions of the wound at each visit to document how the wound is progressing.

Large wounds (> 8–10 cm) may take many months to heal. Once the wound is clean and starting to heal, it may be useful to consider covering the wound with a split-thickness skin graft or a flap to hasten wound healing (see the appropriate chapters for more details).

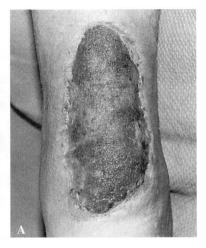 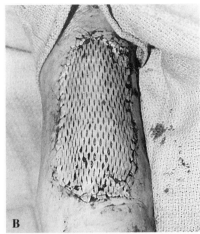

A, Large (12 × 6 cm) chronic wound on the back of the calf. *B*, Wound covered with a split-thickness skin graft to promote closure.

Bibliography

1. Nwomeh BC, Yager DR, Cohen IK: Physiology of the chronic wound. Clin Plast Surg 25:407–414, 998.
2. Stadelmann WK, Digenis AG, Tobin GR: Impediments to wound healing. Am J Surg 176(Suppl 2A):39S–47S, 998.

Chapter 19

SOFT TISSUE INFECTIONS

Soft tissue infections can be difficult to treat. All health care providers, especially those practicing in rural settings, must be able to differentiate between infections that need treatment with antibiotics alone and infections that require incision and drainage or more radical debridement. Serious consequences can result when a severe infection requiring operative management is misdiagnosed as a minor infection.

Cellulitis vs. Abscess

Cellulitis is a diffuse infection of the soft tissues with no localized area of pus amenable to drainage. The affected area is described as indurated (i.e., warm, red, and swollen). It is also painful. A component of lymphangitis (infection involving the lymphatics) is indicated by red streaking, progressing proximally from the affected area.

An **abscess** is a localized collection of pus, often with a component of surrounding cellulitis (with the above signs). One sign of an abscess is an area of fluctuance; that is, when you apply gentle digital pressure over the area, you can push and feel a "give," indicating the presence of fluid underneath. Another sign is that an abscess often seems to "point;" that is, the skin starts to thin from the pressure of the fluid underneath.

The distinction between cellullitis and abscess is important. The main treatment for an abscess is incision and drainage (cutting into the abscess and widely opening the abscess cavity). Cellulitis does not warrant this intervention.

Gangrene

The term *gangrene* is used to describe tissues that are dead. There are two subtypes of gangrene: dry and wet. The distinction is important.

Dry gangrene describes tissues that are generally black and dried out, with a distinct border between dead tissue and surrounding healthy tissue. Sometimes dry gangrenous tissues fall off on their own (dry gangrenous toes can fall off with minimal manipulation). However, debridement is usually required, but it is not emergent. Dry gangrene usually places the patient at no health risk as long as it does not become infected (see below).

In contrast to dry gangrene, **wet gangrene** can be a significant health risk. It connotes active infection (noted by pain, swelling, redness, and drainage of pus) in the tissues surrounding the obviously dead tissue. Urgent debridement is required to prevent further tissue loss and worsening soft tissue infection.

Necrotizing Fasciitis

Necrotizing fasciitis is a serious, life-threatening infection of the fascia (the thin connective tissue overlying the muscle and under the skin and subcutaneous tissue). The popular press calls it the disease of "flesh-eating bacteria."

Necrotizing fasciitis is not common, but it must be considered in evaluating a patient with a soft tissue infection that seems to be progressing rapidly to surrounding tissues. This diagnosis should be considered when the patient is "sicker" than you would expect for simple cellulitis.

The skin is swollen but often without many signs of cellulitis. The skin simply does not look "right." You may be able to feel subcutaneous air in the soft tissues, or you may see air in the soft tissues on x-ray (no air is present in normal soft tissues on x-ray).

The patient is often quite ill, with high fever, low blood pressure, general weakness, or even shock, and the infection spreads quickly. Radical debridement and even amputation may be necessary to save the patient's life.

Treatment requires aggressive operative debridement (opening the soft tissue spaces, as with an abscess) to remove affected tissue, intravenous antibiotics, close monitoring of the patient, and aggressive treatment of septicemia. Hyperbaric oxygen also may be indicated but does not replace aggressive operative treatment. Patients with necrotizing fasciitis should be treated by a surgeon with critical care expertise.

Evaluation of Patients with Soft Tissue Infection

History

Antecedent Trauma

Ask about traumatic injury to the area before the signs of infection developed.

Cuts from glass and punctures from metal objects should raise concern about the presence of a foreign body in the soft tissues.

History of an animal bite should raise concern about specific bacterial organisms that may require a particular antibiotic (see discussion of specific treatments below).

Medical Issues

Infections in patients with diabetes are often worse than you expect, and more difficult to treat. You must treat these infections aggressively, and be sure to control the patient's blood sugar.

Ask about the patient's tetanus immunization status, and give a booster as indicated.

Physical Examination

The classic signs of infection are redness, warmth, swelling, and pain.

Look closely for puncture wounds or other signs of trauma.

Try to distinguish between a localized collection of pus that needs drainage and diffuse infection. Check for fluctuance, as previously described.

Determine whether the induration is spreading to surrounding areas. Do red streaks extend proximally from the affected area?

Feel for crepitus (subcutaneous air) in the soft tissues, which is a sign of necrotizing fasciitis. Press on the soft tissues. If air is present under the skin, it will feel as if you are pressing on crinkled layers of cellophane or popping air bubbles beneath the skin.

Assess the patient for fever, chills, low blood pressure, generalized weakness, and malaise.

Check for enlarged lymph nodes in the surrounding area (groin or armpit, as appropriate).

Determine whether a fluctuant area is present over a pulse point (e.g., in the groin over the femoral artery or on the volar aspect of the elbow over the brachial artery).

Additional Studies

Additional studies for all patients should include a complete blood count with a white blood cell count and X-ray evaluation of the infected area.

If the infectious process overlies a pulse point, the underlying artery may be involved, resulting in a **pseudoaneurysm** (an outpouching of the artery). Before any surgical intervention, you must evaluate the vessel with an ultrasound/duplex scan.

If a pseudoaneurysm is present, a surgeon with vascular expertise must be involved in the patient's care. If you incise and drain the abscess without proper equipment and expertise, you will open the blood vessel, which may result in massive blood loss and death of the patient.

What to Look for on the X-ray

• Foreign bodies

• Unsuspected fractures/dislocations

• Underlying bone infection (bone edges appear irregular because bone has been destroyed by infection)

• Air in the soft tissues (when previous incision and drainage have not been done), which strongly indicates necrotizing fasciitis. Localized air may be present in the soft tissues in the immediate vicinity of an incision and drainage site, but diffuse air in the tissues is a sign of a necrotizing infection.

General Treatment

The patient must be evaluated carefully to distinguish among simple cellulitis, an abscess in need of incision and drainage (I & D), or necrotizing fasciitis in need of emergent radical debridement.

If the patient is stable with normal blood pressure and has no fluctuance, the probable diagnosis is cellulitis. Treatment with antibiotics and warm compresses is indicated. Watch for signs of progression, which may indicate an underlying abscess or need for a change in antibiotic therapy.

If the patient is stable but fluctuance is present, the abscess requires simple I & D. In addition, a short course of oral antibiotics may be useful.

If the patient is quite ill, with evidence of an abscess or possible signs of necrotizing fasciitis or wet gangrene, he or she requires intravenous antibiotics, intravenous fluids, and urgent operative intervention.

Guide to Antibiotics

Antibiotic administration is often the cornerstone of the treatment of soft tissue infections. The following are general guidelines:

1. Remind the patient that more than one dose of an antibiotic is needed to see any significant difference.

2. Follow the patient closely because changes in antibiotic therapy may be needed. In addition, an area that you thought was merely cellulitis may show signs of an abscess at a later time.

3. Whenever possible, send a specimen of any drainage from the area to the lab for aerobic and anaerobic culture and Gram stain. The results of these studies help to guide your choice of antibiotic therapy.

Basic Skin Infections

The infecting organisms are usually staphylococci or streptococci. Treat with an extended penicillin (a drug related to penicillin that covers penicillin-resistant organisms) or a first-generation cephalosporin.

Animal Bites

Pasteurella spp. are associated with cat and dog bites. Treatment requires an antipseudomonal antibiotic (e.g., amoxicillin/clavulanate or cefuroxime). On the hand, cat bites have a much higher incidence of subsequent infection than dog bites (80% vs. 5%, respectively).

Human Bites

Eikenella spp., other anaerobes, and streptococci are associated with human bite infections. If the patient is seen early after the injury before signs of infection have developed, treat with amoxicillin/clavulanate. Once signs of infection are present, intravenous antibiotics such as amoxicillin/sulbactam or ticarcillin/clavulanate are indicated. The pathogens associated with human bites can cause serious infections that must be followed closely and treated aggressively, especially in bites to the hand (see chapter 36, "Hand Infections," for specific information).

Seawater and Shellfish Injury

If the affected area has the typical signs of cellulitis, treatment should cover bacteria of the *Vibrio* species. Appropriate agents include tetracycline or an aminoglycoside.

Freshwater Injury

Aeromonas hydrophila is associated with freshwater infection. A fluoroquinolone or trimethoprim/sulfamethoxazole should be used.

Enlarged Lymph Nodes in the Affected Area

The presence of enlarged lymph nodes may indicate cat-scratch disease, *Mycobacterium marinum* infection, sporotrichosis, or nocardial infection. An infectious disease specialist should be involved in the treatment of such patients.

Concerns about Foreign Bodies

If a foreign body is present in the infected tissues, the infection probably will not resolve until it is removed. However, a foreign body in soft tissues without cellulitis does not have to be removed unless it is causing symptoms.

Incision and Drainage of an Abscess

1. Do *not* be timid. You want to open the abscess cavity fully to prevent the abscess from reforming.

2. Local anesthetic often does not work well in infected tissues, but a block can be quite useful. Sometimes no anesthetic is required, or you may need only light sedation (see chapter 3, "Local Anesthesia," for more details).

3. Make a longitudinal incision through the most fluctuant part of the abscess. Do not make the incision too small. It is often useful to excise an ellipse of skin, because the opening must be large enough to drain the abscess completely and allow you to pack the cavity with gauze.

4. Use the tips of a clamp to explore the abscess cavity gently and to ensure that it has been completely opened.

5. Send a specimen to the microbiology lab for evaluation.

6. Pack the wound with gauze.

Postoperative Care

1. The gauze packing should remain in place for 1 day.

2. Remove the gauze. Then repack the cavity with saline-moistened gauze and cover with dry gauze. The dressing should be changed 2–3 times/day until the wound has healed.

3. The patient may wash the area with gentle soap and water at each dressing change. Showering is permitted.

4. Antibiotics should be continued until the surrounding cellulitis resolves (probably for a few days).

Temporizing Measure for an Abscess in Need of Drainage

Sometimes you cannot perform the I & D without general anesthesia because of pain in the area and the extensive nature of the abscess. If you have to wait to get to the operating room for formal exploration, you can initiate treatment without anesthesia and prevent the patient from becoming more symptomatic.

An abscess can be decompressed by placing a large needle (18 gauge is adequate) into the cavity and aspirating the pus with a syringe. This technique relieves some of the pressure building up in the abscess pocket and helps to prevent the infection from worsening before definitive I & D is performed. Send a small amount of the aspirated fluid to the microbiology lab for analysis.

Bibliography

1. Gilbert DN, Moellering RC, Sande MA (eds): The Sanford Guide to Antimicrobial Therapy, 29th ed. Vermont, Antimicrobial Therapy Inc., 1999.
2. Stevens DL: Cellulitis and abscesses. In Root RK (ed): Clinical Infectious Diseases. New York, Oxford University Press, 1999, pp 501–503.
3. Swartz MN: Cellulitis and subcutaneous tissue infection. In Mandell GL, Bennett JE, Dolin R (eds): Principles and Practice of Infectious Diseases, 5th ed. New York, Churchill Livingstone, 2000, pp 1037–1057.

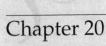

Chapter 20

BURNS

KEY FIGURES:
Rule of 9's adult, child

Burns can be serious injuries and are a major cause of morbidity and disability worldwide. This chapter describes techniques that give the best chance of survival and reduce the risk of long-term disability. When treating patients with a severe burn, you must be prepared to provide extensive care over many days or even weeks. If you cannot meet this commitment, consider transferring the patient to a facility that specializes in the care of burns.

Important Functions of Skin

Intact, uninjured skin plays a vital role in maintaining health. A burn causes significant damage that compromises the ability of the skin to perform its key functions (see table below).

Table 1. The Physiologic Consequences of Burn injury

Skin Function	Consequence of Burn Injury and Required Intervention
Contributes to temperature regulation by preventing heat loss	Patient is prone to lose body heat. You must keep patient covered and warm at all times to prevent hypothermia.
Keeps bacteria and microorganisms from invading body	Patient is at high risk for infection. Antibiotic ointments are used on burn wound, but no systemic antibiotics are indicated unless signs of specific infection are present. Check tetanus immunization status; give booster if needed.
Prevents water loss	Patient loses tremendous amount of fluid into burned skin. Burn also causes release of factors that make all body tissues, not just skin, "leaky" to protein as well as water. Intravascular volume can be greatly depleted by large burn (> 20% body surface area) Common cause of death from large burn is renal failure due to inadequate fluid resuscitation during first 24–48 hrs after acute burn (see "Basic rules for fluid resuscitation" below for prevention strategies)

Mechanism of Injury

A burn can be caused by thermal (heat) injury, electricity, or caustic chemicals. Aside from the resultant skin damage, each mechanism has associated complicating factors of which you should be aware.

Thermal Injury

Thermal injury is the most common cause of burns. In addition to damage to the skin, you must be alert for the possibility of **inhalation injury**—a burn to the patient's airway (pharynx, trachea, even lungs). Failure to diagnose inhalation injury can result in airway swelling and obstruction, which, if untreated, can lead to death.

Signs that may indicate inhalation injury include singed nasal hairs, carbon particles in the sputum, hoarseness, and elevated carbon monoxide (CO) levels in the blood. If you can test for CO, do so. Another way to tell whether the blood contains a significant amount of CO is to look at its color. Blood is bright red when CO is present.

Optimally, bronchoscopy is used to assess edema of the airways and signs of burns in the oropharynx, pharynx, or lower airways.

If signs of airway swelling or burns are present, an endotracheal tube should be placed to protect the airway. Because the swelling worsens over the first 24–48 hours after acute injury, it is best to intubate early. It may be impossible to get the endotracheal tube in place once significant airway swelling has occurred.

Electrical Injury

Electrical burns cause injury by a combination of thermal injury and direct effects of the electrical current (cell membrane instability and de-naturation of cell proteins).

It is often difficult to assess the magnitude of injury because the only visible indication may be damaged skin at the entrance and exit sites. *Significant deep tissue injury often is present along the course of the electrical current through the body.*

Muscle is often the most seriously injured tissue. You must be on the alert for compartment syndrome (swelling of muscle groups that can lead to muscle necrosis). In patients with significant muscle damage, myoglobin is present in the urine, which appears purplish or red. Myoglobinuria requires aggressive treatment to prevent renal failure. The patient should be given sodium bicarbonate in intravenous fluids to make the urine more alkaline, and urine output should be maintained at over 50 ml/hr by giving intravenous fluids as well as intravenous furosemide or mannitol.

Because the heart is a muscle, be alert for cardiac dysfunction. Arrhythmias are common. Patients should be monitored closely and arrhythmias treated appropriately.

Chemical Injury

Chemicals cause damage by reacting with the tissue proteins in a manner that leads to tissue death. Chemical injury is different from thermal injury in that *chemicals can continue to cause damage until they are removed or neutralized.*

In general, the chemical agents are either acids or bases. Basic solutions tend to penetrate deeper into the tissues and thus cause more damage than acidic solutions.

The key to initial treatment is to remove all clothing that may have contacted the chemical and to irrigate the injured area continuously with water for at least 2 hours or longer.

Try to find out the exact chemical that caused the injury. Poison control centers located in almost every state are useful sources of information about the best way to treat various chemical injuries. A useful web address is:

www.medwebplus.com/subject/Poison_Control_Centers.html

It is difficult to estimate the depth of injury from a chemical at initial presentation. Close observation and daily examination of the burn wound are vital for proper treatment.

No matter what the inciting incident, patients with a burn are evaluated and treated in the same manner as outlined below.

Initial Treatment

1. Remove all clothing from the affected area.
2. Immediately cover the burned areas with saline-moistened gauze. Use saline that is lukewarm—*not* too cool.

Special Considerations

If the patient has been injured by hot tar: Tar is not absorbed; do *not* try to remove it by scraping and pulling. Such actions serve only to worsen the burn and injure additional skin. Simply apply petrolatum-based antibiotic ointments to the area (Neosporin or Bacitracin), and the tar will separate as the burns heal.

If grease is present on the burned tissues: Grease often can be removed by gently rubbing with the same petrolatum-based antibiotic ointments.

For **chemical burns**, the area should be rinsed continuously with water for several hours instead of merely applying saline-moistened gauze.

Intravenous access should be obtained for delivering fluids.

Check the tetanus immunization status, and give a booster if needed.

The patient should *not* be given intravenous antibiotics initially. They are used only in the presence of signs that the burn wound has become infected or for treatment of other diagnosed infections (e.g., pneumonia).

Once you have evaluated the extent of the injury, apply a topical agent to the burned areas and cover with sterile gauze. For large burns (> 20% BSA), consider transfer to a burn unit if available (see below).

Table 2.   Commonly Used Agents for Burn Wounds

Agent	Applications Per Day	Indications/Precautions
Bacitracin, Neosporin, or triple antibiotic ointment	1–2	Useful for face burns* or burns over relatively small areas. Do not come in large enough containers for use on large burns.
Silver sulfadiazene (Silvadene)	1–2	Most commonly used agent for burn wounds. Comes in large containers for use on large burns and can be used on all parts of body except face. Does not cause pain upon application. Major side effect is decrease in white blood cell count, which necessitates stopping its use. Do not use in patients allergic to sulfa drugs.
Mafenide acetate (Sulfamylon)	1–2	Comes in large containers. Better burn wound penetration than Silvadene, but painful when applied to burn. Also may cause electrolyte disturbances. Best used for small areas only. Especially indicated for burns on ears to protect cartilage from getting infected. Do not use in patients allergic to sulfa drugs.
Silver nitrate (0.5%)	Several (at least 4 times/ day)	Can be used on large burns and is not painful to apply. Should be applied in wet, bulky dressings. Does not penetrate burn wound as well as Silvadene and may cause severe drop in serum sodium concentration; you must monitor electrolytes closely. Annoying problem is that silver nitrate turns everything it contacts black (e.g., skin, clothing, bedding).

* Keep out of the eyes. Use only ophthalmic preparations for the eyes or areas immediately around the eyes.

Determining Percent of Total Body Surface Area (BSA) Burned

Adults

The rule of nines

- Each entire arm: 9%
- Each entire lower extremity: 18%
- Anterior trunk: 18%
- Posterior trunk: 18%
- Head/neck: 9%
- Genital area: 1%

Children

Modification of the rule of nines

The adult proportions are slightly different in children because of the relatively large size of a child's head in relation to the rest of the body:

• Infant head: ~20%

• Each lower extremity decreased to ~10%

• Other areas remain essentially the same

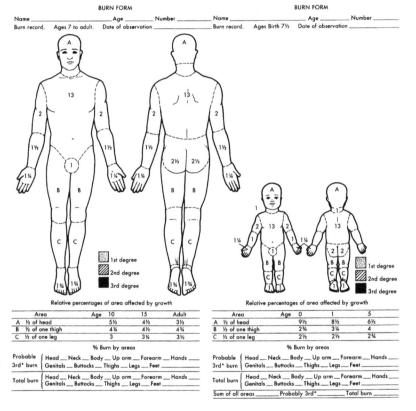

Rule of nines in adults and children. Modification of Lund and Browder chart for determining body surface area. (From Jurkiewicz MJ et al (eds): Plastic Surgery: Principles and Practice. St. Louis, Mosby, 1990, with permission.)

Determining Depth of Burn

It is often difficult to determine the exact severity of the burn at the initial examination. Therefore, reevaluation of the patient once the burns have been cleansed and again 24 hours later is vital.

Burns are classified as first-, second-, or third-degree, depending on the depth of injury. A first-degree burn implies injury to the superficial surface of the skin; it is similar to a sunburn. A second-degree burn involves varying levels of the dermis, and a third-degree burn completely destroys the dermis and may injure even the underlying subcutaneous tissue.

The burn injury is often not uniform. There may be areas of first-, second-, and third-degree burn on different parts of the body. This variation should be noted in your examination. The distinction among burn types is important. In general, the deeper the burn, the greater the amount of intravascular fluid that is lost into the burned tissues and the greater the overall physiologic injury.

Table 3.   Burn Wound Classification

Burn Depth	Appearance	Pain	Sensation
Superficial (first-degree)	Erythema	+	Yes
Partial-thickness (second-degree)*	Blisters, hairs (if present) stay attached	+++	Yes
Full-thickness (third-degree)	Thick, leathery feel Pale color Hairs, if present, do not stay attached May see thrombosed veins	0	No (nerve endings are destroyed)

* Partial-thickness burns can be superficial or deep. A superficial partial-thickness burn may have a thin blister, and the skin is soft and pink. A deep partial-thickness burn appears white but some hair follicles are still attached. It feels softer than a full-thickness burn. A deep partial-thickness burn often behaves like a full-thickness burn.

Basic Rules for Fluid Resuscitation

A burn injury results in dramatic loss of fluids from the intravascular space. To prevent kidney damage or failure, the patient requires a large amount of fluids compared with the baseline state. In patients with second- and third-degree burns affecting > 15–20% BSA, proper fluid resuscitation is vital for survival.

Estimating Fluid Needs for the First 24 Hours after Injury

The Parkland Formula is a good way to estimate fluid needs. The patient must be monitored closely for blood pressure, heart rate, and urine output. Adjustments in fluid rate should be based on these parameters. If necessary and if available, central venous pressure or Swan-Ganz catheter monitoring should be used because they provide more precise measurements of circulatory status. Urine output should be at least 20–30 ml/hr for adults and 1–2 ml/kg/hr for infants or children. Increase output by giving additional intravenous fluids, *not* diuretics.

Parkland Formula

$$4 \text{ ml} \times \text{patient wt (kg)} \times \%\text{BSA} = \text{fluids for first 24 hr}$$

One-half of this amount is given over the first 8 hours after injury; the rest is given over the next 16 hours.

The intravenous fluid of choice in adults is **Ringer's lactate**. Normal saline is the next best option. Do not use dextrose solutions for the initial fluids. In children, use Ringer's lactate, but also administer 5% dextrose in one-fourth normal saline solution ($D_5\frac{1}{4}NS$) for maintenance glucose needs.

Example: A 70-kg man has sustained a 55% BSA burn, of which 10% is first-degree, 20% is second-degree, and 10% is third-degree. Fluids required for the first 24 hours:

$$4 \text{ ml} \times 70 \text{ kg} \times (20 + 10)\%\text{BSA} = 8400 \text{ ml}$$

(I told you that we were talking a lot of fluid!) The total BSA that you calculate includes second- and third-degree burns; first-degree burns are not included.

Give 4200 ml over the first 8 hours, then 4200 ml over the next 16 hours. The amount of fluid given per hour is also an important point:

- If the patient presents immediately after the burn, give 4200/8 = 525 ml/hr for the first 8 hours, then 4200/16 = 262 ml/hr for the next 16 hours.

- If the patient presents 2 hours after the injury, give 4200/6 (fluid must be given over 8 hours after injury, *not* after presentation) = 700 ml/hr over the next 6 hours, then 4200/16 = 262 ml/hr for the next 16 hours.

Pain Control

Few injuries are more painful than a burn. Thus, an important part of the management is adequate pain control. Everything related to a burn injury and its treatment is painful. Keep this in mind, and do *not* skimp on pain medications. Morphine is often the medication of choice. For patients with large burns, intravenous injection is the best way to administer the medication. Absorption of subcutaneous or intramuscular injections is not reliable. Oral pain medications may be indicated with a small burn wound, but they are not useful in patients with significant burn injury.

Morphine

Intravenous morphine is the pain medication of choice. An adult can be given 2–3 mg at a time, titrated to pain control. Do *not* give too much, because excessive morphine can cause the patient to stop breathing.

Guideline for dosing: do not administer more than 0.1 mg of morphine per kg of patient weight (0.1 mg/kg) over a 1–2-hour period. This rule applies to both children and adults.

Sedation

Intravenous sedation can be given along with pain medication. It is especially useful during the initial evaluation and before dressing changes. Sedation may decrease the need for pain medication and alleviates the anxiety often associated with painful procedures. Be cautious, and monitor the patient closely because sedatives also can depress the respiratory drive.

A short-acting agent such as midazolam (Versed) is quite useful. If none is available, diazepam (Valium) is another option. See chapter 3, "Local Anesthesia," for detailed dosing information.

Subsequent Care of Burn Wounds

Patients with a large burn have difficulty in maintaining body temperature. During dressing changes, the patient may become quite hypothermic if precautions are not taken. If possible, warm the room, use warming lights, uncover parts of the wound individually instead of removing all of the dressings at the same time, and use lukewarm, not cold saline.

Examine the burns daily to look for signs of infection (e.g., induration, blanching erythema, increased redness/warmth).

First-degree Burns

Clean daily with gentle soap and water.

Apply a gentle moisturizer (aloe, cocoa butter, something without perfumes) or antibiotic ointment once or twice daily.

First-degree burns require several days to heal.

Second-degree Burns

If the blisters are intact, it is usually best to leave them alone. The area under the blister essentially represents a sterile environment and promotes healing. An exception is the blister that is so tight that it interferes with the circulation of surrounding tissues. Such blisters should be opened and the loose skin removed.

If the blisters have opened, the skin should be removed gently. This procedure usually requires a pair of forceps and a pair of scissors. Removing the skin should not hurt.

Apply antibiotic ointment—usually Silvadene on the body, Bacitracin on the face—twice daily, and cover with dry gauze.

Clean the burn wound with saline, and remove the old ointment before applying new ointment.

Dressing and cleansing the wound are often quite painful. Be sure to give pain medication before changing the dressings.

Superficial second-degree burns usually heal within 10–14 days, whereas deep second-degree burns often take 3–4 weeks. Deeper burns are also prone to thick, hypertrophic scarring. Therefore, unless the area is very small (< 4–5 cm in diameter), tangential excision (see below) is often recommended for deep second-degree burns.

Third-degree Burns

Apply antibiotic ointment—usually Silvadene on the body, Baci-tracin on the face—twice daily, and cover with dry gauze.

Clean the burn wound with saline and remove the old ointment before applying new ointment.

Full-thickness burns take at least 4 weeks to heal and often heal with a hypertrophic scar. Except for small (< 4–5 cm in diameter) third-degree burns, tangential excision and split-thickness skin grafting usually are recommended

Fluids after the First 24 Hours

Because the capillaries are no longer as "leaky" after the first 24 hours, the fluids are changed from crystalloid (Ringer's lactate) to protein-containing solutions (colloids). Colloids provide improved intravascular volume expansion.

In general, give 0.3–0.5 ml/kg/%BSA over 24 hours.

In addition, 5% dextrose in water or 5% dextrose in 0.45 saline is given to maintain urine output of at least 20 ml/hr.

After this regimen, fluids should be administered according to the patient's overall condition.

Nutritional Concerns

A severe burn injury causes severe metabolic disturbances and a concomitant increase in caloric requirements. Chapter 8, "Nutrition," explains how to estimate caloric needs; for a severe burn injury (> 40% BSA), the basal metabolic rate is multiplied by a factor of 2–2.5, a larger factor than for any other injury. Depletion of nutritional stores is a distinct risk. Caloric requirements reach their peak at approximately 7–10 days after injury and do not return to normal until all burns have healed.

Nutritional support is vital for the treatment of a severely burned patient. If the patient cannot ingest enough calories orally, a nasogastric or other type of enteral feeding tube must be placed to supply calories. If the patient cannot tolerate feedings through the gastrointestinal tract, central intravenous nutritional support should be started.

Tangential Excision

For deep second- and third-degree burns larger than a few centimeters, tangential excision followed by split-thickness skin grafting is recommended. It leads to faster healing, with more stable skin coverage. In tangential excision, only the burned tissue is removed; uninjured tissue is left alone.

Careful tangential excision of the burn and split thickness skin grafting should be done relatively early (within days of the injury) if possible. Usually the procedure is done in the operating room under general anesthesia. A special knife or dermatome (see chapter 12, "Skin Grafts") is used. Be sure to excise only the tissue that is burned. You will know when you have reached healthy tissue because it will bleed. In general, dead tissue does not bleed.

This procedure can cause significant blood loss. Usually only small areas (< 10% BSA) are done at any one time, and blood should be available for transfusion. Patients always lose more blood than you expect. Hemostasis usually can be obtained by holding a gauze pad over the area and applying pressure for a few minutes. Sometimes topical thrombin or epinephrine solutions can be applied as well.

The wound is then ready for split-thickness skin grafting (see chapter 12, "Skin Grafts," for details).

Caution: Tangential excision should be done only by a practitioner with special surgical skills who is comfortable performing skin grafting. Unless only a small area (e.g., part of the arm) is involved, this procedure can be quite difficult to perform safely.

Specific Injuries

Hand Burns

See chapter 34, "Hand Burns," for detailed information. Simple techniques can prevent permanent loss of hand function.

Electrical Burns of the Mouth in Children

Electrical burns of the mouth usually occur when the child bites down on an electrical cord. Such injuries usually involve a burn of the lip commissure (where the upper lip meets the lower lip).

The eschar (scab) that forms at the commissure separates after 10–14 days. Separation may be accompanied by significant bleeding from the labial artery. You should warn parents about this potential event. They can control the bleeding by holding gauze over the area and pinching the lip at the commissure. The bleeding should stop after 5–10 minutes of pressure, but medical treatment may be needed.

Burns on the Dorsum of the Foot

Second-degree burns on the top of the foot initially may seem insignificant and, in fact, often heal with local care alone. However, improper management may result in a more extensive tissue loss than you expect. Exposure or injury to the underlying tendons may result and can be quite problematic to treat.

Proper Treatment

1. Apply the usual antibiotic ointment and dressings, as described above.

2. The patient should wear no shoes or boots on the injured foot until the burn is healing well.

3. The foot should be **kept elevated at all times**.

4. The patient should not put weight on the affected foot until you are sure that the burn is healing properly.

Referral to Burn Center

A burn center is a tertiary care center that specializes in the multidisciplinary care of patients with acute burn injuries. Burn centers serve an important purpose and are responsible for improved outcomes in severely injured burn patients. Only second- or third-degree burns should be referred. If you are lucky enough to have one available, the following criteria may be applied for referral:

1. Burns of the genitalia, face, hands, and feet

2. Burns involving over 10% BSA in patients younger than 10 years or older than 50 years

3. Burns involving over 20% BSA in patients of any age

4. Inhalation injury

5. Other significant trauma

6. Third-degree burns involving over 5–10% BSA

7. Multiple medical problems as well as significant burn injury

Do not be reluctant to transfer. Burn patients are seriously ill and have the potential for developing many complications. They are best treated at centers that specialize in burn care.

Even if you decide to transfer the patient to a burn center, you should not hesitate to start the appropriate treatment. The first few hours after an injury are critical, and measures such as fluid resuscitation, burn dressings, and pain control must be initiated and implemented appropriately while awaiting transfer.

Frostbite

Frostbite is an injury caused by prolonged exposure to cold temperature that results in freezing of soft tissues and formation of ice crystals. Ice crystals form not only inside cells but also inside the smallest of blood vessels, causing occlusion. Occlusion ultimately leads to tissue loss.

Initial Treatment

This information applies to patients who present at the time of injury. Some patients do not seek treatment for several days or weeks after injury. The treatment that follows is *not* for delayed presentation (see next section for treatment after the acute thermal process has resolved).

Rapid Rewarming

1. The first line of treatment for patients with acute frostbite injury is rapid rewarming of the tissue. Rewarming should be done only when you are certain that the tissue will not again be exposed to cold.

2. Immerse the affected part in warm water (104–108°F or 40–42°C). Use of hotter water may cause a burn injury, whereas use of cooler water may not provide the benefits of rewarming. It usually takes about 20–30 minutes to rewarm the tissues.

3. Rewarming *hurts*. Give the patient pain medication, preferably intravenous morphine.

4. Do not massage the affected tissue.

After Tissues are Rewarmed or if Patient Presents Days after Injury

1. Unroof only those blisters with clear fluid.

2. Blisters filled with blood should be left alone. They are signs of deeper tissue injury.

3. Gently elevate the affected area to decrease swelling.

4. Apply aloe vera to the affected areas, and cover with a gauze dressing.

5. Antiplatelet medications may be useful (e.g., aspirin, 80–325 mg/day).

6. Use gentle range-of-motion exercises to prevent joint stiffness.

7. For hand injuries, remember to splint the hand in neutral position.

8. Change the dressing daily, or prescribe whirlpool treatments, if available.

9. Check the patient's tetanus toxoid status, and treat appropriately.

10. Antibiotics are used only if signs of infection are present in the surrounding soft tissue.

Note: The cornerstone of treatment of a frostbite injury is to allow the injured tissues to demarcate. The dead tissue turns black, gradually shrivels, and eventually falls off. After dermarcation, you will debride only the tissue that does not survive the injury.

During the first few days or even weeks after the initial injury, tissue that at first appeared unlikely to survive may actually heal. By waiting for the tissues to demarcate, you can tell definitively which tissue is dead, and you will not remove more tissue than necessary. Another indication for surgical debridement of injured tissue is development of an infection that does not resolve with antibiotic therapy.

Long-term Effects

1. Joint stiffness and arthritis are common.

2. The affected area may be permanently sensitive to cold temperatures.

3. In children, frostbite injures the growth plate of the bones and may result in diminution of bone growth.

Bibliography

1. Luce EA: Electrical injuries. In McCarthy JG (ed): Plastic Surgery. Philadelphia, W.B. Saunders, 1990, pp 814–830.
2. Robson MC, Smith DJ: Cold injuries. In McCarthy JG (ed): Plastic Surgery. Philadelphia, W.B. Saunders, 1990, pp 849–866.
3. Salisbury RE: Thermal burns. In McCarthy JG (ed): Plastic Surgery. Philadelphia, W.B. Saunders, 1990, pp 787–813.

Chapter 21

FRACTURES OF THE TIBIA AND FIBULA

KEY FIGURES:

Calf anatomy	Longstanding open
How to do fasciotomy	fracture
Gastrocnemius and	Gastrocnemius flap
neighboring structures	

Fractures of the tibia and fibula are a special concern because missing early warning signs can result in a useless leg.

The tibia and the fibula are the two long bones of the calf. Fractures of these bones often result from a sport-related injury or motor vehicle accident. Most fractures of the tibia and fibula (tib-fib fractures) heal without complication, and the patient is able to resume his or her normal activities.

However, potentially serious complications can develop, and you must be aware of their early warning signs. With this knowledge, you can intervene before permanent tissue damage develops. Early intervention may make the difference between a normally functioning patient with a well-healed fracture and disaster.

Case Example

An 18-year-old boy was playing football and collided with another player, injuring his right leg. He tried to keep playing, but because the pain was so intense he could not place any weight on the leg. He sat out the rest of the game and then came in for evaluation.

The calf was swollen and tender, and the x-ray showed a minimally displaced mid-shaft tib-fib fracture. No orthopedic surgeon was available. After finding the fracture in *Campbell's Orthopaedics*, you placed him in a cast, gave him crutches and pain medications, and sent him home.

He returns a few days later in horrible pain. You remove the cast. His calf is very tight and swollen, and except for the lateral aspect he has no sensation in his foot. When you move his ankle, the pain intensifies in his calf. You check for pulses in his feet, and they are present.

A general surgeon takes one look at the patient, and immediately sends him to the operating room. Incisions are made in the calf, and much of the calf muscle is dead.

The boy's leg will never function as it did before the injury. He will have a life-long disability.

What happened? First you need some basic background information.

Closed vs. Open Fractures

Fractures are usually classified as closed or open.

A **closed fracture** means that the skin around the fracture site is intact. In terms of bone healing, closed fractures have a favorable prognosis because of the low risk for infection of the bone (osteomyelitis) at the fracture site. However, complications may arise, as illustrated by the case example.

In an **open fracture**, also called a compound fracture, the skin around the fracture site has been punctured. Open fractures are more serious injuries because it generally takes greater forces to disrupt the skin and fracture the bones. An open fracture greatly increases the risk for the development of osteomyelitis, and osteomyelitis increases the risk for poor healing.

The quality of the soft tissue around the fractured bones plays a role in fracture healing. Feel your own calf. The anterior surface of the tibia is covered only by skin; there is not much padding around this bone. Significant injury to the skin around the tibia can result in exposure of the bone and thus a greater risk for poor healing of the fracture.

The higher the energy of the injury, the more significant the injury to the soft tissue and the greater the potential for problems. Falling off a step results in a low-energy injury; being hit by a car results in a high-energy injury.

Essential Elements of the Physical Examination

1. Is the skin intact? (open vs. closed fracture)
2. If the skin is punctured, what can you see in the wound? Foreign material must be removed, and dead muscle or skin should be cut out. If the fracture site is exposed, soft tissue coverage may be needed.

3. What is the vascular status of the leg? Check capillary refill. Check the pulses on the top of the foot (dorsalis pedis) and behind the medial malleolus (posterior tibial artery). If capillary refill or pulses are not present, the patient may have a serious arterial injury.

4. What is the neurologic status of the leg? Evaluate the patient for evidence of nerve dysfunction or injury. Check sensation in the following areas:
   • The first web space on the dorsum of the foot between the great toe and the second toe: deep peroneal nerve
   • The plantar surface of the foot: posterior tibial nerve
   • The lateral aspect of the foot: sural nerve
   Check active ankle motion and toe motion:
   • Plantarflexion of the ankle and toes (pointing of toes and foot): posterior tibial nerve
   • Dorsiflexion of the ankle and toes (bringing the toes and foot upward toward the front of the calf): anterior tibial nerve
   • Eversion (elevating the lateral side of the foot): peroneal nerve

5. What are the radiographic findings? A single break in each of the bones usually heals with fewer complications than when the bones are broken into many pieces (a comminuted fracture). A large number of fragments indicates a higher-energy injury, which is associated with a higher rate of complications.

6. Evaluate the patient for signs and symptoms of compartment syndrome. If they are present, you have a surgical emergency on your hands (see below).

Compartment Syndrome

A compartment syndrome develops when pressure builds up within a fixed, well-defined space. The increase in pressure prevents venous and lymphatic outflow, and fluid build-up leads to a further increase in pressure in the tissues. High pressures can cause tissue injury and death.

High pressures also prevent blood and nutrients from reaching the tissues, causing further injury. Without appropriate intervention to relieve pressure build-up, a vicious cycle develops. This is essentially the definition of a compartment syndrome.

Muscle and nerve are the tissues most prone to injury. If a compartment syndrome remains untreated even for a few hours, the result is muscle death, which translates into tissue loss and permanent disability.

The death of muscle tissue can also be a very serious problem for the patient's overall health. A muscle breakdown byproduct, myoglobin, is released into the bloodstream and can cause permanent kidney damage. Thus a compartment syndrome not only endangers normal function; it can also threaten the patient's life. For these reasons, the treatment of a compartment syndrome is a surgical emergency.

Anatomy of the Calf

The anatomy of the calf puts it at increased risk for the development of a compartment syndrome. The muscles of the calf are segregated into four well-defined compartments, surrounded by tight, unyielding fascia. Build-up of pressure in one compartment cannot decompress into another uninjured compartment. In the thigh, on the other hand, the separation of the muscle compartments is not as tight and well-defined. An increase in pressure of the anterior thigh muscle compartment can be absorbed by the posterior compartment. This dissipation of pressure does not occur in the calf.

Understanding the nerves and muscles in each of the four compartments of the calf facilitates examination of an injured leg.

Table 1. Compartments of the Calf

Compartment	Nerve	Motor Function	Sensory Distribution
Anterior	Deep peroneal	Dorsiflexion of foot and toes	Dorsal first web space
Lateral	Superficial peroneal	Eversion of foot	Dorsal aspect of foot except for area noted above
Posterior	*	Plantarflexion of foot	*
Deep posterior	Posterior tibial	Inversion of foot, plantarflexion of toes	Plantar surface of foot

* The sural nerve runs in the subcutaneous tissue of the posterior calf skin; it does not run in the posterior compartment of the calf. The sural nerve provides sensation to the lateral aspect of the foot. This is often spared in the patient with a pending compartment syndrome.

In patients with a tib/fib fracture, the force of the injury leads to bleeding at the fracture site and in the muscle, along with additional swelling of the muscle and soft tissues in the calf. Swelling may impair venous return, which can start the vicious cycle leading to the development of a compartment syndrome.

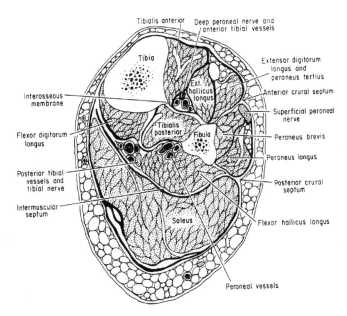

Axial section through the middle third of the calf showing the four compartments. (From Jurkiewicz MJ, et al (eds): Plastic Surgery: Principles and Practice. St. Louis, Mosby, 1990, with permission.)

Signs and Symptoms

It is important to be aware of the potential development of compartment syndrome and to warn patients about the early warning signs. The key is to catch the problem early so that intervention can prevent permanent damage. An untreated compartment syndrome can lead to severe morbidity, extremity loss, and potentially life-threatening complications. The following signs and symptoms should be kept in mind:

- Severe pain in the calf, out of proportion to that expected from the injury

- Significant calf tightness

- Pain with passive stretch of a muscle group; for example, pain in the front of the calf with pointing of the toes and plantarflexing the ankle, or pain in the back of the calf with dorsiflexion of the ankle.

- Tingling or numbness in the foot, along the peroneal and posterior tibial distribution, but *not* necessarily along the lateral aspect of the foot.

Note: Pulses in the foot and ankle may be completely *normal* even with a significant build-up of pressure in the calf compartments.

Prevention

It is vital that the patient keep the leg elevated and not let it dangle in a dependent position. If you have any concerns about the patient's ability to follow these recommendations, the patient should be admitted to the hospital for leg elevation and close observation.

Be careful not to cast the leg too tightly. A tight cast can increase tissue pressure. If swelling in the calf is significant or if you do not have much experience making a cast, consider putting the leg in a splint for the first few days. A splint (sometimes called a backslab in rural areas) is a plaster half-cast placed over padding on the posterior aspect of the calf onto the foot. It is held in place by a loosely applied Ace wrap.

If the patient complains at all that the cast seems too tight, bivalve the cast. Make cuts in the cast along the medial and lateral sides, and separate the underlying padding. This technique may relieve symptoms of pressure. If bivalving the cast does not relieve the symptoms, remove the cast and reevaluate the leg to be sure that a compartment syndrome has not developed.

In patients with an open fracture, do not close the skin if it seems tight. It is better to have an open wound in need of coverage than to risk the development of a compartment syndrome by tightly closing the skin.

Have a high index of suspicion. Remember: a compartment syndrome can occur even with an open fracture and even when the patient has normal pulses.

Treatment

The key to treatment is to open the involved compartments before permanent tissue damage has occurred. Treatment is emergent. You should not wait for many hours or days for a specialist to be available. Each compartment must be individually opened (see diagrams and descriptions).

Often, when you open the compartment, the bulging muscle initially looks purple and dead. Give the tissue a few minutes; it often becomes pinker and healthier-looking. Muscle that remains dark and purple, however, is dead and should be excised.

The incisions should be left open. Saline dressings are a good choice for wound care.

Further surgery is needed for wound closure. Wait at least 3–4 days for the swelling to lessen. A split-thickness skin graft (STSG) is almost always required for wound closure. If you attempt to close one of the incisions primarily, be sure that there is no tension on the skin closure.

Adequate stabilization of the fracture is also required. Usually temporary stabilization can be attained with a posterior splint. If an orthopedic surgeon is available, more definitive stabilization should be done.

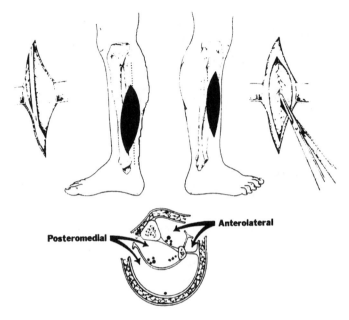

Adequate treatment of a compartment syndrome requires two incisions on the calf. One incision is made along the medial aspect of the calf, 2–3 cm posterior to the medial edge of the tibia. This incision allows access to the two posterior compartments. The second incision—on the lateral aspect of the calf, immediately in front of the fibula—allows access to the anterior and lateral compartments. (From Cameron JL (ed): Current Surgical Therapy, 4th ed. St. Louis, Mosby, 1992, with permission.)

Back to our case example. As you may have guessed, he developed a compartment syndrome that was not recognized.

Open Fractures

The ultimate treatment of open fractures requires specialists, but as a nonspecialist you can take steps to improve the patient's chances for a good outcome until specialty care is available.

Open fractures of the lower leg are a major cause of morbidity because of the high propensity for development of osteomyelitis and inadequate bone healing.

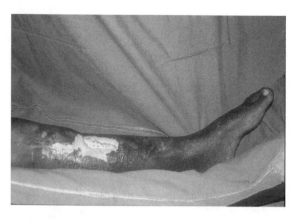

Leg of a patient who sustained an open tib-fib fracture 1 year earlier. No soft tissue coverage was provided at the time of injury. The soft tissue never healed over the bone, and the exposed bone is dead. The patient is in constant pain and cannot walk without assistance.

With poor healing of the fracture, the patient may not be able to walk without assist devices (cane or crutches), may have chronic pain, and often is unable to work. Amputation may become necessary to control infection and improve overall function.

The underlying fracture must be anatomically reduced in a stable position to allow healing of the soft tissues. Healthy soft tissue coverage is vital to healing of the fracture.

Basic Treatment

The goal is to achieve a healed bone, surrounded by healthy soft tissue. Intravenous antibiotics should be started immediately. Both gentamicin and a first-generation cephalosporin (e.g., cephalexin) should be given.

Thoroughly wash out the wound under anesthesia as soon as possible after injury. Be sure to remove all foreign material and dead tissue, and copiously irrigate the wound with saline.

In patients with significant contamination or soft tissue injury, it is best to pack the wound with gauze moistened with antibiotic solution or saline and to immobilize the leg in a splint. Return the patient to the operating room in 24–48 hours to wash out and debride the wound again and to stabilize the fracture.

The patient should keep the leg slightly elevated to minimize swelling. Be sure to watch out for signs and symptoms of compartment syndrome.

If soft tissue can be closed over the bone, do so very loosely. Because of swelling, a tight closure actually increases the chances for further tissue loss, making the wound more difficult to manage. If muscle around the fracture can be sutured together to cover the bone, do so. If the skin cannot be closed, place a STSG over the muscle. This technique is much preferable to tight skin closure.

If only a small area of bone (< 1–1½ cm in diameter) is exposed, the wound may heal secondarily with dressing changes. For larger wounds, a local muscle flap or distant flap is required to cover the fracture and promote proper healing. Flaps require surgical expertise (see below). Optimally, the fracture site should be covered within the first week after injury.

Local Muscle Flaps

Local muscle flaps should be undertaken only by someone with surgical skills. Several muscles in the calf can be used as a local flap to cover an exposed tib-fib fracture site. Muscle flaps also bring robust circulation to the fracture site and thereby improve healing of the injured bone.

The use of muscle flaps has markedly decreased the morbidity associated with open fractures. Studies have shown that muscle flaps promote fracture healing; the average time for proper healing decreases from 9 to 5 months. The risk of developing osteomyelitis also decreases from 40% to 5%, and the amputation rate decreases from almost 30% to 5% when muscle flap coverage of an exposed bone or fracture is done within the first week after injury.

Proximal and Middle Third of the Calf: Gastrocnemius Flap

The gastrocnemius muscle is the most superficial muscle of the posterior aspect of the calf. It accounts for most of the muscle mass at the top of the calf. The gastrocnemius muscle originates from the distal femur and joins the underlying soleus muscle to form the Achilles tendon.

The main vascular supply enters the gastrocnemius muscle proximally near the knee joint. The muscle can be divided from the Achilles tendon and underlying soleus muscle without interfering with its blood supply. It should be divided longitudinally at its midline so that you take only one-half of the muscle.

The gastrocnemius muscle then can be easily moved to cover wounds in the middle and proximal third of the calf. Sometimes the origin of the muscle has to be divided to allow increased movement into the wound. Usually the medial gastrocnemius is used. If the lateral muscle is used, it must swing around the fibula, which decreases the range of the flap.

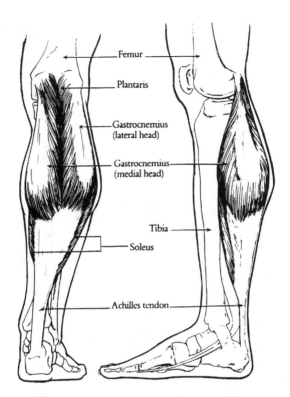

The gastrocnemius muscle and neighboring structures are depicted in posterior and medial views of the leg. The tendon of the gastrocnemius muscle joins with the tendon of the soleus muscle to form the Achilles tendon. (From Strauch B, et al (eds): Grabb's Encyclopedia of Flaps. Boston, Little, Brown, 1990, with permission.)

Operation

1. General or spinal anesthesia is required.

2. Use a tourniquet, if available, for the dissection.

3. Be sure that the wound is adequately debrided and that all dead tissue or bone is completely removed.

4. Do not take overlying skin with the muscle. An STSG is placed over the muscle at the end of the procedure.

5. Extend the open wound onto the medial calf skin to visualize the underlying muscle. Try not to leave skin bridges because they have diminished circulation and may become necrotic.

6. Identify the gastrocnemius muscle. It is the most superficial muscle (closest to the calf skin).

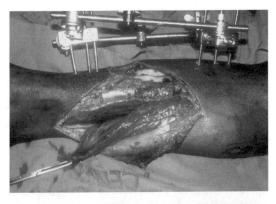

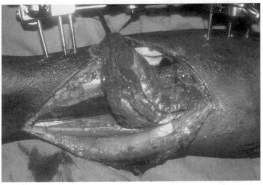

Patient with an exposed, open tib-fib fracture. The injury is less than 48 hours old, and the bone is being covered with a gastrocnemius flap. Note the external fixator, which is stabilizing the fracture.

7. Separate the gastrocnemius muscle from the overlying skin and underlying soleus muscle. This procedure often can be done bluntly or with electrocautery. Be gentle.

8. You will see the vascular pedicle coming into the deep surface of the muscle around the knee. Do not divide or injure these vessels.

9. In the back of the calf, the medial and lateral parts of the muscle come together in the midline. The muscle fibers form a V, whose point marks a natural plane between the two halves of the muscle. The muscle can be divided along this line and then detached from the Achilles tendon using electrocautery.

10. Try to bring the muscle around to the defect. The proximal muscle may need to be freed to allow sufficient length. This procedure can be done safely, but be careful not to injure the vascular pedicle.

11. Once the muscle is freed and seems to reach the wound, remove the tourniquet and ensure hemostasis.

12. The muscle should turn pink and look healthy when the tourniquet is removed. If it remains dark purple, the vascular pedicle has been injured and you are in trouble. Another flap option, perhaps a soleus flap (see below under mid-calf injury) or a distant flap, is necessary.

13. The muscle should be sutured loosely to the wound edges with absorbable sutures. Avoid a tight closure, which may interfere with the circulation to the muscle. Make sure that the blood vessels to the muscle are not kinked.

14. Place a suction drain (if available) or a Penrose drain under the muscle flap and at the donor area. These drains should be brought out through the incisions. They prevent blood and other fluids from accumulating under the muscle flap and under the skin flap that was created when the muscle was dissected free.

15. Place an STSG over the muscle.

16. Place the leg in a posterior splint, and keep it gently elevated.

Postoperative Care

1. The leg should remain elevated and immobilized in either a splint or, if an orthopedic surgeon is available, some type of internal or external fixation device. The leg should not be in a dependent position for at least 7 days after surgery.

2. The dressing should be changed daily. Antibiotic ointment and saline-moistened gauze or a wet-to-wet dressing is best to use over the skin graft.

3. Remove the drains after 2–3 days.

4. The flap initially will be quite swollen. Swelling improves dramatically over the first 2–3 weeks and continues to improve over the next several months.

5. After 7 days, when the wounds are healing well, the patient can gradually let the leg dangle for increasing amounts of time. Start with 15 minutes 2 times/day. When the leg is dependent, it should be gently wrapped with an Ace wrap to prevent swelling.

Middle and Possibly Distal Third of the Calf: Soleus Flap

The soleus muscle lies immediately deep to the gastrocnemius muscle and joins with the gastrocnemius distally to form the Achilles tendon.

The soleus flap is most useful for wounds in the middle of the calf. Although sometimes it can be used for wounds of the lower third, it is not as reliable in the lower leg.

The soleus muscle has a somewhat segmental blood supply without one dominant vessel (as seen in the gastrocnemius muscle). The vessel that enters the top half of the muscle can nourish the whole muscle. In addition, a few smaller vessels in the distal portion of the muscle can nourish the entire soleus if the proximal vessel is divided.

The flap is based most commonly and reliably on its proximal, main blood supply, but at times it can be based on the smaller, distal vessels. Judge which vessel to use by looking at the surrounding damage in the leg. In patients with proximal calf soft tissue damage, it may be prudent to base the flap on the distal vessels. If the injury has injured the distal tissues, base the flap on the proximal vessel.

Operation

1. General anesthesia or spinal anesthesia is required.

2. Use a tourniquet, if available, for the dissection.

3. Be sure that the wound is adequately debrided and that all dead tissue or bone is completely removed.

4. Extend the open wound onto the medial calf skin to visualize the underlying muscles. Try not to leave skin bridges, which have diminished circulation and may become necrotic.

5. Identify the gastrocnemius muscle, which is the most superficial muscle (closest to the skin). The plane of dissection is between the gastrocnemius muscle and underlying soleus muscle. Keep the gastrocnemius muscle attached to the overlying skin as you separate it from the underlying soleus. This procedure often can be done bluntly or with electrocautery. Be gentle to avoid tearing of blood vessels.

6. Bluntly separate the soleus muscle from the muscles of the deep posterior compartment, taking care to avoid damage to blood vessels coming off the posterior tibial artery. Determine which way the flap will be based and divide the vessels that are unnecessary.

7. Determine whether the blood vessel on which you want to base the flap is sufficient to supply circulation to the flap. Place a small vascular (noncrushing) clamp across the vessels that you plan to divide before doing so. If the muscle turns purple with the clamp in place, the blood vessel you are basing the flap on will not supply enough circulation to the flap.

8. Divide the muscle from the Achilles tendon (if basing the muscle proximally) or near its origin (if based on distal vessels).

9. Bring the muscle to the exposed fracture site. The muscle may need to be freed from the tissues around the pedicle to allow sufficient length. This procedure can be done safely, but you must be careful not to injure the vascular pedicle.

10. Once the muscle is freed and seems to reach the wound, remove the tourniquet and ensure hemostasis.

11. The muscle should turn pink and look healthy when the tourniquet is removed. If it remains dark purple, the vascular pedicle has been injured and you are in trouble. A distant flap is required to cover the wound.

12. The muscle should be sutured loosely to the wound edges using an absorbable suture. Tight closure may interfere with the circulation to the muscle. Make sure that the blood vessels are not kinked.

13. Place a suction drain (if available) or a Penrose drain under the muscle flap and in the area from which the muscle was taken. These drains should be brought out through the incisions. They prevent blood and other fluids from accumulating under the flap or at the donor site.

14. Place an STSG over the muscle.

15. Place the leg in a splint, and keep the leg gently elevated.

Postoperative Care

Follow the steps described above for the gastrocnemius flap.

Distant Flaps

In high-energy wounds, the muscles in the calf may be too damaged to use for coverage of the fracture site. In this case, a distant flap is required to achieve healing of the fracture and soft tissues.

Although cumbersome for the patient, a cross-leg flap can be quite useful if you have no access to a reconstructive specialist (see chapter 14, "Distant Flaps," for details).

The other option is a free flap, which is preferred if specialist help is available. Free flaps, however, are beyond the ability of clinicians without microsurgical skills. Transfer of the patient is required.

Bibliography

1. Byrd HS, Spicer TE, Cierney G: Management of open tibial fractures. Plast Reconstr Surg 76:719–730, 1985.
2. Cohen BE: Gastrocnemius muscle and musculocutaneous flap. In Strauch B, Vasconez LO, Hall-Findlay EJ (eds): Grabb's Encyclopedia of Flaps. Boston, Little, Brown, 1990, pp 1695–1702.
3. Hertel R, Lambert SM, Muller S, et al: On the timing of soft-tissue reconstruction for open fractures of the lower leg. Arch Orthop Trauma Surg 119: 7–12, 1999.
4. McBryde AM, Mays JT: Compartment syndrome. In Cameron JL (ed): Current Surgical Therapy, 6th ed. St. Louis, Mosby, 1998, pp 974–979.
5. Tobin GR: Soleus flaps. In Strauch B, Vasconez LO, Hall-Findlay EJ (eds): Grabb's Encyclopedia of Flaps. Boston, Little, Brown, 1990, pp 1706–1711.
6. Yaremchuk MJ, Gan BS: Soft tissue management of open tibia fractures. Acta Orthop Belg 62(Suppl 1):188–192, 1996.

Chapter 22

SKIN CANCER

KEY FIGURES:

Typical melanoma	Incisional biopsy
Basal cell carcinoma	Excisional biopsy
Squamous cell carcinoma	Shave biopsy
Punch equipment	Lazy S incision
Punch biopsy	

The most commonly performed plastic surgical procedures involve the removal of suspicious, possibly cancerous skin lesions. This undertaking usually is not highly technical and, particularly for lesions located on areas other than the face, often does not require special surgical expertise. In areas where few or no specialists are available, it is reasonable for a clinician with basic surgical skills to initiate treatment. However, you should have certain important background knowledge before removing a suspicious lesion. Lack of this knowledge may have negative consequences for your patient.

This chapter presents the basics concerning the most commonly encountered skin cancers and the proper techniques for excising a suspicious skin lesion. In addition, a brief explanation of what to do for the patient diagnosed with a specific type of skin cancer is included.

What Makes a Skin Lesion Suspicious

Several characteristics should make you suspect cancer may be present. An open wound that, despite proper care, just will not heal or one that temporarily heals and then opens again warrants further investigation. Red, raised lesions that do not go away, increase in size, or have small blood vessels at their base should raise suspicion. Skin cancer may develop at the site of a preexisting mole, but not all moles are precancerous.

When to be Concerned about a Mole

If a patient reports a change in what had been a stable mole (i.e., one that has not changed in appearance for many years), biopsy/excision should be done. These changes include but are not limited to:

- Increase in size
- Change in color
- Ulceration/bleeding
- Irritation

Commonly Encountered Skin Cancers

Melanoma

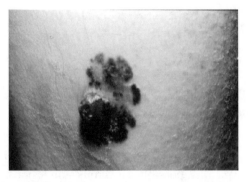

Appearance of a typical melanoma. (From Fitzpatrick JE, Aeling JL (eds): Dermatology Secrets. Philadelphia, Hanley & Belfus, 1996, with permission.)

Melanoma is potentially the most serious of all skin cancers because of its propensity for metastatic spread. There is still no successful adjuvant therapy (such as chemotherapy or radiation treatment); surgery remains the primary mode of treatment. The incidence of melanoma is increasing worldwide.

The thickness of the lesion and the depth of skin penetration determine the need for subsequent surgery as well as the patient's prognosis. This is why proper excision is important and should not be taken lightly.

Etiology

The risk for developing melanoma is related to the patient's history of sun exposure and genetic background. People with fair skin, who sunburn easily, have a higher incidence of melanoma than darker-skinned people, who rarely sunburn.

What It Looks Like

Although sun exposure is a causative factor for the development of melanoma, the lesions are not necessarily found on sun-exposed areas. Melanoma can occur anywhere on the body, including the palms of the hands, soles of the feet, perineal area, and under fingernails or toenails.

Most melanomas arise from preexisting moles. Classically, a melanoma is described as looking like a very dark brown or black mole, but color is not the only characteristic that should raise suspicion. Other characteristics of a pigmented mole that are considered to be worrisome (but *not* diagnostic) for melanoma include:

- Asymmetry

- Irregular shape

- Border irregularity—the edges of the mole are ragged instead of smooth

- Color variability—a benign mole tends to have a uniform color. A worrisome mole will have some portions lighter or darker than the predominant color. Also, a dark mole that has lost some of its pigmentation is worrisome.

- Diameter > 6 mm—moles > 6 mm are at a significant risk for melanoma and should be excised. (However, if a mole of this size has been present for years, is light brown in color, and has not changed at all in appearance, it probably does not have to be removed.)

Note: Many elderly people develop very dark brown/black moles that appear to be "stuck on" or glued to the skin surface. They do not look like typical moles, which are embedded in the skin. These lesions, known as **seborrheic keratoses**, are benign despite their dark pigmentation. However, if any of the above mentioned signs is associated with one of these lesions, it should be removed.

Basal Cell Carcinoma

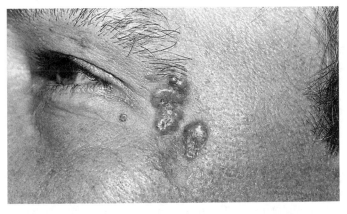

Appearance of a typical basal cell carcinoma.

Basal cell carcinoma (BCC) is the most common type of skin cancer. It occurs primarily on sun-exposed skin and often looks like a small ulcer or nonhealing area with raised edges and a red base. BCCs usually do not metastasize, but they can recur if not adequately excised. They also have a propensity to burrow into deeper tissues, which can make complete excision difficult.

Squamous Cell Carcinoma

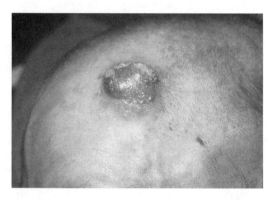

Appearance of a typical squamous cell carcinoma.

Squamous cell carcinoma (SCC) is less common than BCC but more common than melanoma. SCC almost always arises on sun-exposed areas, often in an area with previous skin damage. It usually appears as an ulcerative lesion with crusting, but it can be a raised, solid, reddish lesion. SCC can metastasize to lymph nodes, but metastasis is not as common as with melanoma.

SCC can develop in a chronic wound (i.e., a longstanding pressure sore or a burn that never achieved a stable scar). Such lesions involve a higher incidence of metastatic spread than usually is associated with SCC. They are more aggressive tumors.

What to Do When Someone Presents with a Suspicious Lesion

Start with a Good History

History of skin cancer, either personally or in the family. Melanoma and even some forms of BCC may run in families. Patients with a personal history of skin cancer are at a higher-than-normal risk for developing another similar skin cancer.

History of sun exposure. This question is not aimed only at finding out whether the patient spends hours in the sun trying to tan, but also applies to patients whose work or hobbies keeps them outdoors in the sun. As noted above, sun exposure is a causative factor for most primary skin cancers.

History of the lesion. How long has the lesion been present? Has it changed recently? A longstanding, stable lesion (i.e., one that has not changed for several years) is less worrisome than a lesion of short duration that has changed in appearance.

Weight change or other change in overall medical status. Weight loss, general fatigue, or simply not feeling well can be signs of metastatic spread if no other reasons can be found.

Physical Examination

Note the specific characteristics of the lesion, such as size, color, and ulceration.

Examine the entire patient for other suspicious lesions. It is vital to do a thorough examination so that other lesions are not missed. With melanoma on an extremity, you should be particularly concerned about lesions proximal to the one under suspicion. Proximal lesions indicate a more aggressive stage of disease.

Check for enlargement of lymph nodes in the area where the lesion would drain. Enlargement may imply lymphatic spread of cancer.

Table 1.   Lymph Node Drainage Areas

Location of Suspicious Lesion	Area to Check for Enlargement of Draining Lymph Nodes
Hand/arm	Axilla (armpit)
Foot/leg	Groin/inguinal area
Face	Cervical (neck) area
Trunk	Axilla and inguinal areas; these lesions have multiple drainage sites

Check for enlargement of the liver, which also can be a sign of metastatic spread.

How to Make the Diagnosis: Biopsy

A definitive diagnosis requires removing the entire lesion (or just a representative portion) and sending it to a pathologist for formal evaluation.

Biopsy Techniques

Incisional Biopsy

An incisional biopsy removes a small, representative sample of the lesion, not the entire lesion. It should include the full thickness of skin into the underlying subcutaneous tissue.

Excisional Biopsy

The entire lesion with a rim of surrounding, normal-appearing tissue is removed with an excisional biopsy. Again, the full thickness of the involved skin is removed. The resultant defect is larger than with an incisional biopsy and usually is closed primarily. However, depending on the size of the lesion, other choices for wound closure may be more appropriate.

Shave Biopsy/Excision

A shave biopsy removes the lesion with only the top layers of skin, which seem to be grossly involved with the lesion. This is more correctly called a shave excision. Because only the top layers of skin are removed rather than the full thickness of skin, the defect will heal well with local wound care alone.

When to Do Which Biopsy Technique

Table 2.   Indications for Each Type of Biopsy Technique

Technique	Lesion Characteristics	Reasoning Behind Biopsy Choice
Excisional biopsy	< 1–2 cm	Wounds of this size usually are easy to close and may allow treatment with one procedure.
Incisional biopsy	Large lesions: > 3 cm on body or > 2 cm on face	Large wounds may be difficult to close. Incisional biopsy allows you to make the diagnosis and plan further treatment. It is often good to make the diagnosis before making a large wound, especially on the face.
Shave biopsy/ excision	Only for obviously benign lesions, seborrheic keratitis	Unless you are well trained in recognizing skin cancers, you probably should not perform shave excisions. Especially on a pigmented lesion with any chance of being melanoma, shave excision is not recommended because it makes thickness measurements (important for staging and treatment decisions) impossible.

How to Do the Biopsy

General procedures common to all techniques:

- The excision can be done using **clean technique** for gloves and gauze, but the instruments and suture material should be **sterile**.

- Place the patient in **as comfortable a position as possible**, sitting or reclining as appropriate. Because some patients faint or feel light-headed during the procedure, it is best for them to be reclining.

- Administer **local anesthetic** (usually lidocaine; see chapter 3, "Local Anesthesia"). Use as small a needle as possible, and inject slowly. Injection of local anesthetics hurts. If bicarbonate is available, add it to the solution before injection.

- Do not inject directly into the lesion; inject into the **surrounding normal tissues**.

- "Paint" the area, i.e., apply an **antimicrobial solution** to the lesion and surrounding skin before making any incisions.

- The biopsy specimen should be taken to the pathologist in a **small container with formalin**. There should be at least enough formalin in the container to cover the lesion.

Incisional Biopsy

An incisional biopsy needs to be only a few mm in width and should be taken from an area representative of the entire lesion. Stay away from areas with a lot of crusting. It is usually best to take the biopsy toward the periphery of the lesion, because the center of a large lesion is often necrotic tissue, which may not yield a diagnosis on pathologic evaluation. It is useful to include a rim of normal-appearing skin at the margin to aid the pathologist. The biopsy specimen should be full-thickness skin, including the upper portion of the underlying subcutaneous tissue.

Punch biopsy procedure.   If you have access to a punch biopsy instrument, use it. This instrument has a sharp, hollow, circular end that easily takes the biopsy for you.

1. The skin around the lesion should be held under some tension.

2. Hold the instrument perpendicular to the lesion.

3. Push the sharp end gently into the lesion; then twist 180°.

4. Remove the instrument.

5. The specimen can be removed by gently grasping the skin surface with a forceps, pulling it upwards, and cutting the subcutaneous tissue attachment on the undersurface of the specimen.

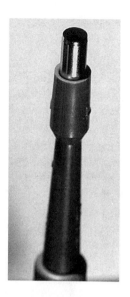

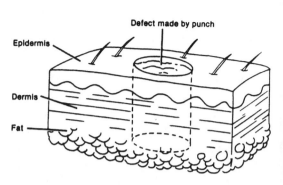

Left, Punch biopsy instrument. (Photo courtesy of Moore Medical Corporation.)

Above, Punch biopsy procedure. The punch should be introduced through the dermis and into the fat. (From Habif TB (ed): Clinical Dermatology, 3rd ed. St. Louis, Mosby, 1996, with permission.)

If you do not have access to punch biopsy instruments, use a scalpel and forceps. Excise a piece of tissue that is a few mm wide by 1 cm (or longer if the lesion is large) in an elliptical fashion (see figure below). An ellipse is the easiest shape to suture closed, but other shapes may be chosen, depending on the characteristics of the lesion. Because the biopsy site is small, the defect can be allowed to heal on its own (with antibiotic ointment and a dry dressing daily) or closed primarily with 1 or 2 sutures.

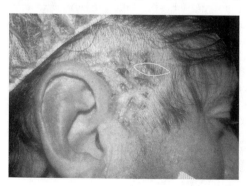

Incisional biopsy. The white ellipse is an example of how to orient an incisional biopsy to include abnormal skin as well as a normal-appearing skin margin. The pathology report showed this lesion to be a BCC.

Excisional Biopsy

Whenever possible, primary closure of the excision site is usually best. However, on some areas (e.g., the calf), even small 1–2-cm excisions can result in a wound that is difficult to close because little redundant surrounding skin is available. If such is the case, you often can treat the wound with local dressings and allow it to heal secondarily. This approach is especially useful on the forehead or lateral cheek (in front of the ear), behind the ear, and on the calf.

If you believe that primary closure is possible, remove the lesion as an ellipse to facilitate closure (see figure below). If you have a marking pen, it is helpful to draw the ellipse or whatever shape you intend to use before making the incision. Usually you should draw the ellipse in the direction of the lesion if one dimension is larger than the other or in the direction of the most redundant skin. If you cannot determine the best direction, excise the lesion as it appears. Once the lesion is removed, the surrounding skin tension will open the wound and show you the best way to finish the ellipse to facilitate closure.

Remember: you want to include a 1–2-mm rim of normal-appearing tissue around the lesion. In general, the length of the ellipse should be 3 times its width.

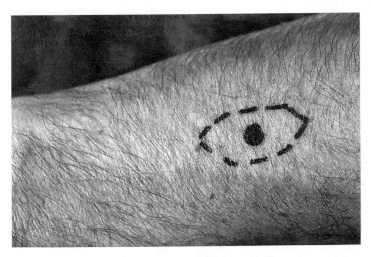

Excisional biopsy. The most common way to excise a lesion is in the form of an ellipse. The long axis should be approximately 2–3 times the diameter of the lesion so that the closure will be smooth. Undermining may be required to obtain wound closure.

Make the incision. If the markings have one limb of the ellipse above the other, do the bottom limb first. This will prevent any bleeding from the top limb from dripping down and obscuring your ability to easily make the lower incision (a lesson learned the hard way by many).

Cut through the skin and dermis and into the subcutaneous tissue. This should be a full-thickness skin biopsy. The thickness of the skin varies over different areas of the body. The back has very thick skin (which is often a surprise to the inexperienced surgeon), whereas the skin of the dorsum of the hand or face is much thinner.

If you have access to an electrodesiccator, use it to treat the resultant wound. This technique stops the bleeding and also treats any remaining abnormal cells if the lesion is a BCC.

If you can almost but not quite suture the wound closed, you can try undermining the surrounding skin (see chapter 2, "Surgical Skills"). I do not recommend more than a few centimeters of undermining.

If you choose primary closure, follow the instructions in the chapter 11, "Primary Wound Closure." Wash the excision site and the surrounding skin with saline. Apply antibiotic ointment and cover with a dry gauze. The gauze can be removed after 24 hours; the suture line should be cleaned and dressed daily. After 2–3 days the suture line can be left open.

If you choose secondary closure, apply antibiotic ointment to the wound and cover with dry gauze. The wound should be dressed and cleansed daily. Wet-to-dry dressings also may be used. Once the wound has formed an eschar (dry scab), no dressings are required. Reassure the patient that leaving the wound open to heal secondarily will *not* necessarily lead to an increased risk of infection, but it may leave a somewhat larger scar than primary closure. However, because closing a wound under tension involves far higher risks for infection and wound-healing problems, secondary closure is more appropriate.

Shave Excision

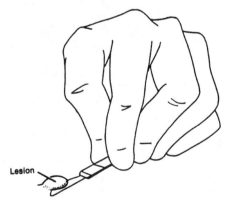

Shave excision. The curved surgical blade is laid flat on the skin surface and drawn smoothly through the base of the lesion. (From Habif TP: Clinical Dermatology, 3rd ed. St. Louis, Mosby, 1996, with permission.)

Performing a shave excision requires a scalpel and forceps. Place the scalpel so that it is flat against the skin with the sharp edge parallel to the skin. Using a back-and-forth sawing motion, pass the knife under the lesion, taking only the top layers of skin. Dermis should remain at the excision site when the lesion is removed.

The resultant defect should be treated with an electrodessicator if possible. The electrodessicator heats the tissues and kills superficial cancer cells if the lesion is BCC. Apply antibiotic ointment to the wound and cover with a dry gauze. Repeat daily until a dry scab forms. The wound can then be left open.

Marking the Tissue Specimen

For all excisions, it is helpful to mark the specimen so that the pathologist can orient the lesion. Place a nonabsorbable stitch at the superior edge of the specimen, and tie it in place. Cut the ends, and note on the specimen slip what the marking stitch represents (i.e., superior margin). Another stitch can be placed along the medial or lateral margin. Cut the suture ends longer than the stitch on the superior margin. Again, be sure to explain what you have done on the pathology slip (i.e., long stitch = lateral margin).

If the lesion is malignant and goes to the edge of the specimen, the pathologist can report which edge of the specimen is involved. This information simplifies the repeat excision.

What the Pathology Report Means in Terms of Further Treatment

If the lesion is benign:

You are done. Remove the sutures when appropriate. If you did an incisional biopsy and part of the lesion remains, you can remove the remainder by using the shave biopsy technique, if the patient so desires.

If the lesion is fully excised BCC or SCC:

You are done. Remove the sutures when appropriate. The patient should be seen again in 3–6 months and then yearly. Look for new lesions, and check the excision site for recurrence.

If the lesion is BCC that was not fully excised:

If you have a close margin (< 0.1 mm) and treated the area with the electrodessicator at the time of the excision, you can either watch closely (see the patient every 3 months for the first year and then semiannually) or re-excise. Repeat excision is recommended if you expect follow-up to be difficult or impossible or if you did not have access to an electrodessicator.

If the lesion is SCC that has not been fully excised:

Re-excise. You should take a bit more grossly "normal" tissue with re-excision of SCC than with re-excision of BCC.

Re-excision of BCC or SCC

The re-excision can be done at the time of diagnosis or after a few weeks when the tissues have begun to heal.

If the defect was closed primarily, the portion of the suture line containing the positive margin should be excised as an ellipse. Remember to take a few mm margin around the suture line to ensure a clear margin (i.e., no residual tumor).

If the biopsy site is healing secondarily, excise the involved margin, making sure to take at least a few mm of grossly normal surrounding skin.

If the positive margin is the deep margin: make sure that you go deeper into the subcutaneous tissues than on the first excision.

If Melanoma is Diagnosed

Patients diagnosed with melanoma should see a specialist. However, if no specialist is accessible, further excision is required. The extent of the re-excision is determined by the depth of the primary lesion. The following is a basic guide to further treatment.

A **lesion < 1.0 mm** is considered a very thin melanoma, but it still needs to be re-excised with a 1-cm margin all the way around the scar. Often such re-excision is curative.

A **lesion of 1.0–4.0 mm** is considered an intermediate-thickness melanoma. Re-excision is required with 1.5–2-cm margins. Often you will not be able to close the resultant defect primarily. A split-thickness skin graft or a local flap may be the best option for closure. In the presence of clinically palpable lymph nodes, lymphadenectomy is recommended. This procedure is beyond the abilities of a nonsurgeon; refer the patient to a specialist.

A **lesion > 4 mm** is considered a thick melanoma and is associated with a high likelihood of metastatic spread at the time of diagnosis. To control local disease, re-excision with 2–3-cm margins is recommended. Split-thickness skin grafting or a local flap often is required. In the presence of clinically palpable lymph nodes, lymphadenectomy is recommended.

Re-excision for Melanoma

A re-excision for melanoma is a more extensive procedure than re-excision for BCC or SCC. It is also more extensive than the initial biopsy. The melanoma re-excision includes skin and subcutaneous tissue down to, but not including, the fascia of the underlying muscle group. This is a much larger chunk of tissue than the initial biopsy. Unless the lesion is in an area with a great deal of redundant tissue (e.g., on the abdomen), a split-thickness skin graft or local flap may be required for closure.

One technique that may facilitate primary wound closure is to perform the re-excision making a "lazy S" incision instead of the usual ellipse (see figure below). With limited undermining of the surrounding skin edges, the lazy S incision often can be closed primarily.

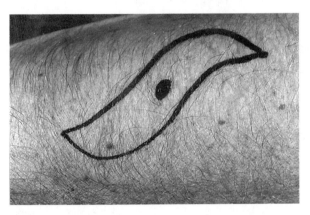

To perform a wide excision for melanoma, it is often useful to use the lazy S technique instead of the usual ellipse.

Reasons for Specialist Intervention

In an attempt to improve overall survival rates, a new technique called **sentinel lymph node biopsy** is recommended for patients with thin and intermediate-thickness melanoma and no clinically palpable draining lymph nodes in an attempt to identify microscopic metastatic lymph node spread. It is hoped that removal of diseased lymph nodes before they become clinically palpable can prevent melanoma cells from metastasizing to a distant site.

Essentially the surgeon injects dye or a radioactive isotope into the area of the primary lesion. The draining lymph node basin is then surgically explored, and the specific lymph node that first takes up the dye/isotope is identified. If a radioactive isotope is used, a Geiger counter-like device is used to find the lymph node; if dye is used, the surgeon looks for a blue lymph node. The lymph node is then removed, and the pathologist examines it thoroughly for melanoma. If no cancer is found, no further treatment is performed. If cancer is present, a formal lymph node dissection is performed. So far this approach shows promise for catching the cancer at the earliest possible stage with the least amount of patient morbidity.

For All Patients with Melanoma

Check for enlargement of draining lymph nodes, and order a chest radiograph to look for signs of metastases. The patient should be followed every 3–6 months for several years to look for recurrence at the excision site, new satellite lesions in the skin heading toward the draining lymph area, enlargement of draining lymph nodes, and enlargement of the liver.

Important Postexcision Instructions for All Patients

Remind all patients that sun exposure is a causative factor in most primary skin cancers. All patients who have been seen for a suspicious skin lesion should be counseled about the importance of staying out of the sun as much as possible. The regular use of a good sunscreen (SPF > 15) must be emphasized.

Bibliography

1. Balch C, Houghton A, Sober A, Soong S (eds): Cutaneous Melanoma, 3rd ed. St. Louis, Quality Medical Publishing, 1998.
2. Goldberg DP: Assessment and surgical treatment of basal cell skin cancer. Clin Plast Surg 24:673–686, 1997.
3. Roth JJ, Granick MS: Squamous cell and adnexal carcinomas of the skin. Clin Plast Surg 24:687–700, 1997.
4. Wagner JD, Gordon MS, Chuang TY, Coleman JJ: Current therapy of cutaneous melanoma. Plast Reconstr Surg 105:1774–1799, 2000.
5. www.skin-cancer.com
6. www.melanoma.net

Chapter 23

CLEFT LIP/PALATE

KEY FIGURES:

Unilateral cleft lip	Cleft lip: preoperative
Bilateral cleft lip	and postoperative
Cleft palate	Pierre Robin syndrome

Also known as "harelip," cleft lip with or without a cleft palate is the most common craniofacial birth defect. It is beyond the scope of this text to describe the specific surgical procedures used to correct this anomaly. In fact, the treatment of cleft lip/palate remains a challenging problem even for plastic and reconstructive surgeons.

All health care providers, especially those in rural settings, should have an understanding of basic background information so that they can educate parents and ensure that the child receives proper treatment.

Definitions

Cleft Lip

A cleft lip results when the developing tissues of the lip do not completely fuse. The lip is divided into two parts, and an incorrect alignment of the lip muscles (orbicularis oris) results.

A cleft lip primarily involves the upper lip, although rare forms of facial clefting can involve the lower lip. The typical cleft lip often involves the nose, with resultant distortion of the nostrils and nasal sill.

Cleft Palate

The palate is essentially the roof of the mouth. It is composed of two parts, the hard palate and the soft palate. The teeth erupt in the anterior hard palate (called the alveolar ridge), and the posterior hard palate serves as the base of the nasal cavity.

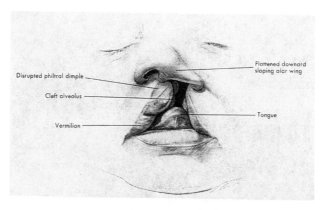

Unilateral cleft lip. The upper lip is twisted and shortened vertically. Cupid's bow is incomplete, the vermilion tapers cephalad, and the white line extends into the vestibule. In this case an alveolar cleft is present, creating a defect in the nasal floor. The alar rim is significantly distorted. (From Jurkiewicz MJ, et al (eds): Plastic Surgery: Principles and Practice. St. Louis, Mosby, 1990, with permission.)

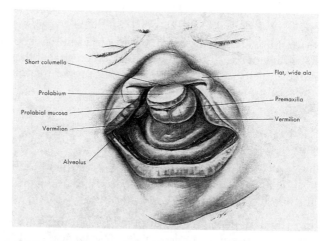

Bilateral cleft lip. Severely shortened columella, wide flattened alae, and jutting, often rotated premaxilla are hallmarks of the deformity. (From Jurkiewicz MJ, et al (eds): Plastic Surgery: Principles and Practice. St. Louis, Mosby, 1990, with permission.)

The soft palate is the posterior portion of the roof of the mouth. The soft palate is mobile and is composed of several muscles important for normal speech and proper function of the eustachian tubes (associated with the middle ear).

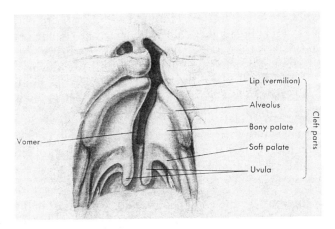

Unilateral complete cleft lip and palate. (From Jurkiewicz MJ, et al (eds): Plastic Surgery: Principles and Practice. St. Louis, Mosby, 1990, with permission.)

Presentation and Incidence

Presentation varies widely. The child may be born with a unilateral or bilateral cleft lip with a normal palate, a cleft palate (soft only or hard and soft) with a normal lip, or a unilateral/bilateral cleft lip with a cleft palate. The most common presentation is left-sided unilateral cleft lip with cleft palate. Male infants are affected more often than female infants.

The majority of affected infants are otherwise healthy and normal intellectually. However, there is a 25% incidence of additional anomalies, including neurologic and cardiac abnormalities as well as club foot. Evaluate the child closely so that other problems are not missed.

Cleft lip/palate is the most common congenital facial abnormality. The incidence in Caucasian populations is 1–1.5/1000 live births; in African and African-American populations, < 0.5/1000 live births; and in Asian and Hispanic populations, 2–3/1000 live births.

Embryologic Development and Etiology

During fetal development the lip and palate are formed during the first trimester (days 30–60 of gestation). A cleft develops when something interferes with the normal processes of fusion and mesodermal penetration of the frontonasal processes and maxillary processes of the face of the embryo. Essentially, instead of growing together to form a normal lip and palate, the embryonic tissues remain separate, causing the cleft to develop.

Parents without clefts who have one child with a cleft lip/palate have a 5% chance of having another child with a cleft lip/palate (compared with the usual 0.14% risk in parents with no family history of cleft). If both one parent and one child have a cleft or if two normal parents have two children with clefts, the likelihood of a cleft in another child increases to 15–20%. These data seem to suggest a genetic component.

The development of cleft lip/palate, however, probably is due to a combination of multiple factors—for example, folic acid deficiency, advanced maternal/paternal age, use of anticonvulsants (phenytoin or phenobarbital), alcohol intake, and possibly smoking. A viral etiology also has been suggested.

It is quite common for the parents of a child with a cleft to give a history that includes none of the above factors. In some rural cultures, a cleft palate is thought to represent a sign of evil or wrong-doing on the part of the family. Parents are often quite guilt-ridden, thinking that they did something to cause the defect. *Therefore, it is important to assure parents that they did nothing wrong to cause the child's abnormality.*

Immediate Concerns

Adequate Nutrition

The initial concern for an infant with cleft lip/palate is ingestion of adequate calories and fluids to maintain health and allow proper growth.

An infant's ability to suck is related to two factors: the ability of the external lips to perform the necessary sucking movements and the ability of the palate to allow the necessary build-up of pressure inside the mouth so that foodstuff can be propelled into the mouth.

Infants with cleft lip/palate have sufficient external lip muscle movements. Therefore, an isolated cleft lip usually does not interfere with the child's ability to suck, although it may take some practice not to lose a lot of milk out of the cleft lip defect.

In contrast, a child with a cleft palate with or without a cleft lip has difficulty sucking properly. The cleft in the palate impedes the proper build-up of pressure inside the mouth. For the same amount of effort, the infant with a cleft palate does not ingest as much milk as a normal infant. This increase in the work of feeding may lead to insufficient intake of calories for proper growth and health.

Helpful Strategies

The child should be fed with the head upright at about a 45° angle.

Usually bottle feeding is needed. If possible, use a nipple made for premature infants because it has a larger opening than normal. An alternative is to cut an X in the tip of a regular nipple to enlarge the opening. The larger-than-normal opening allows more liquid to flow out of the nipple with less suction.

A squeezable bottle also facilitates getting the milk into the infant's mouth.

If you are in an area with access to a pediatric orthodontist, an appliance can be made to fit into the infant's mouth and cover the cleft defect. This appliance, called an obturator, greatly improves the infant's ability to suck and ingest calories with less energy expenditure.

Do not be alarmed when milk comes out of the infant's nose. The palate serves to separate the nasal cavity from the oral cavity. The presence of a cleft in the palate removes this separation so that food and liquids easily pass from the mouth and come out of the nose.

Initial Corrective Operations

Correction of the cleft lip/palate deformity is not a life-preserving medical necessity. However, nontreatment often results from lack of access to specialists rather than a conscious decision to leave the child untreated.

A cleft lip/palate is a challenging deformity to repair. Usually, the lip is repaired at around 3 months of age. In full-term, healthy infants, however, repair may be undertaken at an earlier age.

In utero repair of the cleft lip defect is a subject of ongoing research. Clefts usually can be seen on prenatal ultrasound, and it has been shown that fetal tissues heal without the scars usually seen in infants and adults.

The palate is repaired at a separate operation, usually when the infant is around 12 months of age. In areas with limited access to specialists, however, the lip and palate can be repaired at the same time. In fact, even in the developed world where plastic surgeons are abundant, some authorites believe that simultaneous repair of the lip and palate may yield better results than separate repairs.

Often, if the infant has recurring ear infections, pressure-equalizing (PE) tubes are needed. Usually they are inserted at the time of palate repair.

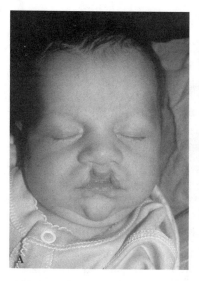 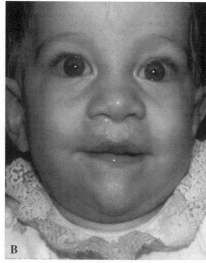

Infant with an incomplete bilateral cleft lip. *A*, Preoperative appearance. *B*, Appearance after one operation.

Other Possible Operations

Unfortunately, even under the best of circumstances, further operations, available primarily to patients in the developed world, may be required for definitive treatment. The combination of cleft lip and cleft palate requires additional surgery more often than cleft lip or cleft palate alone.

Even if the palate is properly repaired, the child may have significant speech difficulties. Often they can be corrected with speech therapy, but approximately 20% of children with a repaired cleft palate require an additional operation to improve palatal function, usually between the ages of 4 and 6 years.

Irregularities of the lip often are noticeable even after repair. Some irregularities that are present when the child is 1–2 years of age are due to tight scarring and improve with time. Revisions usually are delayed until the child is 4–6 years of age.

In addition, significant deformity of the nostrils may require correction, usually when the child is 4–6 years of age. Surgery on the nose can be done at the same time as lip revisions.

Most clefts of the anterior hard palate (alveolar ridge) are repaired when the canine tooth on the side of the cleft begins to erupt, usually around age 7–8 years.

Optimally, a pediatric dentist or orthodontist should be continually involved with the care of children with cleft palate to get the teeth in as normal a position as possible.

If the maxilla (upper jaw) does not grow normally, corrective surgery may be indicated. The procedure, called a Le Fort I osteotomy, usually is delayed until the child is much older, often in the later teen years.

Table 1.   Overview of Operations that May be Required for Cleft Lip/Palate

Approximate Age	Operation	Comments
3 mo	Cleft lip repair	Should be delayed for small children (< 10 lb or 4 kg) to decrease risks from anesthesia.
12 mo	Cleft palate repair	Can be delayed to 18 mo because of airway concerns, but should be done before infant starts to talk.
3–12 mo	PE tubes	Depending on number of ear infections, PE tubes can be placed at time of lip repair or palate repair.
4–6 yr	Improvement of palatal function	Improves child's speech; about 20% of children with cleft palate repair require additional surgery.
4–6 yr	Lip revision, minor nostril corrections	These procedures can be done at the same time.
7–8 yr	Repair of anterior (alveolar) hard palate	Usually done when canine tooth begins to erupt; can be done successfully in older child (10–12 yr old).
> 17–18 yr	Le Fort I osteotomy: upper jaw surgery	Maxilla usually does not grow normally in child born with cleft palate and may need to be cut and repositioned to correct relationship of upper jaw to lower jaw (mandible).
> 17–18 yr	Rhinoplasty; more complex nose surgery than performed before	Nose may need significant work to achieve more normal appearance and function. Procedure may include cartilage grafts, bone repositioning, and correction of deviated septum.

PE = pressure-equalizing.

Visiting Surgeon Programs

Skilled plastic surgeons and other health professionals in several international programs travel to remote areas and perform cleft lip/palate repair and other reconstructive procedures. These high-volume initiatives serve tens of thousands of patients. There is no need for rural families to lose hope for their child.

Listed on the following page are just a few organizations that you can contact to gain more information or to arrange a visit to your area.

Table 2.   Visiting Surgeon Programs

Organization	Contact Information	Background Information

Operation Smile	(757) 321-7645
	Fax: (757) 321-7660
	6435 Tidewater Drive
	Norfolk, VA 23509
	www.operationsmile.org
		Operating since 1982
		Members travel in
		   U.S. and through-
		   out world

Interplast	(650) 962-0123
	Fax: (650) 962-1619
	300-B Pioneer Way
	Mountain View, CA 94041
	www.interplast.org
	e-mail: DirMedServcs
	  @Interplast.org
		Operating since 1969
		Members travel
		   throughout world

American Society
  of Plastic Surgery-
  Reconstructive
  Surgeons Volun-
  teers Program
	(847) 228-9900
	Fax: (847) 228-9131
	444 E. Algonquin Rd
	Arlington Heights, IL 60005
	www.plasticsurgery.org
		Formed in 1988
		Clearinghouse that offers
		  information about many
		  organizations that
		  volunteer time and
		  skills worldwide

Pierre Robin Syndrome

Pierre Robin syndrome is another congenital anomaly to be aware of. These patients may also have a cleft palate, so be sure to evaluate all neonates with a cleft palate for signs of this syndrome.

Pierre Robin syndrome describes an infant with a small, posteriorly displaced mandible that causes the tongue to seem too large for the mouth. During fetal development a cleft palate or a highly arched

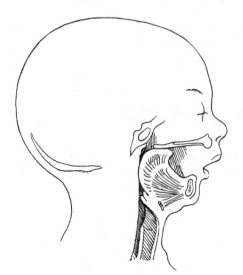

Pierre Robin syndrome. Note the small lower jaw and the resultant position of the tongue in the back of the throat. The tongue can cause potentially life-threatening airway obstruction. (From McCarthy J (ed): Plastic Surgery. Philadelphia, W.B. Saunders, 1990, with permission.)

palate forms to accommodate the relatively large tongue. Early recognition of newborns with Pierre Robin syndrome is mandatory to avoid serious complications.

Immediate Concerns

Affected infants may present with episodes of **severe respiratory distress**. When the infant is in an upright position or with the head forward, the tongue falls forward and the airway opens. If the infant is placed in the supine position (lying down, face up—the usual position in which an infant is placed to sleep), the tongue falls backward and blocks the airway, causing severe respiratory distress. If unrecognized, this syndrome can result in death.

Treatment

- The infant must be monitored closely and kept in the prone (face-down) position for sleep.

- The child should sit upright in a somewhat forward position when eating.

- Occasionally the tongue needs to be stitched to the lower lip to prevent the tongue from falling backward.

- Rarely, in very severe cases, the infant may require a tracheotomy to maintain an adequate airway.

- If the infant has a cleft palate, repair is usually delayed until the child is a few years old because of airway concerns.

- As the infant grows, the mandible grows. Respiratory concerns become less problematic. Usually, no other treatment is required.

Bibliography

1. Mackool RJ, Gittes GK, Longaker MT: Scarless healing. Clin Plast Surg 25:357–366, 1998.
2. Stal S, Klebuc M, et al: Algorithms for the treatment of cleft lip and palate. Clin Plast Surg 25:493–507, 1998.

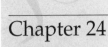

Chapter 24

BREAST SURGERY

In the developed world, breast reconstruction after mastectomy and breast reduction (reduction mammaplasty) are common reconstructive procedures. They require a combination of artistic and technical skills, which can be obtained only through many years of surgical training.

Because of their highly technical nature, no specific procedures are discussed in detail. Instead, this chapter offers basic information.

Breast Reconstruction

Evolution of Procedures

Over the past 25 years, because of advances in plastic surgical techniques, the esthetic quality of breast reconstruction has improved greatly. Before the early 1970s, breast reconstruction was a multistaged procedure in which a distant random flap was transferred to the chest in a series of operations. The results were not always successful, nor were the reconstructed breasts consistently cosmetically pleasing.

Snyderman and Guthrie reported the use of a silicone implant for breast reconstruction in 1971. Their achievement was remarkable because for the first time a breast was reconstructed in a single procedure. Although it was not necessarily a cosmetic triumph, patients were so pleased to have a breast after one operation that they considered the procedure worthwhile.

Implant reconstruction is still a popular option for breast reconstruction, although now saline implants are used. To achieve the best aesthetic result, implant reconstruction is often not a single procedure. Initially, a tissue expander (a modified implant to which the surgeon

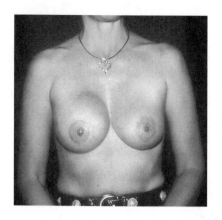

Breast reconstruction with a saline implant. Nipple-areolar reconstruction also has been completed. (Photo courtesy of Nelson Goldberg, M.D.)

can add saline in the office) is placed under the chest wall muscles and skin. The expander is then gradually filled with saline to stretch the tissues of the chest. Thus, an implant large enough to match the opposite breast eventually can be placed. Expansion usually takes several months to complete, and a second operation is required to replace the expander with the permanent implant.

Implant breast reconstruction has its drawbacks. Because the implant is a foreign body, risks include infection, implant deflation, and distortion of the reconstructed breast. It is also difficult to create a droopy breast with an implant. Because of these limitations, other reconstructive options were developed.

In the late 1970s, axial musculocutaneous flaps enhanced a patient's reconstructive options. These flaps (composed of muscle and overlying skin and subcutaneous tissue) could be designed for use in breast reconstruction. The use of a muscle flap allows creation of the reconstructed breast from the patient's *own tissues.*

The **latissimus dorsi flap** (a flap using tissue from the back) became a popular reconstructive option. However, only a relatively small sized breast can be reconstructed with this flap, so an implant may still be needed to attain symmetry in a large-breasted woman. The advantage of this procedure is that even if an implant is needed, the breast can be reconstructed in one operation. The latissimus dorsi flap with or without an implant remains a viable reconstructive option.

In the mid 1980s, Carl Hartrampf popularized the pedicle **TRAM flap** for breast reconstruction. TRAM stands for transverse rectus abdominis (the paired muscles that are vertically oriented on the abdomen and run on either side of the umbilicus) myocutaneous flap. This procedure often is called the "tummy tuck" breast reconstruction.

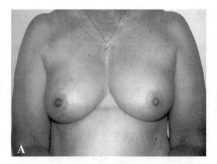

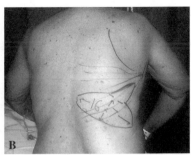

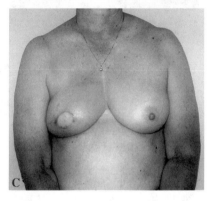

Latissimus dorsi flap. *A*, Patient with Paget's disease of the right breast. *B*, The patient underwent a skin-sparing mastectomy; only the nipple and areolar skin were removed with the underlying breast tissue. The breast was reconstructed immediately with a latissimus dorsi musculocutaneous flap. The flap is drawn on the patient's back. *C*, Final result before nipple reconstruction.

The pedicle TRAM flap is composed of the lower abdominal skin and subcutaneous tissue, which remains attached to the rectus abdominis muscle. The blood supply comes from the superior portion of the muscle. The TRAM flap allows creation of a larger breast (compared with the latissimus dorsi flap) without the need for an implant.

The pedicle TRAM flap is still a popular reconstructive technique, but the procedure does have limitations. Under some circumstances and in some patient populations (diabetics, smokers, and obese patients), an unacceptably high rate of partial flap loss has been noted.

Because of these limitations, researchers performed cadaver dissections to more fully evaluate the blood supply to the TRAM flap. These studies demonstrated that the tissues making up the TRAM flap are better supplied by the deep inferior epigastric artery and inferior rectus muscle (as opposed to the deep superior epigastric artery and superior rectus muscle used in the pedicle TRAM technique). Microsurgeons now perform breast reconstruction using the TRAM as a free flap based on the deep inferior epigastric vascular circulation. Because of its better blood supply, the free TRAM flap overcomes most of the limitations of the pedicle TRAM.

Currently free TRAM breast reconstruction offers the best way to make a large breast in one operation using the patient's own tissues. The drawback is that not all plastic surgeons have the technical skills required to perform microsurgery.

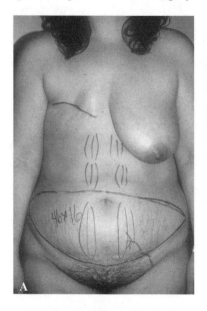
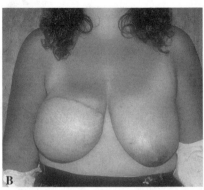

Free TRAM breast reconstruction. *A,* Preoperative markings show the amount of abdominal wall tissue to be removed. The rectus muscles and vascular pedicle also are drawn to show the underlying anatomy. *B,* Completed reconstruction.

Reconstruction of the Nipple and Areolar Complex

The above procedures describe the creation of the breast mound. The nipple and areolar complex usually are reconstructed in a second, relatively minor procedure.

Small flaps of tissue from the breast mound are used to create a nipple. Sometimes a full-thickness skin graft is required as well. A tattoo machine is used to add pigment to the nipple and surrounding skin to complete the reconstruction of the nipple and areolar complex. This procedure often can be done in the surgeon's office.

Timing of Breast Reconstruction

Breast reconstruction can be done at the time of mastectomy (immediate reconstruction) or at almost any time after the mastectomy (delayed reconstruction). The advantage of an immediate reconstruction is that the patient awakens from the mastectomy with a reconstructed breast. Avoidance of an extended period with a flat, scarred chest is an important psychological boost for some patients.

Because of concerns that reconstruction may interfere with surveillance for recurrent breast cancer, general surgeons initially were hesitant to refer patients for immediate breast reconstruction. Studies have shown that these concerns are unwarranted. Immediate breast reconstruction does not interfere with surveillance or mask evidence of recurrent disease.

Some patients may not be appropriate candidates for immediate reconstruction because of the extent of disease or concerns that postoperative radiation or chemotherapy may affect the reconstruction. Delayed reconstruction is always an option and can be performed months or even years after cancer treatments have been completed. The timing of breast reconstruction is ultimately decided on an individual basis after thorough discussion between the patient and her doctors.

Currently, women with breast cancer have many options for breast reconstruction. Depending on the patient's reconstructive needs and expectations, the prognosis for obtaining a matched pair of breasts after mastectomy is excellent.

Breast Reduction

Large, pendulous breasts (D–DDD or even larger cup sizes) can be a source of embarrassment for some women and also may cause significant neck, upper back, and shoulder pain. These symptoms can significantly interfere with their ability to work.

Breast reduction (reduction mammaplasty) decreases the size of the breasts, so that they are more appropriately proportioned to the patient's body habitus. Attaining an aesthetically pleasing result is a high priority.

Classically, this procedure involves large incisions to remove excessive breast tissue and to reposition the nipple and areolar complex. These incisions result in long scars (around the areola, from the areola to the inframammary fold, and along the inframammary fold). These scars can be problematic as well as noticeable. Other complications of breast reduction include loss of nipple sensation, inability to breast feed, and loss of the nipple/areolar complex. Despite these risks, most women who undergo breast reduction are quite pleased with the results.

To obviate the need for such large incisions and to decrease the risks for other complications, liposuction is beginning to be included in the operative technique. Currently, plastic surgeons are developing other modifications to decrease the risks inherent in breast reduction.

Gynecomastia

Gynecomastia is the term for abnormal enlargement of the male breast. It is commonly encountered in pubescent males or older men because of hormonal considerations. Gynecomastia associated with puberty usually resolves within a few years; no surgery should be considered until the patient is at least 19 or 20 years of age.

When evaluating a patient with gynecomastia, be sure to get a thorough medical history. Medications associated with gynecomastia include cimetidine, spironolactone, digitalis, and reserpine. Be sure to inquire about recreational drug use because marijuana also has been implicated.

You must examine the patient's testicles to rule out the presence of a testicular tumor, which may produce hormones responsible for breast enlargement. Especially with unilateral enlargement or when a a discrete breast mass is palpable, you must rule out the possibility of an underlying breast cancer. (Yes, men can get breast cancer). Blood tests to evaluate the levels of various hormones also should be done.

Gynecomastia is quite challenging to treat. Simple mastectomy used to be the treatment of choice, but esthetic considerations make it a poor option. Currently, liposuction with or without additional formal excision of breast tissue (using a small incision along the areola) is the treatment of choice and has resulted in a markedly improved esthetic outcome.

Bibliography

Breast reconstruction
1. Hartrampf CR, Scheflan M, Black PW: Breast reconstruction with a transverse abdominal island flap. Plast Reconstr Surg 69:216–225, 1982.
2. Maxwell GP: Latissimus dorsi breast reconstruction: An aesthetic assessment. Clin Plast Surg 8:373–387, 1981.
3. Schusterman MA: The free TRAM flap. Clin Plast Surg 25:191–195, 1998.
4. Slavin SA, Schnitt SJ, Duda RB, et al: Skin-sparing mastectomy and immediate reconstruction: Oncologic risks and aesthetic results in patients with early-stage breast cancer. Plast Reconstr Surg 102:49–62, 1998.
5. Snyderman RK Guthrie RH: Reconstruction of the female breast following radical mastectomy. Plast Reconstr Surg 47:565, 1971.
6. Spear SL, Majidian A: Immediate breast reconstruction in two stages using textured, integrated valve tissue expanders and breast implants: A retrospective review of 171 consecutive breast reconstructions from 1989–1996. Plast Reconstr Surg 101: 53–63, 1998.

Breast reduction/Gynecomastia
7. Hammond DC: Short scar periareolar inferior pedicle reduction (SPAIR) mammaplasty. Plast Reconstr Surg 103:890–901, 1999.
8. Hidalgo DA: Improving safety and aesthetic results in inverted T scar breast reduction. Plast Reconstr Surg 103:874–886, 1999.
9. Lejour M: Vertical mammaplasty: Update and appraisal of late results. Plast Reconstr Surg 104:771–781, 1999.
10. Rosenberg GJ: Gynecomastia. In Spear SL (ed): Surgery of the Breast: Principles and Art. Philadelphia, Lippincott Williams and Wilkins, 1998, pp 831–841.

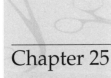

Chapter 25

FACIAL FRACTURES

KEY FIGURE:
Ivy loops

Definitive treatment for most facial fractures requires advanced surgical skills and special equipment. However, certain interventions that may improve patient outcome do not require special skills. This chapter provides basic information about the initial evaluation and treatment of patients with a facial fracture. In addition, an easy-to-perform procedure specifically for the treatment of a mandible (lower jaw) fracture is described to assist the provider with no access to specialty care.

Initial Patient Evaluation

The type of injury that results in a facial fracture can cause other significant injuries. When examining a patient with a possible facial fracture, you must be vigilant not to overlook a potentially life-threatening injury.

If the patient was reported to have lost consciousness or if the patient has any signs of altered level of consciousness, you must rule-out a **cerebral injury**.

Patients with a facial fracture also may have a **cervical spine injury**. Be careful with positioning of the patient's head and neck until you are sure that the cervical spine is not injured.

Be sure the patient is breathing easily and has a **stable airway**. Patients with a fractured lower jaw or severe fracture of the midface (cheekbones, nose, and/or upper jaw) may have difficulty with breathing. Difficulty with breathing can result from blockage of the airway by bleeding from the fracture site or by displaced bones.

Patients with **injury around the eye**, should have a thorough eye exam.

See chapter 5, "Evaluation of the Acutely Injured Patient," for more specific information.

Diagnosis

Physical Exam

Most patients who sustain any type of facial trauma have significant soft tissue swelling. However, swelling alone does not signify a fracture. Feel along the jaws, cheeks, orbital rim, and base of the nose. You are looking for bony instability or a "step-off" irregularity of the bones, which indicates a fracture.

If the fracture involves **tooth-bearing bone**, patients often report that their teeth do not seem to meet correctly or that the teeth do not feel "right" during biting down. Check to see whether the patient can adequately open and close his or her mouth.

Examining the Patient's Bite

- Use a tongue depressor to pull each cheek away from the teeth.
- Have the patient gently close the mouth and bring the teeth together.
- Examine the vertical midline between the upper and lower central incisors. Does it line up?
- Look along the lateral side of the molars. Are the molars lined up equally, or do you see space between the upper and lower teeth on one side but not the other?
- Ask the patient whether any findings you note are new or old. New changes probably represent the result of a fracture involving tooth-bearing bone.
- If the jaw is fractured, look inside the mouth for a laceration of the gum overlying the fracture. If the gum is torn, the fracture is an open fracture that requires treatment with antibiotics.

Patients with a **fracture of the cheek bone or orbit** often report numbness of the inner cheek and upper lip on the side of the fracture. The numbness is due to injury of the infraorbital nerve (V_2) as it emerges from the bone under the inferior orbital rim. Normal sensation often returns within 1–2 months of injury. The eyelids on the side of the injury show significant swelling, and the conjunctiva may be blood-stained.

Radiologic Studies

The best way to evaluate the mandible is with a **Panorex radiograph** that shows the entire upper and lower jaws.

If you have access to a **computed tomography (CT) scanner**, order a face scan with axial and coronal views. CT is the best way to diagnose a fracture of the other facial bones. **Note:** To allow coronal views, the patient must hyperextend at the neck or lie prone with the neck bent. The cervical spine must be cleared of injury before obtaining coronal views on a CT scan of the face.

Plain radiographs of the face should be obtained if you cannot get a CT scan. When interpreting the radiographs, begin by looking at the maxillary sinuses (the large paired sinuses on either side of the nose). Usually, the sinuses are areas of black (air), surrounded by white bone and located on either side of the nose. If fluid is present in the sinus, it looks white instead of black. The presence of fluid may be due to a fracture and should alert you to check the radiographs carefully for a fracture on the same side of the face.

Basic Initial Treatment

If the patient has a **fracture of the jaw with laceration of the overlying mucosa**, start antibiotics—usually penicillin. The patient also should rinse the mouth with salt water several times each day to decrease bacterial content. These interventions are necessary to decrease the chance for infection of the bone.

To decrease swelling: When the patient is lying in bed, the head should be elevated with pillows or by raising the head of the bed. The patient should avoid bending and heavy lifting, which can worsen facial swelling. The application of cool compresses to the face also helps to decrease swelling.

If the patient has a **significant facial fracture**, especially with involvement of tooth-bearing bone, it is best to transfer the patient to a facility where specialty help is available. If transfer is impossible, most midface fractures will heal, although the patient's appearance may be altered significantly.

Patients with a **mandibular fracture and reasonably aligned teeth** who can open and close the mouth easily can be treated with a soft diet for 4–6 weeks.

In contrast, patients with an **unstable mandibular fracture** (i.e., with mobile bone segments or inablity to open and close the mouth effectively) have a significant amount of pain and are unable to eat. This type of injury heals poorly without reduction of the fracture and immobilization of the jaws. Without proper treatment, the patient may be left with permanent pain and difficulty in eating.

Specific Treatment for Mandibular Fracture When No Specialty Care Is Available

If there is a dead or decayed tooth at the fracture site, remove it.

To decrease pain and infection risk and to improve the chance for bone healing, the jaws should be wired together. Intermaxillary fixation stabilizes the fracture(s), brings the bones into proper alignment, and promotes healing.

Placement of Ivy loops is a relatively easy way to achieve intermaxillary fixation and requires little special equipment.

Ivy Loops Procedure

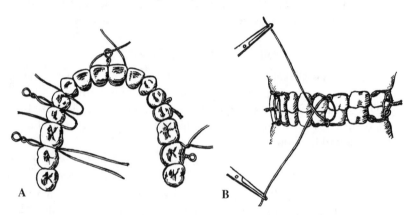

A   B

Placement of Ivy loops for intermaxillary fixation. (From McCarthy JG (ed): Plastic Surgery. Philadelphia, W.B. Saunders, 1990, with permission.)

1. General anesthesia with nasal intubation is the best choice.

2. Cut a 24-gauge wire (or whatever you have) into at least 6 pieces, each 6 inches (15 cm) in length. Be careful, because the ends of the wire can easily pierce through the glove into your finger.

3. Bend the piece of wire in half. Grasp the midsection of the wire with a needle holder, and twist the wire 2–3 times, making a small loop at the bend in the wire.

4. Pass both ends of the wire between two teeth that seem to be stable and are located distal to the fracture. Be sure that matching stable teeth are available on the opposite upper or lower jaw. The wire goes through the gum from outside (the side nearest the cheek) to inside (the side nearest the tongue). The loop should be along the outer surface of the teeth.

5. Take one end of the wire and wrap it around the tooth in front by passing it through the gum, going from inside to outside.

6. Wrap the other end of the wire around the tooth behind in the same manner. Both wire ends should be on the outside of the teeth.

7. Pull on the ends to keep the wire snug along the teeth.

8. Pass one wire end through the loop.

9. Bring the wire ends together, and manually twist them in clockwise direction once or twice.

10. Use a needle holder to grasp the twisted wire a few centimeters away from the gum. Pull up on the needle holder, and twist the wire in a clockwise fashion until the wire seems snug. Look closely at the wire while doing so. If the appearance of the wire changes from shiny to dull, stop—or you will break the wire and have to start again.

11. Repeat this process on the corresponding teeth on the opposite jaw and on teeth on the other side of the fracture. You will need to place the wires around at least 4 pairs of teeth.

12. Use a wire cutter to shorten the twisted wire ends to a length of 1 cm. Bend the wire into the surface of the gum so that the wire ends do not cut into the cheek mucosa.

13. When all of the wires have been placed, bring the patient's jaws together and try to line up the teeth. Be sure that the tongue is not caught between the teeth.

14. Use additional wire to connect each pair of loops and thereby bring the top and bottom jaws together. This technique immobilizes the jaws and fracture sites. Twist the wire (as previously described) in place.

15. The jaws should stay wired together for approximately 6 weeks. To ensure adequate nutrition, the patient should eat pureed foods and drink lots of liquids. Most patients lose weight. Encourage patients to ingest sufficient calories. Be sure to discourage smoking. Poor nutrition and tobacco use impair fracture healing.

16. The teeth should be carefully brushed at least 1–2 times each day, and the mouth should be rinsed with salt water after meals and before going to bed.

17. When pain is no longer present at the fracture site (usually after 4–6 weeks), remove the connecting wires and allow the patient to eat nothing harder than soft foods for an additional 2–3 weeks.

18. If the patient develops pain at the fracture site, reconnect the jaws for another 2–3 weeks.

19. If, after removing the connecting wires, the patient can eat and the fracture site remains pain-free, remove the wires from the teeth.

Note: When the connecting wires are first removed, the patient's ability to open the mouth will be limited. This problem will improve over the subsequent days and weeks.

Bibliography

1. Manson PN: Facial Injuries. In McCarthy JG (ed): Plastic Surgery. Philadelphia, W.B. Saunders, 1990, pp 867–1141.
2. Markowitz BL, Sinow JD, Kawamoto HK Jr, et al: Prospective comparison of axial computed tomography and standard and panoramic radiographs in the diagnosis of mandibular fractures. Ann Plast Surg 42:163–169, 1999.
3. Plaiser BR, Punjabi AP, Super DM, Haug RH: The relationship between facial fractures and death from neurologic injury. J Oral Maxillofac Surg 58:708–712, 2000.
4. Sinclair D, Schwartz M, Gruss J, McLellan B: A retrospective review of the relationship between facial fractures, head injuries, and cervical spine injuries. J Emerg Med 6:109–112, 1988.

Chapter 26

THE NORMAL HAND EXAM

KEY FIGURES:

Volar landmarks	Intrinsic muscles
Sensory innervation	Vascular supply
FDS motor function	Finger rotational
FDP tendon function	deformity
Thumb opposition	

For most people, good hand function is essential for day-to-day living, as well as the ability to support a family. Especially in areas that have a weak economic safety net, even minor hand injuries can have a disproportionately devastating effect on individual well-being.

Effective, early treatment of hand injuries can produce dramatic benefits in the final outcome of hand function. Conversely, lack of proper early treatment may cause a seemingly trivial injury to result in severe limitation of hand function and permanent disability.

The first step in providing optimal care of a hand injury is to know the basic principles of normal hand function, which are described in this chapter. The following chapters explain how to evaluate an injured hand and detail the treatment of specific hand injuries.

Anatomic Definitions

It is important to describe the hand in anatomic position: the arms are at the patient's sides with the palms facing forward so that the little finger is **medial** (also described as **ulnar**), next to the body, and the thumb is **lateral** (also described as **radial**), away from the body. The **dorsal** surface is the back of the hand, where the extensor tendons are located, and the **volar** surface is the palmar/front surface of the hand, where the flexor tendons are located.

Proximal means closer to the heart, and **distal** means farther away.

The **thenar eminence** represents the soft tissue bulk on the volar surface of the hand just proximal to the thumb; it includes the intrinsic muscles to the thumb.

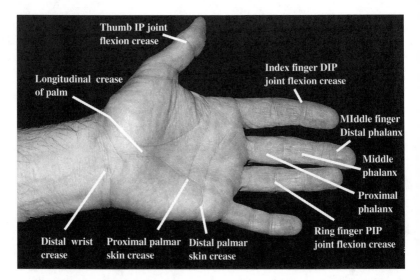

The volar (palmar) surface of the hand. IP = interphalangeal, DIP = distal interphalangeal, PIP = proximal interphalangeal.

The **hypothenar eminence** represents the soft tissue bulk on the volar surface of the hand just proximal to the little finger.

The **phalanges** are the bones of the fingers.

The **metacarpophalangeal (MCP) joint** is the joint where the fingers and thumb join the hand (essentially, the knuckles).

The **proximal interphalangeal (PIP) joint** is the finger joint closest to the MCP joint.

The **distal interphalangeal (DIP) joint** is the finger joint farthest from the MCP joint.

The thumb has only the **interphalangeal (IP) joint**.

The **carpal tunnel** is the space in the center of the proximal palm between the thenar eminence and hypothenar eminence. The nine flexor tendons to the fingers and thumb and the median nerve traverse this tunnel into the hand. The boundaries of the carpal tunnel are bone on the deep, medial, and lateral sides; the roof is the strong transverse carpal ligament (a fascial layer of the hand).

Skin creases are landmarks that help to describe where to place an incision or where a lesion on the volar surface of the hand is located. Location often is described in relation to the various skin creases on the volar surface of the hand.

The Normal Hand

A good understanding of the normally functioning hand is necessary for adequate evaluation of a hand injury. Seemingly insignificant injuries, such as a simple laceration, may involve damage to more tissue than just the skin. If this additional tissue damage is missed, significant morbidity can result, with a devastating effect on the patient.

If you identify an abnormality that may not make sense in light of the injury, there may be another explanation besides trauma. An abnormality may be a normal variant. For example, a patient without a palpable radial pulse may have congenital absence of the radial artery rather than an arterial injury. When these variants occur, they often involve the other hand as well. It is always a good idea to check the other hand for comparison.

Sensory Exam

Three major nerves are responsible for sensation to the hand: the radial, ulnar, and median nerves.

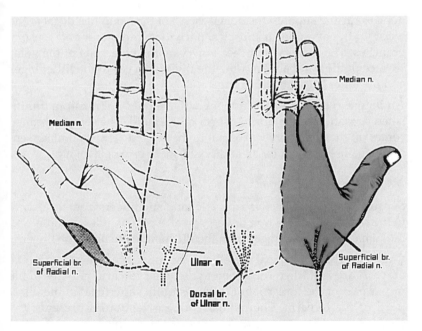

Sensory innervation of the hand. (From Jurkiewicz MJ, et al (eds): Plastic Surgery: Principles and Practice. St. Louis, Mosby, 1990, with permission.)

Radial Nerve

Sensory distribution: dorsal aspect of the radial two-thirds of the hand and thumb; dorsal aspect of the thumb, index, middle, and radial half of the ring finger to the PIP joint.

Course in the forearm: the radial nerve runs in the muscles of the dorsal aspect of the forearm and becomes superficial (near the skin) approximately 4–5 cm proximal to the wrist on the lateral border of the forearm. At this site the nerve is especially prone to injury.

Ulnar Nerve

Sensory distribution: dorsal and volar aspects of the ulnar side of the hand; dorsal and volar sides of the medial half of the ring finger and the entire little finger.

Course in the forearm: the ulnar nerve runs deep to the muscles on the medial side of the forearm, adjacent to the ulnar artery in the distal half of the forearm. An injury to the ulnar artery should alert you to test specifically for an ulnar nerve injury. Approximately 8 cm proximal to the wrist, the nerve sends off a sensory branch that travels under the dorsal skin and supplies the dorsal aspect of the hand. Just distal to the wrist, in the hypothenar muscles, it divides into motor and sensory branches. The sensory branches innervate the ulnar side of the volar surface of the hand and become the digital nerves to the little finger and the ulnar half of the ring finger.

An injury to the ulnar nerve at the wrist should not result in diminished sensation to the dorsal aspect of the hand. The sensory branch comes off the main nerve proximal to the injured area. If all ulnar sensation is missing, look for an additional, more proximal injury.

Median Nerve

Sensory distribution: volar aspect of hand and fingers from the thumb to the radial half of the ring finger; dorsal aspect of index, middle, and radial half of the ring finger from the PIP joint to the tip of the finger.

Course in the forearm: at the elbow, the median nerve is next to the brachial artery. It then runs deep to the volar forearm muscles in the upper part of the forearm but becomes quite superficial in the distal third of the forearm. The palmaris longus tendon, if present (it is absent in 10–15% of people), is just overtop of the nerve and offers some protection near the wrist. The nerve then goes through the carpal tunnel to give off its sensory and motor branches in the hand. The sensory branches become the digital nerves to the thumb, index finger, long finger, and radial half of the ring finger.

Motor Exam

Many people do not realize that a large part of hand and finger movement is governed by muscles and tendons originating in the forearm. To move the hand and fingers requires proper functioning of both muscles originating in the forearm (**extrinsic muscles**) and muscles originating in the hand itself (**intrinsic muscles**).

If limitation in movement is due to dysfunction of an extrinsic muscle, you must determine whether the injury involves the distal tendon or the nerve supply. Dysfunction of the intrinsic muscles usually is due to an injury to the nerve supply.

If the hand or fingers do not flex (bend) or extend (straighten) appropriately and with adequate strength compared with the noninjured hand or fingers, you must determine the precise cause so that appropriate treatment can be given. This process is detailed and methodical. However, with practice and an understanding of what you are testing, the motor exam takes only a few minutes to complete.

Extrinsic Muscle/Tendon Evaluation

The **flexor digitorum superficialis (FDS)** inserts into the middle phalanx of each finger. It is tested by blocking the finger MCP joint and asking the patient to flex the PIP joint. To block the MCP joint, hold the proximal phalanx in extension just distal to the MCP joint, so that the MCP joint is unable to bend when the patient tries to flex the finger.

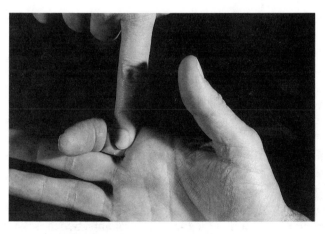

Testing flexor digitorum superficialis function.

The **flexor digitorum profundus (FDP)** inserts into the distal phalanx of each finger. It is tested by blocking the finger PIP joint and asking the patient to flex the DIP joint. To block the PIP joint, hold the middle phalanx in extension just distal to the PIP joint, so that the PIP joint is unable to bend when the patient tries to flex the finger.

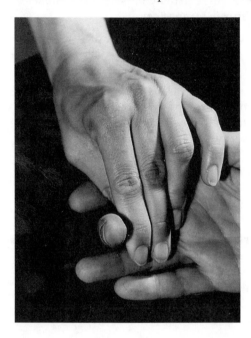

Testing flexor digitorum profundus function.

The **flexor pollicis longus (FPL)** is the primary flexor of the thumb interphalangeal (IP) joint. It is tested by holding the thumb MCP joint in extension and asking the patient to flex the thumb IP joint.

The **wrist flexors** include the flexor carpi radialis, flexor carpi ulnaris, and palmaris longus (PL; weak effect). When the patient flexes the wrist, you should be able to feel these tendons under the skin. In a small percentage of the population, the PL is absent. Compare with the uninjured hand.

The **extensor pollicis longus (EPL)** is the primary extensor of the thumb IP joint. Test the patient's ability to extend the thumb IP joint.

The **finger extensors** are responsible for extension of the MCP joints of the fingers (not thumb). Please note: the finger extensors are not responsible for extension of the the finger IP joints, which is the function of the intrinsic muscles (see ulnar nerve below).

The **wrist extensors** are the extensor carpi radialis and extensor carpi ulnaris. Check function by testing for wrist extension.

Evaluation of Extrinsic Muscle/Intrinsic Muscle Nerve Supply

Radial Nerve

Hand: no motor innervation to the intrinsic muscles.

Forearm: innervates the forearm muscles that provide extension of the wrist, thumb, and all finger MCP joints.

Median Nerve

Hand: primarily thumb opposition (bringing the thumb tip to meet the tip of each finger).

Forearm: innervates the muscles that flex the thumb, wrist (FCR), all PIP joints, and DIP joints of the index and middle fingers.

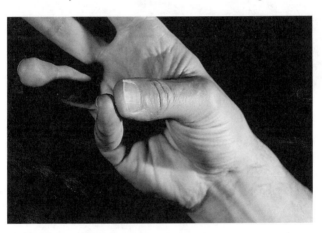

To test function of the motor branch of the median nerve, bring the thumb and little finger together in opposition. Keep the thumb IP joint at 0° so that you do not confuse action of the flexor pollicis longus with action of the thenar muscles.

Ulnar Nerve

Hand: the ulnar nerve provides the dominant innervation to the intrinsic muscles of the hand: flexion of the MCP joints and extension of the IP joints of the fingers and adduction of the thumb. It is best to check the first dorsal interossei (the muscle along the index metacarpal bone in the thumb web). Ask the patient to abduct the index finger against resistance. Alternatively, you may ask the patient to hold a piece of paper between adjacent fingers that are fully extended.

Forearm: innervates the muscles that flex the wrist (flexor carpi ulnaris) and DIP joints of the ring and little fingers.

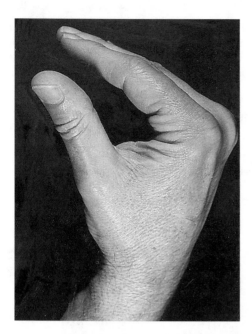

Metacarpophalangeal joint flexion and interphalangeal joint extension. The intrinsic muscles are innervated primarily by the ulnar nerve.

Vascular Evaluation

Two main arteries supply the hand: the radial artery and the ulnar artery. Both are branches of the brachial artery. In the hand the radial artery and ulnar artery come together and meet, forming the palmar arch. The digital arteries come off the palmar arch to supply circulation to the fingers.

Radial Artery

Most people are familiar with the radial artery, which health care providers palpate to check heart rate. The radial artery usually can be felt on the lateral aspect of the volar surface of the wrist, just below the thenar eminence. Check for presence of a pulse, and compare with the other side. In some patients anatomy varies from the norm, and this variance is often symmetrical. Always check the opposite hand.

Ulnar Artery

The ulnar artery is actually the more important of the two arteries supplying circulation to the hand. It usually supplies most of the blood to the hand. The ulnar artery can be felt on the medial aspect of the volar surface of the wrist, just below the hypothenar eminence. It is often more difficult to feel than the radial artery pulse. Check for presence of a pulse, and compare with the other hand.

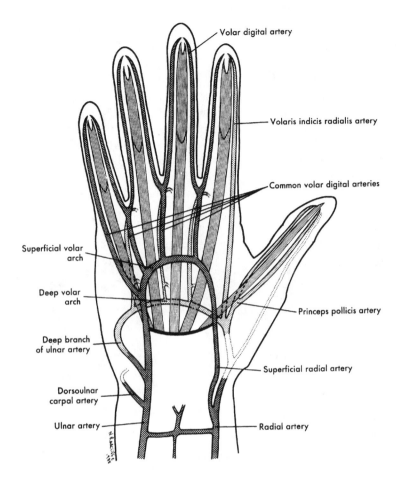

Blood supply to the hand. The superficial arch and the deep arch are separated by tendinous structures. The superficial arch is formed primarily by the ulnar artery, the deep arch by the radial artery. This arrangement is seen in most, but not all dissections. (From Jurkiewicz MJ, et al (eds): Plastic Surgery: Principles and Practice. St. Louis, Mosby, 1990, with permission.)

Capillary Refill

A well-vascularized finger generally has a pink hue under the nail. If the area under the nail is blue or very pale, circulation may be impaired. These findings also may be a sign that the patient is very cold or hypovolemic; be sure to compare with the uninjured hand. To test capillary refill, pinch the fingertip, which should blanch (i.e., turn pale). Then release the pressure. The color should return to normal within 2–3 seconds. A period longer than 2–3 seconds may imply an arterial injury (i.e., difficulty with getting blood to the finger). A period shorter than 2–3 seconds may imply a problem with the venous circulation (i.e., difficulty with draining blood from the finger).

Alignment of the Fingers with Movement

You should evaluate the patient for a rotational deformity of the finger, which indicates significant bone or joint injury. When the patient actively flexes the finger IP joints in tandem, the nails and fingertips should be well aligned. When MCP flexion is added, the fingers should not criss-cross; they should point gently toward the thenar eminence. As always, compare with the other hand because some people may have mild rotational deformities in the uninjured state.

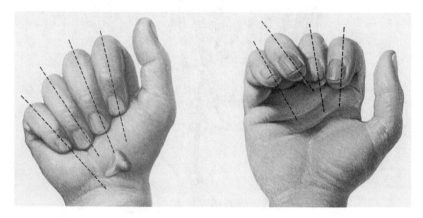

Left, Normally all fingers point toward the region of the scaphoid when a fist is made. *Right,* Malrotation at fracture site causes the affected finger to deviate. (From Crenshaw AH (ed): Campbell's Operative Orthopedics, 7th ed. St. Louis, Mosby, 1994, with permission.)

This evaluation is important in examining a patient with a phalangeal or metacarpal fracture. At rest, with the fingers straight, the fingers may look well positioned. However, when their alignment is checked with motion, the fingers may criss-cross, which suggests that the fracture requires greater reduction. If the fracture is not reduced properly and the rotational deformity becomes permanent, hand function may be limited.

Bibliography

1. Ariyan S: The Hand Book. New York, McGraw-Hill, 1989.
2. Lampe EW: Clinical Symposia: Surgical Anatomy of the Hand. 40th anniversary issue 40(3), 1988.

EVALUATING THE INJURED HAND

Patients with hand injuries have many different presentations, ranging from a swollen, tender finger or a small laceration on the palm of the hand to a severely mangled hand. This chapter explains how to evaluate patients with a hand injury. It is important to do a complete exam of every injured hand so that no important injuries are missed.

As usual, **the first priority is to control life-threatening hemorrhage**. Apply point pressure over the wound. This does not mean to place gauze in the wound and wrap the area with an Ace bandage. It means to place a wad of gauze over the injured area and to apply firm point pressure to the injured site with two fingers. The pressure may need to be maintained for several minutes before the bleeding stops. In patients with arterial bleeding, exploration is required.

If the patient has a **rapid, exsanguinating hemorrhage** that cannot be controlled with point pressure, place a tourniquet or blood pressure cuff proximal (closer to the heart) to the injury. If a blood pressure cuff is used, it must be inflated to at least 50 mmHg above the patient's systolic pressure.

Caution: Tourniquets hurt and place the tissues at risk for ischemic injury. Optimally, the tourniquet should not be left in place for more than 15–20 minutes. If a tourniquet is needed, so is urgent operative exploration.

For **patients with a non–life-threatening injury**, the following elements are crucial to the evaluation of an injured hand.

Important Elements of the History

As discussed more thoroughly in chapter 6, "Evaluation of an Acute Wound," it is important to obtain a good history from the patient.

Information about what caused the injury may have important implications for treatment.

Nature of Injury

Human bites are very dirty wounds. Never close a human bite to the hand. Such injuries require specific antibiotics, and surgical exploration and wash-out in the operating room may be necessary.

Animal bites. About 80% of cat bites become infected compared with 5% of dog bite wounds. Remember to ask about the animal's rabies vaccination status.

Glass wound. Did the glass shatter? Are foreign bodies retained in the wound?

Knife/sharp object wound. The object may have penetrated more deeply than you think.

Dirty wound. Worry about particulate matter in the wound, and check tetanus immunization status.

Burn. Is injury due to thermal, chemical, or electrical burn? Each has different implications. See chapters 20, "Burns," and 34, "Hand Burns."

Component of a crush injury. Crush mechanisms involve a more extensive injury than you may initially expect. See chapter 35, "Hand Crush Injury and Compartment Syndrome."

Other Important Questions

1. Is the injured hand the **dominant hand**? If the injury involves the dominant hand, treatment outcome is especially important. This consideration may affect which treatment modalities you select.

2. What is the patient's **tetanus immunization status**? Update as needed. See chapter 6, "Evaluation of an Acute Wound," for tetanus booster recommendations.

3. Did **pulsatile bleeding** occur at the time of injury? Pulsatile bleeding (blood squirting out with some force as opposed to a continuous ooze) implies an arterial injury and usually mandates surgical exploration.

4. Was any **deformity** noted immediately after injury? Ask about an immediate deformity that has since disappeared. Many patients are able to reduce (realign) a dislocated joint right after the injury so that it appears normal at the time of exam. However, the injured finger may still require protective splinting even if it appears to be in its normal position.

5. Does the patient have a history of **previous trauma** to the hand? A previous injury may be the cause of an abnormal exam instead of the acute injury. Be sure to ask whether the functional deficit or contour abnormality identified on the exam was present before the current trauma.

Physical Examination of the Injured Hand

Remove immediately all rings that the patient is wearing. Injury to a hand often leads to significant swelling. The rings may become quite tight, possibly to the point that they cut off circulation to the finger. If the ring is tight, lubricating jelly or antibiotic ointment is often useful. If this strategy is unsuccessful, the ring may need to be cut off with a ring cutter or strong wire cutter.

Full evaluation of the injured hand may necessitate **anesthesia** to control the pain so that the patient can cooperate with the exam. See chapter 3, "Local Anesthesia," for specific information. *Be sure to test sensation distal to the injury before administering local anesthetic.* Once you have given the anesthetic, it is too late to test for sensory function.

Vascular Exam

Active Bleeding

Is the wound actively bleeding during the exam? If so, is the bleeding pulsatile, with bright red blood (probable arterial injury), or continuous, with darker blood (probable venous injury)?

Capillary Refill

Check for capillary refill of the digits distal to the injury. Is the tissue pink, indicating sufficient circulation, or is it bluish or pale, indicating inadequate circulation to the distal tissue?

Radial and Ulnar Pulses

Make sure that the radial and ulnar pulses are intact, even if capillary refill of the hand seems normal. Missing an arterial injury can have serious consequences (see chapter 33, "Nerve and Vascular Injuries of the Hand").

Note what happens when you press on either the radial or ulnar artery. Does the pulse of the other artery disappear? In patients with an injury to the radial artery in the mid-forearm, for example, you may still feel a pulse in the radial artery at the wrist. In most people the radial and ulnar arteries come together in the hand to form the palmar arch. Because of this anatomic arrangement, blood from the ulnar artery flows through the palmar arch. From the palmar arch blood travels into the digital vessels and into the distal radial artery. Thus patients with injury to the proximal radial artery may still have a palpable radial pulse at the wrist. If you press on the ulnar artery to occlude its flow and the radial pulse also disappears, injury to the radial artery is indicated.

Sensory Exam

Test sensation distal to the injury. It is best to determine whether the patient can differentiate between a sharp stimulus (pinprick) and a dull stimulus (light touch of a dry cotton swab). Patients who cannot feel the sharp stimulus probably have a nerve injury.

Motor Exam

Unless you see an obvious muscle injury, the purpose of testing the function of a specific muscle group is to evaluate for a specific underlying nerve injury or tendon injury (see below).

Table 1. Muscle Functions and Associated Nerves

Muscle Function	Associated Nerve
Extension of finger IP joints, finger adduction/ abduction, or abduction of the first dorsal interosseous muscle	Ulnar nerve
Thumb opposition	Median nerve
Wrist flexion	Median nerve primarily; some contribution from ulnar nerve
Wrist extension	Radial nerve

IP = interphalangeal.

Tendon Exam

1. Depending on the site of injury, make sure that nearby flexor and extensor tendons are intact. Remember that there are two flexor tendons to the fingers.
2. Flexion of the metacarpophalangeal (MCP) joints and extension of the interphalangeal (IP) joints are under intrinsic muscle control; they are *not* controlled by flexor or extensor tendons.
3. Note whether you can see cut tendon ends in the wound.

Exam for Fracture or Dislocation

Obvious Deformity

Most finger dislocations and fractures are quite obvious, but this is not always the case. Sometimes the finger is just slightly swollen. The patient may report that right after the injury the finger looked "funny," but the patient was able to "pop it back" into position.

Rotational deformity when the patient flexes the fingers strongly implies a fracture or dislocation in need of reduction.

Open Wound

Is the joint visible in the wound? Is the capsule intact? Is a fracture visible? An open fracture (fracture associated with skin laceration) has a higher rate of infection and improper healing than a closed fracture.

Whenever you have any doubt about the possibility of a fracture or dislocation, order a radiograph.

Soft Tissue Coverage

Is there enough healthy tissue to allow wound closure or at least to cover exposed tendons, bones, nerves, or blood vessels?

Foreign Bodies

Check to be sure that no pieces of foreign material are present in the wound (e.g., grass, glass, metal, dirt). Some foreign materials can be seen on a radiograph. Foreign debris should be removed before the wound is closed to prevent infection.

Physical Exam of an Unconscious Patient

Although it is impossible to do a complete hand exam on an unconscious patient, certain parts of the exam can be performed:

1. Examine the wound, and evaluate the hand's vascular status, as described above.

2. For a gross estimate of the status of the flexor tendons, grab the patient's forearm and shake the hand gently. Then allow the hand to fall backward so that the palm faces up. The fingers should assume a gently flexed posture, with the little finger slightly more flexed than the ring finger, the ring finger more flexed than the middle finger, and the middle finger more flexed than the index finger. The thumb also should assume a slightly flexed position. If any finger assumes a more extended posture than expected, flexor tendon injury is indicated.

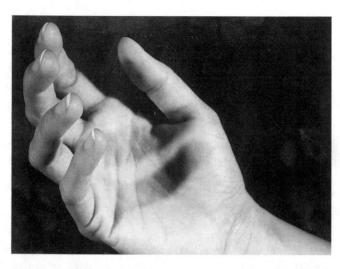

The resting posture of an uninjured hand in an unconscious patient. Note that all of the fingers are in a slightly flexed position.

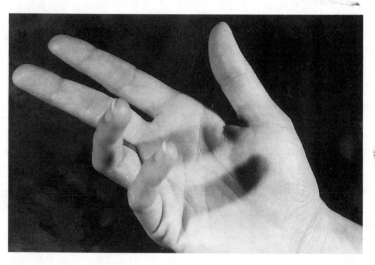

An unconscious patient with a forearm injury involving the flexor tendons to the index and middle fingers. Note the difference in hand posture compared with the uninjured hand (above). The affected middle and index fingers are in an extended position.

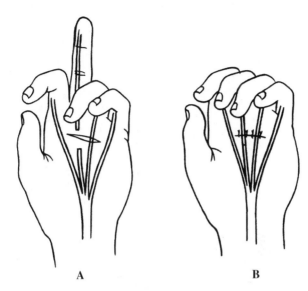

A   B

Same process as in the two previous photographs, but the tendon injury is located in the hand. (From Crenshaw AH (ed): Campbell's Operative Orthopaedics, 7th ed. St. Louis, Mosby, 1994, with permission.)

Bibliography

1. Ariyan S: The Hand Book. New York, McGraw-Hill, 1989, pp 91–172.
2. Walton RL, Chick LR, Petry J, Borah G: Hand injuries: General principles. In Jurkiewicz MJ, Krizek TJ, Mathes SJ, Ariyan S (eds): Plastic Surgery: Principles and Practice. St. Louis, Mosby, 1990, pp 605–643.

Chapter 28

HAND SPLINTING AND GENERAL AFTERCARE

KEY FIGURES:

Neutral position for basic splinting
Neutral position splint
Splint for flexor tendon injury
Splint for extensor tendon injury

Thumb spica splint
Ulnar gutter splint
Finger immobilization
Proper elevation of injured hand

Splinting

The hand and fingers often need a period of immobilization after injury to allow the tissues to heal properly. For most hand injuries, a splint rather than a cast is the method of choice.

Splint vs. Cast

A cast immobilizes the injured hand by completely surrounding it with hard, inflexible materials (plaster or fiberglass). The inflexibility of a cast can cause serious problems if the injured tissues swell or if the cast is placed too tightly. Potential problems include skin loss due to pressure on the skin from the tight cast or possibly development of a compartment syndrome (see chapter 55, "Hand Crush Injury and Compartment Syndrome") if the tightness compromises blood circulation to the extremity.

A splint is essentially a half cast used for immobilization. The extremity is not completely bound by inflexible materials. Therefore, a splint is safer than a cast because it usually can accommodate tissue swelling without becoming too tight.

Materials

Place cotton gauze between each finger to absorb perspiration.

Rolls or sheets of plaster of Paris are used to make the splint. Fiberglass rolls also can be used but are much more expensive than plaster rolls. Fiberglass is used in the same way as plaster for creating a splint.

Padding is important. You need cotton padding to protect the hand and forearm from the heat of the plaster (splint materials become quite warm as they dry and can burn unprotected skin). The padding also prevents the splint from rubbing or putting too much pressure on the skin.

An Ace or other soft wrap is needed to hold the splint in place.

How to Make the Splint

1. Measure the required length of the splint. To immobilize the hand and fingers adequately, the splint should be long enough to cover from the mid-forearm to the fingertips.

2. Place four layers of cotton padding between the patient's skin and the plaster.

3. Cut another layer of cotton padding to place on the outer side of the plaster. This outer layer makes it easier to remove the splint to reexamine the hand and allows the splint to be reused.

4. Use approximately 12 layers of plaster of Paris of a width appropriate for the extremity. The splint should be a bit wider than the extremity; cut it if necessary.

5. Wet the plaster with lukewarm water, and squeeze out the excess water. The plaster should be damp, not soaking wet. Do *not* use hot water. Because the plaster heats as it dries, hot water increases the risk of burning the patient.

6. Place the four layers of cotton padding on the plaster, and place the splint on the patient's extremity. Be sure that the cotton padding is directly against the patient's skin. This rule sounds simple, but it is easy to make a mistake.

7. Place the single layer of cotton padding on the outside of the plaster.

8. Secure the splint in position with an Ace or other soft wrap. *Do not wrap tightly.* If the Ace wrap is tight, it will become inflexible, making the splint as potentially dangerous as a cast. Wrap the extremity lightly—just tight enough to secure the splint in position.

9. Hold the splint in the appropriate position (see below) until it dries. It will take a few minutes for the plaster to cool and dry.

Position and Contour of the Splint

The contour of the splint is determined by the hand injury.

Neutral Position

The neutral position is used for basic splinting of an injured or infected hand. The purpose of the splint is to allow the hand to rest in a safe position—that is, a position that will not lead to hand dysfunction if stiffness results. The wrist is placed in 20° of extension, the metacarpophalangeal (MCP) joints are positioned in 70° of flexion, and the interphalangeal (IP) joints should be straight. The splint usually is placed on the volar side of the hand. *Exception:* a burn on the volar surface of the hand may require a dorsal splint.

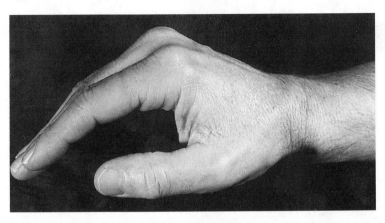

The neutral position is a safe position for immobilization of an injured hand. The IP joints are straight, the MCP joints are flexed, and the wrist is slightly extended.

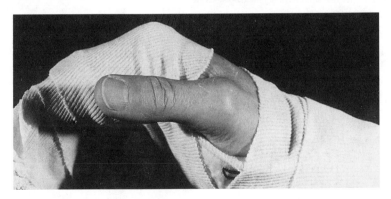

Splinting the hand in neutral position. The splint usually is placed on the palmar surface of the hand and forearm.

For a Flexor Tendon Injury

The splint should hold the hand in a position that prevents extension of the hand and finger. For this reason, the splint is placed on the dorsal side of the hand. The wrist is flexed 20–30°, the MCP joints are positioned in 70° of flexion, and the IP joints are flexed slightly at

10–20°. Do not put anything rigid (anything that prevents passive flexion of the fingers) on the volar side of the hand or fingers.

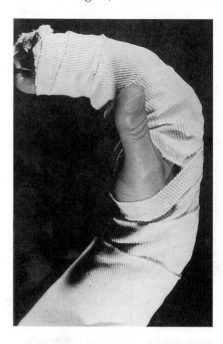

Splinting the hand with a flexor tendon injury. The splint is on the dorsal surface of the hand. The wrist and MCP joints are flexed.

For an Extensor Tendon Injury

The splint is used to prevent flexion of the hand and fingers. For this reason, the splint is placed on the volar side of the hand. The wrist should be placed in 20° of extension, the MCP joints are positioned in 10–15° of flexion (they should not be completely straight), and the IP joints should be straight. (See figure on following page.)

For an Injury to the Thumb

If the thumb is the only injured part of the hand, it is possible to immobilize the wrist and thumb with a thumb spica splint and leave the fingers free. The patient thus can use the hand for light activities. The splint is placed on the radial side of the forearm and brought over the thumb, all the way out to the tip. The thumb should be slightly abducted (positioned away from the rest of the hand). Mold the plaster so that it wraps half-way around the thumb to keep it immobilized. (See figure on following page.)

For a flexor tendon injury, the wrist should be slightly flexed; for an extensor tendon injury, the wrist should be slightly extended, as described above. The thumb IP joint should be held straight for either injury.

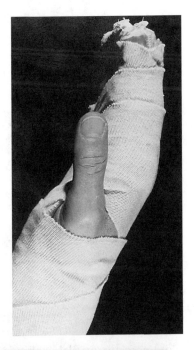

Splinting the hand with an extensor tendon injury. The splint is on the palmar surface of the hand. The wrist is extended, and the MCP joints are almost, but not quite, at 10–15° of flexion.

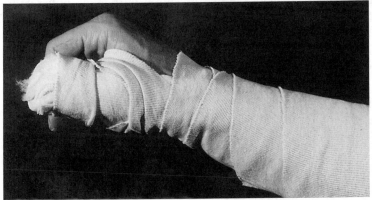

Thumb spica splint. The thumb and wrist are immobilized, but the rest of the fingers are free.

For an Injury to the Little Finger

If the little finger is the only involved finger, it is possible to immobilize the wrist and little finger with an ulnar gutter splint and leave the rest of the hand free. The patient thus has more use of the hand. The splint is placed on the ulnar side of the forearm and hand and then extended just beyond the little finger. Mold the plaster so that it partially wraps around the little and ring fingers. The ring finger is included to add extra protection to prevent accidental movement of the little finger. The wrist, MCP joints, and IP joints should be positioned as with flexor or extensor tendon injury, depending on the exact nature of the injury to the little finger.

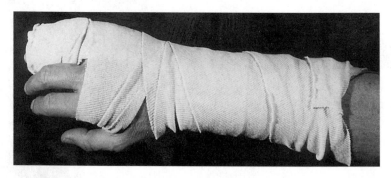

Ulnar gutter splint for the little finger. The little and ring fingers as well as the wrist are immobilized. The thumb and index and middle fingers are free.

For Injury to a Single Finger

Commercially available aluminum splints with foam rubber padding can be shaped to the proper position to immobilize a single digit. This type of splint is indicated for immobilization of a phalangeal fracture or dislocation. If such splints are not available, plaster with padding or a tongue depressor cut to the appropriate size also can be used.

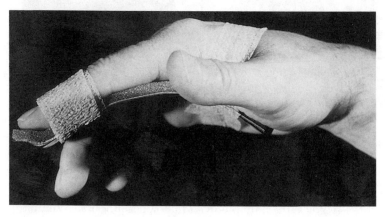

When only one finger needs to be immobilized, an aluminum splint is quite useful.

General Aftercare

Basic aftercare recommendations should be explained thoroughly to all patients, no matter what their injury. More specific instructions, tailored to each injury, are given in subsequent chapters.

Elevation of the Extremity

Elevation is the cornerstone of the treatment of hand injuries. Hand elevation decreases swelling and thus improves wound healing. Hand elevation also significantly decreases pain.

When the patient is resting or reclining, elevating the affected hand by placing it on a pillow is usually sufficient. Be sure that the hand is higher than the elbow.

When the patient is walking, the hand should be held up and not allowed to dangle by the side. I generally do not recommend arm slings, because patients tend to become too dependent on them and do not move their shoulder. This tendency can lead to shoulder stiffness, which may become problematic.

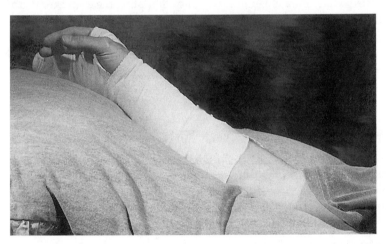

Proper elevation of the injured hand at rest. The hand should be higher than the elbow to promote drainage and decrease swelling.

Dressings

The specific type of dressing depends on the injury. (See chapter 9, "Wound Care," for specific details.)

Motion

It is your responsibility to tell the patient when it is permissible to start moving the hand and fingers. Specific information is given for different hand injuries in subsequent chapters. Once patients are allowed to start moving the injured hand and fingers they should be given instructions for various ways to exercise the hands.

Passive Range-of-motion Exercises

The patient (or another person) gently moves the finger joints passively (i.e., without use of the patient's own muscle contractions).

Active Range-of-motion Exercises

The patient should actively flex and extend the entire finger by using the muscles of the forearm and hand. To exercise the distal IP joint and prevent stiffness, the patient should hold the finger straight at the proximal IP joint and actively move the distal IP joint.

The above exercises can be easier to do if the patient places his or her hand in warm water for a few minutes before attempting the exercises. Warmth allows the fingers to move more easily by making the tissues more supple. The patient can even do the exercises while the hand is soaking.

Duration of Splinting

Unless you tell the patient to remove the splint to clean the hand or to do gentle range-of-motion exercises, the splint should be removed only under your supervision. However, be sure to show the patient how to wrap the splint in place so that it can be loosened if the patient feels that the splint is tight.

Specific information about how long to splint the hand after various hand injuries is discussed in subsequent chapters.

Smoking

Vigorously counsel the patient not to smoke during the healing process. Smoking considerably reduces blood circulation in the hand and thus may lead to unnecessary tissue loss, delayed bone and tendon healing, and poor functional outcome.

Bibliography

1. Coppard BM, Lohman H: Introduction to Splinting: A Critical-Thinking and Problem-Solving Approach. St. Louis, Mosby, 1996.
2. Falkenstein N, Weiss-Lessard S: Hand Rehabilitation: A Quick Reference Guide and Review. St. Louis, Mosby, 1999.

Chapter 29

FINGERTIP AND NAIL BED INJURIES

> **KEY FIGURES:**
> Digital tourniquet   Thenar flap
> Bone rongeur   Repair of nail bed
> Fingernail with hematoma

Hand injuries are commonly encountered by health care providers throughout the world. In the United States alone, the hand is involved in approximately 10% of all accident cases seen in the emergency department.

Hand injuries are particularly important to treat, because good hand function frequently is necessary to hold a job and support a family. Specific injuries and their basic evaluation and treatment are discussed in this and subsequent chapters.

Although specialists are required for optimal final treatment of some injuries, often the care given by the first-line provider has a dramatic effect on the ultimate outcome. Accurate evaluation and proper initial basic care can significantly improve outcome and decrease disability.

You should be aware of the basics of treatment in case you find yourself the only health care provider around.

Fingertip Injuries

Fingertip injuries are probably the most commonly encountered hand injury. The best treatment is usually the simplest. A fingertip injury can cause short-term disability but generally should not affect long-term hand function. Improper treatment, however, can result in a stiff finger and reduce long-term hand function.

Initial Care

It is often useful to start by giving a digital block with either lidocaine or bupivacaine (see chapter 3, "Local Anesthesia"). The block allows you to examine and evaluate the finger completely. Although the wounds may not be large, fingertip injuries are often quite painful. It may be necessary to place a digital tourniquet to control slow bleeding from the wound, which prevents a thorough examination.

Digital Tourniquet

A digital tourniquet is easy to create and makes exam and repair much simpler. Do not keep the tourniquet in place for more than 25–30 minutes. The tourniquet can be made from a surgical glove that is one size smaller than the patient's hand:

1. Cut off the ring or little finger from the glove; then cut off its tip.
2. Put the piece of glove on the injured finger.
3. Roll the cut end of the glove from distal to proximal to force the blood out of the finger and to control bleeding.

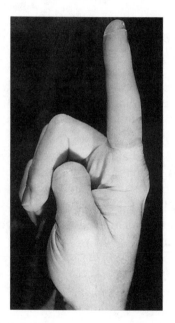 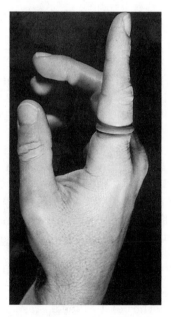

Digital tourniquet. *Left*, Cut off the finger from a glove and place it on the injured finger. *Right*, Roll the glove proximally to create the tourniquet.

Clean the wound with gentle soap and water, and irrigate it with saline.

Remove all foreign material and dead tissue. To remove grease, Bacitracin or another petrolatum-based antibiotic ointment is often useful.

Treatment

If the skin can be sutured together, use a few loose, simple sutures. A tight closure can lead to further tissue loss.

If no skin is available for closure and no bone or tendon is exposed, the wound can be left open and treated with dressings.

If only a few millimeters of bone are exposed, try to shorten the bone, using a bone rongeur (see figure below) or other instrument. Shorten the bone enough that it can be covered by soft tissue. Because the profundus flexor tendon inserts on the proximal half of the bone, do not be too aggressive.

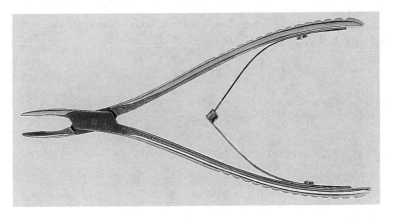

Bone rongeur. (Photo courtesy of Moore Medical Corporation.)

4. **If a segment of the fingertip has been amputated**, the skin can be defatted and used to cover the soft tissue as a full-thickness skin graft. To defat the skin, take a pair of scissors and cut away the fat on the undersurface of the skin. See chapter 12, "Skin Grafts," for a more detailed description of this technique. Although the graft may not survive, it will serve as a biologic dressing and may decrease pain and hasten healing.

5. **If more than a few millimeters of bone have been exposed**, see "Complicated Fingertip Injuries" later in this chapter.

General Aftercare

Apply antibiotic ointment and a simple dry dressing 1–2 times/day.

Clean with gentle soap and water with each dressing change.

If the wound was closed with sutures, after a few days the dressings can be stopped.

If the wound was left open, continue the dressing changes until the wound has healed. If the wound becomes covered with a grayish material, change to a wet-to-dry saline dressing for a few days, until wound appearance improves.

Encourage the patient to use the finger and hand to prevent joint stiffness. Active and passive range-of-motion exercises also should be encouraged.

Initially, acetaminophen alone may be insufficient to control pain. Fingertip injuries can be quite painful for the first several days.

Strongly encourage the patient not to smoke. The use of tobacco products significantly slows the healing process of fingertip wounds.

The patient should keep the affected hand elevated to decrease swelling and pain and to promote healing.

More Complicated Fingertip Injuries

Open Fracture of the Distal Phalanx

Open fractures involve a soft tissue wound around the fracture site. They are more serious than closed fractures because of the higher risk for infection.

When the fracture does not involve the distal interphalangeal (DIP) joint, it usually can be treated by manipulating the fracture into alignment and closing the soft tissues. Closing the soft tissues serves to splint the bone.

If the fracture involves the joint surface, full reduction (proper alignment of the pieces) is necessary to preserve joint motion. Full reduction requires special skills and equipment (often K-wires or screws) that belong to the realm of the hand surgeon. Without the intervention of a hand surgeon, the wound will heal, but the patient probably will be left with a very stiff joint and little normal motion.

The wound should be cleansed thoroughly, and the patient should be given oral antibiotics for several days. The antibiotics prevent bone infection (osteomyelitis), which can become a chronic problem and may be quite difficult to treat.

The finger should be immobilized in a splint that prevents the patient from moving only the DIP joint. The DIP joint should be in an extended position. The proximal interphalangeal (PIP) and metacarpophalangeal (MCP) joints should be free. The splint should be used until the fingertip is no longer tender (probably 7–10 days). No other stabilization of the bone usually is required.

Subungual Hematoma

Many injuries, especially those with a crush component (as when the patient hits a finger with a hammer), result in a subungual hematoma (blood clot under the nail). Treatment depends on the size of the hematoma.

A **small subungual hematoma (< 50% of the nail surface)** usually heals on its own, but the pressure of the blood under the nail can be extremely painful. Heat the tip of a needle or the end of a paper clip until it is red hot. Then use it to puncture the nail, and let the accumulated blood escape. Alternatively, an electrocautery unit can be used to make the drainage hole in the nail.

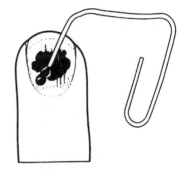

Drainage of a subungual hematoma. (From Simon RR, Brenner EE (eds): Emergency Procedures and Techniques, 3rd ed. Baltimore, Williams & Wilkins, 1994, with permission.)

In patients with a **large hematoma (≥ 50% of the nail surface)**, the usual recommendation is to remove the nail. Often there is a significant laceration in the nail bed, which can be repaired once the nail is removed. See "Nail Bed Injuries" later in this chapter for further details.

Fracture of the Bone with Nail Bed Injury

Fracture of the bone with nail bed injury is considered an open fracture. The patient should be given oral antibiotics for a few days.

If more than just a few mm of bone is exposed:

A skin graft will not heal over exposed bone, and in the finger, little local tissue is available to cover the bone reliably. A distant flap, such as a chest flap or cross-arm flap, may be required to cover the bone.

Another useful flap for a small wound (1–2 cm at most) is the thenar flap.

Thenar Flap

A thenar flap involves bending the injured finger to the thenar eminence at the base of the thumb (by the MCP flexion crease). The injured finger is essentially sutured into the palm so that the finger and the skin flap from the thenar eminence grow together. Later, the finger is separated with its newly acquired tissue.

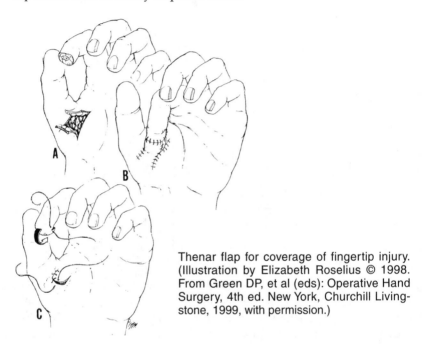

Thenar flap for coverage of fingertip injury. (Illustration by Elizabeth Roselius © 1998. From Green DP, et al (eds): Operative Hand Surgery, 4th ed. New York, Churchill Livingstone, 1999, with permission.)

Indications.   A thenar flap is used to cover a fingertip injury when bone is exposed and preservation of finger length is important. Thenar flaps should be done only in patients younger than 30 years. Significant joint stiffness may result if they are used in older patients.

The thenar flap is best used to provide coverage for the index and middle fingers. The ring and little fingers do not reach the thenar area very well. A similar type of flap can be designed over the hypothenar eminence for coverage of injuries of the ring and little fingers.

Procedure.   A thenar flap can be done under local anesthesia using a wrist block. The following steps are essential:

1. Observe where the injured finger makes contact with the thenar eminence just proximal to the MCP joint of the thumb.

2. Mark the three sides of a proximally based flap (i.e., the skin should stay attached at the side closest to the wrist). The flap should be slightly longer and wider than the defect.

3. Incise the three sides of the flap, and raise the flap with subcutaneous tissue attached to the skin. Do not go too deeply; you may injure the digital nerves of the thumb.

4. Suture the flap loosely to the fingertip.

5. A full–thickness skin graft can be sutured to the donor site, or the donor area can be allowed to heal on its own with dressings.

6. Apply a dorsal splint to keep the affected finger flexed into the palm. The splint prevents the patient from accidentally extending the finger and thereby pulling the finger off the flap.

7. Divide the flap (i.e., cut through area where the skin remains attached to the palm) after 10–14 days. Sew the edge of the flap to the open wound of the finger very loosely. Do not worry about achieving perfect skin closure; small gaps between the flap and fingertip will heal with dressings.

8. Antibiotic ointment and dry dressings should be used as needed postoperatively.

Nail Bed Injuries

The nail bed is often involved with injuries to the fingertips. Unfortunately, even with the most precise repair, the nail may not grow back with a completely normal appearance. Be sure to warn the patient about this risk.

Nails grow slowly. A normal, uninjured nail takes approximately 100 days to reach full length (to the end of the finger). With injury to the nail bed or fingertip, growth is delayed by almost 1 month.

As noted above, if a nail bed injury is associated with a fracture of the distal phalanx, treat the injury as an open fracture.

If a subungual hematoma is > 50% of the nail surface, a significant laceration usually is found in the nail bed. Repair of the laceration warrants removal of the nail for formal exploration.

Repair of an injured nail bed can be quite difficult because the tissues are very delicate and friable. Recent studies have shown that if the nail and surrounding nail margin are intact, removal of the nail and repair of nail bed lacerations are unnecessary in both children and adults. But you must still drain the hematoma.

If a subungual hematoma is accompanied by injury to the margin of the nail, the nail should be removed to allow proper repair of the nail bed and its surrounding tissues. A digital block and a digital tourniquet make the procedure much easier. Nail bed tissue is *highly* vascular.

Removing the Nail

1. Use a digital block. This procedure hurts!
2. Place the digital tourniquet once the finger is anesthetized. Alternatively, you can wait to place the tourniquet until the nail has been removed.
3. Place a small hemostat clamp just beneath the nail (between the nail and nail bed).
4. Gradually spread the clamp (open its jaws) to free the nail completely from the underlying nailbed.
5. Gradually advance the clamp proximally, until it is under the proximal portion of the nail (where it emerges from under the skin).
6. Grab the nail with the clamp, and pull. It may take some effort.
7. Clean the nail, and save it in saline-moistened gauze or a cleansing solution (e.g., Betadine). The nail may be useful for splinting the nail bed repair.

Repair

1. Use as small an absorbable suture as you can find (6-0 chromic is best) to repair the nail bed. Some type of magnification often is helpful. (See figure on following page.)
2. Nail bed tissue is highly friable and difficult to sew—much like suturing wet toilet paper. Take small amounts of tissue, and do not pull up on the needle as you pass through the tissue. Take your time. This procedure can be frustrating.
3. Once the repair has been completed, place the nail back on the nail bed to serve as a splint. Be sure to slide the proximal part of the nail under the skin fold at the base of the nail. This technqiue prevents the skin fold from scarring down to the nail bed.
4. If necessary, place a single stitch through the nail and the distal fingertip skin to hold it in place. Remove this stitch after a few days.
5. The injured nail will be pushed off by the growth of the new nail.

Nail bed lacerations are often multiple and uneven. (From Foucher G (ed): Fingertip and Nail Bed Injuries. London, Churchill Livingstone, 1991, with permission.)

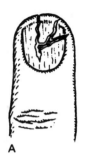 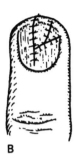

A   B

Aftercare

Place a small amount of antibiotic ointment around the nail, and cover the fingertip with light gauze.

After 1 or 2 days the fingertip can be left open without a dressing.

The hand should be kept elevated at all times. The finger will start to throb if the hand is dependent.

Encourage the patient to move all the joints of the finger to prevent stiffness.

Remember pain medication. Fingertip and nail bed injuries are quite painful.

Strongly encourage the patient to refrain from using tobacco products, which significantly delay healing.

Bibliography

1. Hart R, Kleinert H: Fingertip and nail bed injuries. Emerg Med Clin North Am 11: 755–765, 1993.
2. Lee L: A simple and efficient treatment for fingertip injuries. J Hand Surg 20B:63–71, 1995.
3. Roser SE, Gellman H: Comparison of nail bed repair versus nail trephination for subungual hematomas in children. J Hand Surg 24A:1166–1170, 1999.
4. Seaberg DC, Angelos WJ, Paris PM: Treatment of subungual hematomas with nail trephination: A prospective study. Am J Emerg Med 9:290–310, 1991.

Chapter 30

FINGER FRACTURES AND DISLOCATIONS

KEY FIGURES:
Rotational deformity
Buddy taping
Reduction of metacarpal fracture

Because we use our hands for so many things, finger fractures and dislocations are common injuries. Unless they are associated with significant soft tissue injury, definitive treatment is not emergent. Often the initial evaluation and necessary splinting can be done by a nonspecialist.

This chapter describes basic treatments for finger fractures and dislocations that can be done by all health care providers. For the best possible outcome, however, more highly technical procedures may be required. Whenever possible, patients with all but the simplest injuries should be referred to a hand specialist for definitive treatment.

An occupational therapist also should be consulted to help with rehabilitation once the fracture or dislocation has been properly treated.

In areas where specialists are not available, the basic interventions discussed in this chapter can help the patient attain an acceptable functional outcome.

Definitions

To **reduce** a fracture or dislocation means to restore the proper anatomic and functional alignment of the bone or joint. For most hand injuries, functional status is most important to the patient.

An **open** fracture or dislocation implies a wound in the soft tissues overlying the bone injury. In a **closed** injury the surrounding skin is intact. This distinction is important. An open fracture or dislocation has a high risk for infection. To prevent this complication, careful and thorough wash-out of the wound is required. The patient also should be given antibiotics (the oral route is usually sufficient, but extent of injury is the determining factor) for at least 48 hours after the repair. A closed fracture or dislocation is not associated with a high risk of infection; thus, the patient does not require treatment with antibiotics.

Finger Fractures

Compared with leg fractures, finger fractures may seem to be insignificant injuries. However, finger fractures can be quite problematic. Without proper treatment, a finger fracture can lead to significant limitation in hand function and disability.

Anesthesia

Administer a digital block before attempting to reduce a fracture. Use a combination of lidocaine and bupivacaine whenever possible to help with postprocedure pain control.

Distal Phalangeal Fractures

The distal phalanx is the most commonly fractured bone of the finger. Distal phalangeal fractures are classified into three types: tuft fractures, shaft fractures, and intraarticular fractures.

Tuft Fractures

A tuft fracture involves the most distal portion of the bone. It usually is caused by a crush mechanism, such as hitting the tip of the finger with a hammer. A tuft fracture is often an open fracture because of its common association with injury to the surrounding soft tissues and/or nail bed. Even without injury to surrounding soft tissue, the fracture is considered open in the presence of nail bed injury.

Treatment

1. The soft tissue wound should be cleansed thoroughly, and all foreign material should be removed.
2. In patients with a subungual hematoma > 50% of the nail surface, consider removing the nail to allow repair of the nail bed (see chapter 29, "Fingertip and Nail Bed Injuries").
3. Soft tissues should be sutured loosely in an interrupted fashion. Use 4-0 nylon or chromic material. Repair the nail bed with 5-0 or 6-0 chromic sutures. Repair of soft tissues usually leads to adequate reduction of the fracture.
4. Cover the suture line with antibiotic ointment and dry gauze. The dressing should be changed daily.
5. Keep the finger elevated as much as possible.

6. Strongly advise the patient to avoid smoking. Tobacco products slow the healing process.

7. Provide pain medication. Tuft fractures are often quite painful and tender for several days.

8. The patient may wear a protective splint or bulky dressing over the fingertip and distal interphalangeal (DIP) joint to prevent movement. The splint also protects the finger from accidental reinjury. However, do *not* immobilize the entire finger with the dressing or splint. Complete immoblization leads to unnecessary finger stiffness.

9. Once the finger is less tender (usually within 10–14 days), encourage the patient to gradually resume normal use of the finger.

Shaft Fractures

Shaft fractures involve the central portion of the distal phalanx. They also are associated often with soft tissue or nail bed injuries. As described above, repair of any soft tissue usually leads to adequate reduction of the fracture.

For further bone stabilization, a 20-gauge needle can be passed manually from the end of the fingertip into the bone segments. This procedure should be done before repair of any soft tissue injury (if present). The needle easily passes through the soft tissues into the bone if it is pushed firmly with a twisting motion. Bend the top part of the needle (the hub) so that it does not protrude too far from the end of the fingertip.

Basically, shaft fractures are treated like tuft fractures. If a needle is used to stabilize the fracture, remove it when the fingertip is no longer tender.

Intraarticular Fractures

Intraarticular fractures involve the joint surface of the distal phalanx at the DIP joint. The patient may present with a mallet deformity (inability to extend the DIP joint fully) if the fracture involves the bony insertion of the extensor tendon. In this setting, treat the finger like a mallet finger, as described in chapter 32, "Tendon Injuries of the Hand."

If there is no evidence of mallet deformity, the joint surface should be aligned as meticulously as possible to ensure optimal function. Such injuries are best referred to a hand specialist. If no specialist is available:

1. Manipulate the finger to align the bone pieces as precisely as possible.

2. Immobilize the DIP joint in 0–10° of flexion for 10–14 days. You can use a plaster splint or make a splint from a tongue depressor. Alternatively, the 20-gauge needle technique (described above) can be used to immobilize the DIP joint.

3. However you immobilize the joint, be sure to allow motion of the proximal interphalangeal (PIP) joint.

4. When the finger is no longer tender, the patient should start moving the joint both passively and actively in hope of regaining functional range of motion at the DIP joint.

Middle and Proximal Phalangeal Fractures

Middle and proximal phalangeal fractures are classified according to whether they involve the joint surface.

Extraarticular Fractures

Extraarticular fractures affect the part of the bone that is not involved with the joint surface. The main concern is whether a rotational deformity is present when the patient attempts to bend the fingers. See chapter 26, "Normal Hand Exam," for discussion of rotational finger alignment.

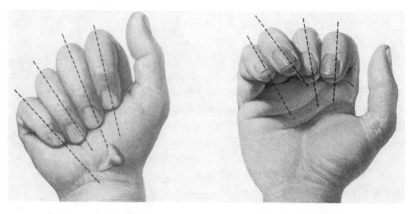

Any malrotation associated with metacarpal or phalangeal fractures must be corrected. *Left,* Normally all fingers point toward the region of the scaphoid when a fist is made. *Right,* Malrotation at the fracture site causes the affected finger to deviate. (From Crenshaw AH (ed): Campbell's Operative Orthopaedics, 7th ed. St. Louis, Mosby, 1987, with permission.)

If no rotational deformity is present, the finger can be treated by buddy taping for 2–3 weeks until the finger is no longer tender. Buddy taping is used to initiate gentle movement of the injured finger while maintaining proper bone alignment. The injured finger is taped to the adjacent finger, and the patient is instructed to use the hand as normally as possible.

Table 1.   Which Fingers to Use for Buddy Taping

Injured Finger	Finger Used for Buddy Taping
Index	Long
Long	Index
Ring	Long
Little	Ring

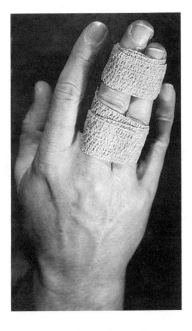

Buddy taping. To promote protected motion of the injured finger, secure it to an adjacent noninjured finger.

If a rotational deformity is present, give a digital block, and try to align the bone by manipulating the finger. Then place the finger in a volar splint.

If the fracture involves the proximal phalanx, the splint should immobilize the PIP joint in 0° of flexion and the metacarpophalangeal (MCP) joints in 70° of flexion. If the fracture involves the middle phalanx, the splint should immobilize both the DIP and PIP joints in 0° of flexion. The splint should be worn for 2–3 weeks until the tenderness over the fracture site has resolved.

After removing the splint, buddy-tape the finger for an additional 1–2 weeks. This approach initiates gentle movement of the affected finger and improves motion of the joints.

Fractures with a rotational deformity should be treated by a hand specialist if one is available.

Intraarticular Fractures

Intraarticular fractures involve the portion of bone that makes up the joint surface. Proper reduction is required to obtain adequate range of motion and finger function once the bone has healed. Intraarticular fractures usually require operative exploration for proper bony stabilization (with pins or screws) and thus should be treated by a hand specialist if one is available. If no hand specialist is available, try the treatment described for extraarticular fractures.

Metacarpal Fractures

Metacarpal fractures are included in this chapter because they can affect the position and function of the affected finger. A poorly aligned metacarpal fracture can cause a rotational deformity.

Metacarpal fractures may occur anywhere along the bone. Many require some type of pin fixation or stabilization for optimal treatment. Therefore, you should consult a hand specialist whenever possible.

If no specialist is available, begin by checking finger rotation. If the fingers maintain proper alignment and the fracture looks reasonably well positioned on radiographs, a short period (2–4 weeks until the fracture site is no longer tender) of cast or splint immobilization may be all that is required.

If a rotational deformity is present, reduction and manipulation must be performed before immobilization.

Fracture Reduction

Before the fracture is reduced a wrist block or a hematoma block should be given for pain control.

Hematoma Block

1. Draw up 3–5 ml of lidocaine in a syringe.

2. Clean the area overlying the fracture with alcohol or povidone-iodine solution. This procedure must be done under **sterile conditions** so that you do not contaminate the area around the fracture site and cause an infection.

3. Insert the needle into the tissues overlying the fracture until the tip of the needle contacts bone. Then back up the needle a few millimeters and inject 1–2 ml of solution.

4. Without completely removing it from the skin, back up the needle and reposition the tip by a centimeter or so. Then inject the rest of the solution.

Reduction Procedure

1. Start by flexing the MCP joint.

2. Apply downward pressure on the dorsal side of the fracture and exert upward pressure at the MCP joint until you feel the bone fragments move into the proper position.

3. Recheck finger alignment to ensure that the rotational deformity has been corrected. Repeat this procedure until proper alignment is achieved.

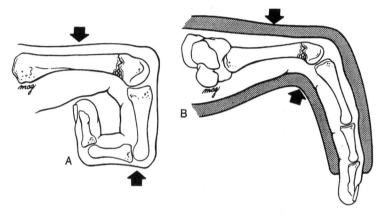

Reduction of a metacarpal fracture. Arrows indicate the direction of pressure application for fracture reduction. (From Green DP, et al (eds): Operative Hand Surgery, 4th ed. New York, Churchill Livingstone, 1999, with permission.)

4. Immobilize the hand with a cast or splint that includes the wrist (20–30° of extension) and MCP joints (60° of flexion). The interphalangeal joints can be left free so that you can monitor for rotational changes in the fingertips.

5. If you place the hand in a cast, be sure to use several layers of padding to protect the skin, and do not wrap the plaster too tightly.

6. The initial swelling from the injury should decrease after a few days. Therefore, the cast may need to be changed 5–7 days after injury to ensure adequate immobilization of the fracture site.

7. The hand should be immobilized for 3–4 weeks. Watch for changes in the position of the fingertips, which may be a sign that the reduction has slipped. If so, repeat manipulation of the fracture is required.

8. When the fracture site is no longer tender, the patient can begin to use the hand for light activity. Gradually increase activity over the next few months, as tolerated by the patient.

Joint Dislocations

For treatment purposes, finger joint dislocations can be classified as either simple or complex. A **simple dislocation** involves no fracture of the bone and can be reduced easily. A **complex dislocation** is not reducible or is associated with fracture of one of the involved bones. The main concern is whether the dislocation is reducible.

Simple MCP Joint Dislocations

Reduction of an MCP joint dislocation demands particular care. An incorrect reduction can change a simple dislocation into a complex one.

Reduction Technique

1. You may need to give a wrist block or gentle sedation for pain control.

2. Flex the wrist to keep the flexor tendons slack.

3. Avoid pulling on the finger and placing extension forces onto the joint.

4. Apply direct digital pressure on the dorsal side of the base of the proximal phalanx, and push the proximal phalanx in a volar direction to reposition the proximal phalanx above the metacarpal head.

After Reduction

The joint will slide into a flexed position once the dislocation has been reduced. The patient is allowed to use the finger, but a splint should be placed on the dorsal surface of the hand (onto the finger) to prevent extension of the MCP joint beyond 0°. The patient should wear the splint until the joint is completely non-tender, usually for 2–3 weeks.

Active and passive range-of-motion exercises should be done for several months to attain full motion in the joint.

Simple Interphalangeal Joint Dislocations

Often the patient presents after the dislocation is reduced. If reduction is required, use the following technique.

Reduction Technique

1. A digital block may be required for pain control.

2. Apply gentle traction to the finger by grasping the finger distal to the affected joint. Gently pull on the finger, and the dislocation should reduce.

After Reduction

The affected joint(s) should be immobilized with a dorsal splint, keeping the joint in 20–30° of flexion for 5–7 days until the tenderness significantly decreases.

The finger then should be buddy-taped for another 2–3 weeks. When the affected joint is completely pain-free, the taping can be stopped.

Joint stiffness may remain for months. The patient should continue range-of-motion exercises until the finger moves normally.

Complex Dislocations

The treatment of a complex dislocation requires operative exploration, the description of which is beyond the scope of this text. Complex dislocations require referral to a hand specialist.

Bibliography

1. Glickel SZ, Barron OA, Eaton RG: Dislocations and ligament injuries in the digits. In Green DP, Hotchkiss RN, Pederson WC (eds): Green's Operative Hand Surgery, 4th ed. New York, Churchill Livingstone, 1999, pp 772–808.
2. Kiefhaber TR, Stern PJ: Fracture dislocations of the proximal interphalangeal joint. J Hand Surg 23A:368–380, 1998.
3. Stern PJ: Fractures of the metacarpals and phalanges. In Green DP, Hotchkiss RN, Pederson WC (eds): Green's Operative Hand Surgery, 4th ed. New York, Churchill Livingstone, 1999, pp 711–771.

Chapter 31

TRAUMATIC HAND AND FINGER AMPUTATIONS

KEY FIGURES:

Care of amputated segment
Amputation of the middle finger
Successful replantation

This chapter outlines the basic principles for the evaluation and treatment of traumatic hand and finger amputations proximal to the distal interphalangeal (DIP) joint. Amputations distal to the DIP joint can be treated as a fingertip injury (see chapter 29, "Fingertip and Nail Bed Injuries").

The procedure to reattach an amputated part is highly technical and tedious. It includes reconnecting blood vessels (both an artery and at least one vein), nerves, and lacerated tendons as well as realigning and stabilizing the bones. A highly trained microsurgeon with access to specialized equipment is required.

If No Properly Equipped Microsurgeon is Available

Your best strategy is to help the wound heal with as little functional disability as possible. You can take steps to prevent, for example, a painful stump, which will interfere with use of the hand.

Basic Wound Treatment

After administering a digital block or wrist block, as indicated by the level of amputation, completely clean and examine both the stump and the amputated part (see chapter 6, "Evaluation of an Acute Wound").

Exposed tendons that have lost their distal insertion sites should be cut off so that the ends of the tendons are covered by soft tissue.

Do not discard the amputated part until you have thoroughly examined the wound. You may be able to use some of the skin from the amputated segment as a skin graft to cover the open wound.

Options for Wound Closure

If enough skin is available, close the wound with a few loose sutures. A tight closure can lead to further tissue loss.

If no skin is available, no bone or tendon is exposed, and the wound is relatively small (< 2 cm), the wound can be left open and treated with local care. An alternative is to use noninjured skin from the amputated segment as a full-thickness skin graft to cover the wound.

If the wound is large and cannot be closed primarily or if bones or intact tendons are exposed, a distant flap (e.g., chest flap, groin flap) is needed for wound closure. (See chapter 14, "Distant Flaps.")

If a nerve is exposed at the end of the stump, place a clamp on the nerve and pull gently. Then cut the nerve back to the point where it exits the soft tissues. This maneuver allows the nerve to retract under healthy skin or soft tissue and thus prevents development of a sensitive or painful stump.

Wound Care

Clean with gentle soap and water or sterile saline daily.

Strongly urge the patient not to smoke.

The patient should keep the affected hand elevated to decrease swelling and pain and to promote healing.

Remember pain medication. Acetaminophen alone may not be enough for the first few days after injury. Amputations can be quite painful.

Apply antibiotic ointment and a simple, dry dressing 1–2 times/day. Wet-to-dry dressings also can be useful.

- If the wound was sutured closed, after a few days the dressings can be discontinued.
- If the wound was left open, continue the dressing changes until the wound is healed.

Encourage the patient to move the finger and hand to prevent joint stiffness. Active and passive range-of-motion exercises also should be encouraged.

If a Properly Equipped Microsurgeon is Available

You can take several important steps before the patient is transferred to the microsurgeon's care. An amputated hand or finger(s) can be replanted even many hours after the injury, but the amputated part must receive proper care.

In addition, the patient must be informed that he or she will not awaken from surgery with a normally functioning hand. Replantation of the amputated segment commits the patient to a long and tedious rehabilitation program to obtain maximal hand function. Be sure to explain this prolonged process to the patient.

Patient Preparation

1. **Administer intravenous (IV) fluids** (normal saline or Ringer's lactate) to keep the patient hydrated. While awaiting surgery, the patient should not be allowed to eat or drink anything except required medications.

2. **Give aspirin** (*not* acetaminophen) at a dose of 80–160 mg, which is equivalent to one baby aspirin or one-half of an adult aspirin. It can be given by mouth or as a rectal suppository. The antiplatelet properties of aspirin may help to prevent clotting of the vessels after the reattachment has been completed.

3. **Give a dose of IV antibiotics.** A first-generation cephalosporin is most appropriate.

4. **Control pain** with IV morphine or a digital block. Give the nerve block only after consultation with the surgeon.

5. **Clean and dress the stump** with saline-moistened gauze (damp, not soaking wet), and wrap the stump lightly with dry gauze to control oozing and to keep the wound clean.

6. **Gently elevate** the affected hand.

7. **Get a radiograph** of the stump as well as the amputated segment.

Care of the Amputated Part

1. **Remove any foreign material** from the exposed soft tissues.

2. **Clean** the amputated part with saline, and **wrap** it in saline moistened gauze (damp, not soaking wet).

3. Place the wrapped segment in a **plastic bag**.

4. Place the bag into a **container filled with ice mixed with saline.** *Do not place the amputated part directly on ice.*

5. Do not forget to get a **radiograph** of the amputated part.

The patient is now ready for transfer.

Bibliography

Merle M, Dautel G: Advances in digital replantation. Clin Plast Surg 24:87–106, 1997.

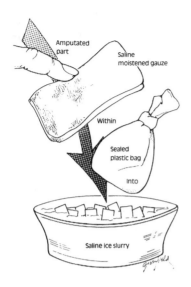

Care of the amputated segment. The amputated segment should be cooled immediately by wrapping it in a moist saline gauze, placing it in a sealed plastic bag, and immersing it in an iced saline container. (From McCarthy J (ed): Plastic Surgery. Philadelphia, W.B. Saunders, 1990, with permission.)

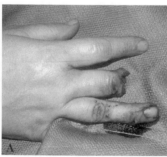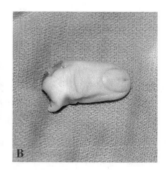

Traumatic amputation of the middle finger. *A,* Hand with missing finger. *B,* Amputated segment.

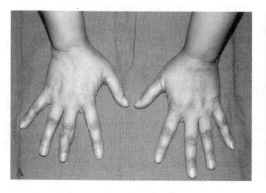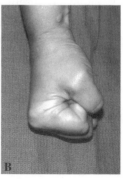

One year after successful replantation. *A* and *B,* Patient has regained excellent function of her hand.

Chapter 32

TENDON INJURIES OF THE HAND

KEY FIGURES:

Extensor surface of hand	Injured finger in
Mallet finger	stack splint
Mallet splints	Repair of open mallet

Most hand specialists believe that the earlier a tendon injury is repaired, the better the final result. However, repair of a lacerated flexor tendon is not a surgical emergency mandating immediate repair.

If the tendon ends are easily identifiable in the wound, you should repair the tendon when you first see the patient. However, if immediate repair is not possible or if you do not have the necessary surgical skills, the tendon can be repaired at a later time when a specialist is available. The overall outcome will not be adversely affected by delayed repair.

The most important point is to thoroughly wash out the wound and loosely close the skin as soon as possible after injury. This treatment prevents wound infection and allows safe performance of definitive repair at a later time (preferably within 7–10 days).

Flexor Tendon Injuries

Suspect a flexor tendon injury if the patient is unable to actively flex the distal (DIP) or proximal interphalangeal (PIP) joint of a finger, the interphalangeal (IP) joint of the thumb, or the wrist.

Partial and complete flexor tendon lacerations should be repaired to prevent disability. Repair requires careful exploration in the operating room (the proximal end of the cut tendon almost always retracts and is therefore difficult to locate) and advanced surgical skills. A clinician with technical expertise in hand surgery should repair flexor tendon injuries; the procedure can be quite challenging.

An important part of the initial treatment after repair of the overlying open wound is to place the hand in a splint. For injury to the flexor tendon of the thumb, use a thumb spica splint. For injury to the flexor tendon of the finger or wrist, immobilize the entire hand by applying a dorsal splint that covers the forearm, hand, and fingers. For more detailed information about splinting, see chapter 28, "Hand Splinting and General Aftercare." The patient should wear the splint until he or she is evaluated by a specialist.

Extensor Tendon Injuries

An extensor tendon injury should be suspected when the patient cannot extend the metacarpophalangeal (MCP) joint of a finger or the thumb, the IP joint of the thumb, or the wrist.

Injury to the extensor tendon mechanism on the dorsal surface of the finger is evidenced by an inability to extend the PIP and DIP joints. Unless the patient has lacerations over each finger, generalized inability to extend the PIP and DIP joints of *all* fingers probably represents an ulnar nerve injury rather than a tendon injury.

In wounds over the dorsal surface of the hand or a finger, the cut ends of the tendon often can be identified with minimal wound exploration. Therefore, an extensor tendon injury often can be repaired on initial evaluation without taking the patient to the operating room.

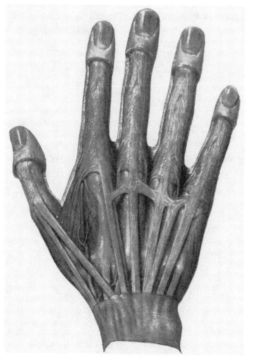

Dorsal view of the hand showing extensor tendons, accessory communicating tendons (vincular accessorium), and extensor expansions. (From Crenshaw AH (ed): Campbell's Operative Orthopaedics, 7th ed. St. Louis, Mosby, 1987, with permission.)

Repair of the Extensor Tendon

Administer local anesthetic either by direct infiltration of the wound or by digital block. Be sure to clean the wound thoroughly.

If you see the tendon ends in the wound, repair the tendon (see below). If you cannot identify the proximal end (usually the harder end to locate), try to extend the involved finger and wrist. If this maneuver is unsuccessful, try to enlarge the wound with a knife by an additional 1–2 cm. Keep the involved part in extension, and see if this maneuver brings the tendon end into view.

If you are unable to locate the tendon ends, surgical exploration by a clinician with hand expertise is needed. Loosely close the skin so that the repair can be done at a later date.

If the tendon ends are identified, sew them together using a nonabsorbable suture such as 4-0 nylon. The tendon can be repaired with a single figure-of-eight suture. Alternatively, place one or two simple sutures in the tendon ends to bring them together.

Caution: When tying the suture(s), do not pull too tightly. You may rip the suture out of the tendon.

Repair the overlying skin laceration with a few simple sutures. Apply antibiotic ointment and dry gauze over the repaired skin. A splint is required to protect the repair.

Table 1.   Splinting of Extensor Tendon Injury*

Location of Injury	Type of Splint
On finger	Volar splint of finger that extends onto palm of hand. It is best to use an aluminum splint or to make a splint from plaster. Finger should be immobilized with MCP joint in 10–15° of flexion and IP joints straight.
On thumb	Thumb spica splint.
Extensor tendon to finger(s) on dorsum of hand or wrist	Volar splint from forearm to fingertips. Wrist should be placed in 20° of extension, MCP joints in 10–15° of flexion, and IP joints straight.
Extensor tendon to thumb on dorsum of hand or wrist	Thumb spica splint.

*See chapter 28 for more information about splinting.

If the extensor tendon is repaired, the patient should wear the splint for 4–6 weeks. An occupational therapist (if available) should see the patient to promote proper tendon healing and hand function.

If the tendon is not repaired, the splint should be worn until the patient can be evaluated by a hand specialist.

Mallet Finger

Mallet finger results from injury of the extensor tendon at its insertion into the distal phalanx. The patient cannot fully extend the finger at the DIP joint. Without adequate treatment, the finger will not completely straighten, which can be quite bothersome. For example, patients will not be able to get objects out of their pocket, a common everyday activity.

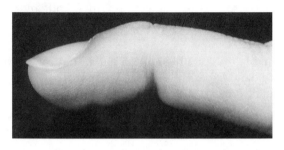

Mallet finger. The patient cannot actively extend the DIP joint.

In contrast to most tendon injuries, a mallet finger can result from a closed injury (no cut to the overlying skin that also injured the tendon) as well as an injury with an overlying skin laceration. A closed mallet injury is caused by sudden, forced flexion of an extended finger. The tendon is torn off the distal phalanx, and sometimes the bone is fractured.

Closed Mallet Deformity

With No Underlying Fracture or a Fracture of < 50% of the Articular Joint Surface

The best treatment is a volar splint—either the commercially available splint (Stack finger splint) or an aluminum foam splint. If neither is available, a splint can be made from plaster or from a piece of a tongue depressor (with cotton padding). The splint should be long enough to immobilize only the DIP joint. The PIP joint should not be immobilized.

Position the DIP joint in slight hyperextension. **Caution:** Be careful not to hyperextend the joint too much because skin necrosis may result. Look at your own finger—you can see the skin blanch (indicating diminished blood circulation) when you overly hyperextend the DIP joint. This effect should be avoided.

If you are unable to get the joint into proper hyperextension with a volar splint, a dorsal splint can be used. Again, immobilize only the DIP joint. You must be careful because of the higher incidence of skin breakdown when the splint is placed over the dorsal surface of the joint.

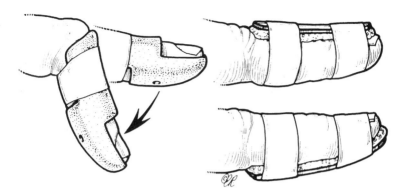

Splints for treatment of mallet finger. (Illustration by Elizabeth Roselius © 1998. From Green DP, et al (eds): Operative Hand Surgery, 4th ed. New York, Churchill Livingstone, 1999, with permission.)

Tape is used to keep the splint in place. The splint is removed only to cleanse the finger (once daily). The patient should keep the joint in extension while the splint is off. The splint stays in place continuously for at least 6 weeks.

After 6 weeks, if the finger is nontender and the patient can actively hold the finger in full extension, the splint can be removed during the day, but only light activity should be allowed. The patient should wear the splint at night for another 4 weeks and when doing strenuous work with the hand.

If after 6 weeks the patient cannot actively hold the finger in full extension, the splint should remain in place continuously for another 4 weeks.

If at any time after the splint is removed the patient notices loss or weakness of full active extension of the DIP joint, the splint should be replaced and worn continuously for another 4–6 weeks.

This treatment regimen can be successful even if the patient does not seek treatment until several months after the initial injury.

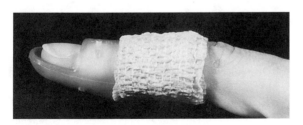

Injured finger in a Stack splint.

With a Facture of > 50% of the Articular Joint Surface

To optimize functional outcome, the fracture should be meticulously reduced and stabilized. This procedure requires operative treatment by a hand specialist. However, if none is available, try the treatment described above. It may be successful.

Open Mallet Deformity

In open mallet deformities, the overlying skin is lacerated as well as the tendon.

Once the finger has been thoroughly cleansed, the skin and tendon can be repaired together with one or two nonabsorbable figure-of-eight sutures (4-0 or 3-0 nylon). Alternatively, if you can see the tendon ends, the tendon can be repaired separately from the skin, but often this approach is not possible. A nonabsorbable suture should be used to repair the tendon.

The splinting regimen is the same as for closed mallet deformity. The skin sutures are removed after 10–14 days, regardless of how the repair was performed.

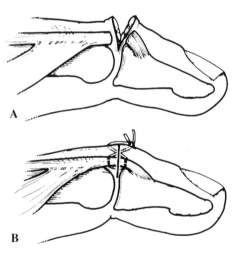

Repair of an open mallet deformity. The extensor tendon and overlying skin are lacerated (A). The skin and tendon can be repaired together with one or two nonabsorbable figure-of-eight sutures (B), which are removed after 10–14 days. The finger must remain splinted for at least 6 weeks. (Illustration by Elizabeth Roselius © 1998. From Green DP, et al (eds): Operative Hand Surgery, 4th ed. New York, Churchill Livingstone, 1999, with permission.)

Bibliography

1. Doyle JR: Extensor tendons: Acute injuries. In Green DP, Hotchkiss RN, Pederson WC (eds): Green's Operative Hand Surgery, 4th ed. New York, Churchill Livingstone, 1999, pp 1950–1987.
2. Ingari JV, Pederson WC: Update on tendon repair. Clin Plast Surg 24:161–174, 1997.
3. Strickland JW: Flexor tendons: Acute injuries. In Green DP, Hotchkiss RN, Pederson WC (eds): Green's Operative Hand Surgery, 4th ed. New York, Churchill Livingstone, 1999, pp 1851–1897.

Chapter 33

NERVE AND VASCULAR INJURIES OF THE HAND

KEY FIGURES:
Digital nerve location on finger
Epineurial repair

Nerves and blood vessels of the hand and fingers usually are quite delicate, and some are quite small. Optimal repair of injuries often requires the microsurgical expertise of a reconstructive surgeon. However, an understanding of basic principles is useful when you find yourself without specialist support.

Nerve Injuries

Nerve Physiology

When a nerve is cut, the distal part of the nerve slowly dies and cannot regrow. The proximal part of the nerve will regenerate. However, without proper treatment, there is no guarantee that the nerve will grow correctly or that function (sensory or motor) will be restored.

The nerve laceration should be repaired by sewing the cut ends together. Repair increases the likelihood that the living proximal part will grow in the proper direction, along the path left by the disintegrating distal part.

Nerves grow at a rate of 1 mm/day once the reparative process begins (usually within a few weeks of injury).

Remind the patient that even if the nerve is repaired, normal sensation and movement will not be apparent immediately after the procedure. It will take many months to know the final outcome.

General Nerve Anatomy

Nerves are made up of axonal fibers running in parallel. These fibers are surrounded by loose connective tissue, called **epineurium**. In larger nerves that have many different axons (some sensory, some motor in function), the connective tissue between the individual axons is called **perineurium**. Sutures should be placed in the loose connective tissue around the axons, *not* in the axonal substance itself.

Digital Nerves

Digital nerves are approximately 2–3 mm in diameter. They run with the digital arteries along the sides of each finger. If you look at your

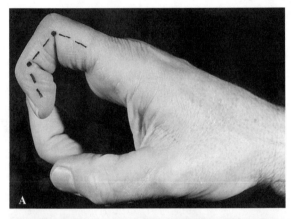

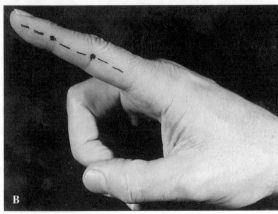

Determining the position of the digital nerve. *A,* Flex the finger and mark the most dorsal aspect of both PIP and DIP flexion creases with a dot. Connect the dots in a straight line. *B,* The course of the digital nerve is illustrated by the dashed line.

finger from the side and completely flex the distal (DIP) and proximal interphalangeal (PIP) joints, the neurovascular bundle runs along a line that connects the flexion creases of these joints.

Digital nerves are purely sensory. If a digital nerve is cut, the patient feels numbness on the corresponding side of the finger. Motor function in the finger should be normal, because it is controlled by the tendons, whose muscles are innervated more proximally in the forearm. Impairment of motor function (other than pain with movement) suggests that tendon injury also is present.

Injury to a digital nerve at any point proximal to the DIP flexion crease should be repaired. In the fingertip (distal to the DIP flexion crease), the nerve divides into its terminal branches, which are too small to repair. With distal nerve injuries, sensation may return without formal nerve repair.

Larger Nerves

Nerves in the forearm and wrist (e.g., median and ulnar nerves at the wrist) are much larger than digital nerves; their diameters range from 5–10 mm. Most have both motor and sensory functions. When you look at the cut ends of the nerve, especially under magnification, you can see that the inner nerve fibers are of various diameters and that some fibers seem to be grouped together within the nerve.

For optimal outcome, the proximal sensory fibers should be sutured to the distal sensory fibers and the proximal motor fibers to the distal motor fibers. Specialists sometimes repair larger nerves with electophysiologic guidance. This technique uses electric stimulators to identify which fibers are sensory and which are motor. Thus, the surgeon can determine exactly which fibers should go together. However, this specialized equipment usually is found only in high-technology hand centers.

Your best strategy is to try to align the nerve, using whatever landmarks you can discern. For example, try to line up the tiny blood vessels in the connective tissue around the nerve and fibers of similar size.

Nerve Repair

For optimal results, use at least twofold magnification (glasses or microscope). The more magnification, the better. Twofold magnification glasses make the image appear twice as large as with the naked eye.

Use the most delicate instruments you have—jewelers forceps, fine needle holders, fine scissors—and the smallest needle you can find (8-0 or 9-0 nylon is best).

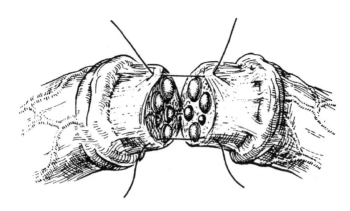

Epineurial repair. Sutures are placed in the connective tissue surrounding the nerve fibers. (From McCarthy JV (ed): Plastic Surgery. Philadelphia, W.B. Saunders, 1990, with permission.)

Place your sutures in the epineurium, not in the nerve fibers. This approach aligns the nerve fibers and allows proper growth.

There should be no tension on the repair. You may need to free the nerve from the surrounding soft tissues to remove tension. You also can change the position of the patient's fingers or wrist to allow the ends to meet more easily. **Caution:** if you bend the finger or wrist during surgery to bring the nerve ends together, it must stay in this position for 10–14 days. If you accidentally straighten the hand in the operating room, you will disrupt the repair.

If you have no magnification and minimal instruments: For a digital nerve, place a single simple suture to bring the ends together. For a larger nerve, 3–4 sutures should be placed.

If you have magnification and very small sutures (8-0 or 9-0): For a digital nerve, place 2–4 simple sutures to bring the ends together. For larger nerves, place as many as you need to get a smooth repair (i.e., nerve fibers should not protrude from the epineurium).

If there is too much tension on the nerve repair despite different positioning techniques, a nerve graft is required. This technically challenging procedure requires referral to a specialist for optimal outcome. Even so, there is no guarantee that a nerve graft will work. To facilitate future exploration and nerve grafting, mark the ends of the nerve by placing a 4-0 or 5-0 nylon or prolene simple suture in the epineurium. Be sure to use a nonabsorbable material, which helps to locate the nerve ends at the next operation. The surgeon performing the subsequent procedure will be grateful.

Postoperative Care

The repair should be immobilized by splinting the hand or finger for a minimum of 10–14 days.

If the finger or hand required special positioning to get the nerve ends to meet during the operation, the patient should begin to open the finger or hand *slowly* (over the subsequent 1–2 weeks) to avoid disruption of the repair.

If a motor nerve is injured, the patient should move the joints of the hand regularly to prevent stiffness. It takes months for the nerve to start working again. Even if the nerve repair is successful, the patient may not regain function if the joints have become stiff from disuse.

If a sensory nerve is injured, remind the patient to be careful around very hot, very cold, or sharp objects to prevent accidental injury to the insensate area.

Vascular Injuries

First, address the risk of exsanguination (bleeding to death), which is a real danger with arterial injuries.

If serious bleeding persists: Apply point pressure over the wound. This does not mean placing gauze in the wound and wrapping the area with an Ace bandage. It means placing a wad of gauze over the injured area and using two fingers to apply firm point pressure to the injured site. You may need to hold the pressure for several minutes before the bleeding stops. If the bleeding is arterial, exploration is needed.

If you cannot control an exsanguinating hemorrhage, place a tourniquet or blood pressure cuff proximal to the injury (closer to the heart). If you use a blood pressure cuff, it must be inflated to at least 50 mmHg above systolic arterial pressure (usually to at least 200–250 mmHg). *Tourniquets hurt* and place the tissues at risk for ischemic injury. The tourniquet should not be left in place for more than 15–20 minutes. If a tourniquet is needed, urgent operative exploration is required.

Patients with a history of pulsatile bleeding (blood squirting out from a hand or forearm wound) must be explored surgically, even in the absence of active bleeding at the time of exam. Failure to tie off or repair the vessel is associated with a high incidence of pseudoaneurysm (outpouching of the vessel). A pseudoaneurysm can be dangerous because of its propensity for rupture in the future.

Digital Artery

Bleeding from a digital artery usually can be controlled by repairing the skin laceration and applying pressure over the injured area. In the rare instance when this approach fails, the vessel can be tied off with a very small suture (5-0 or 6-0 silk or chromic).

Caution: The digital nerve is adjacent to the artery. Do not accidentally place the suture around the nerve as well as the artery. *If you accidentally tie off a digital nerve, the patient will have considerable postoperative pain.*

Radial Artery

Although we palpate the radial artery to check heart rate, it is not the dominant source of circulation to the hand. Many patients with a radial artery injury still have adequate circulation in the injured hand, as evidenced by good capillary refill and normal hand temperature (compared with the other hand). The artery does not necessarily need to be repaired or reconstructed. The vessel can be tied off with minimal morbidity. Remember to tie off both ends of the vessel.

Because a significant amount of pressure pushes blood through an artery, a preferable and more secure way to tie off a larger artery is to use a "stick tie." Both techniques are discussed in the chapter 2, "Basic Surgical Skills."

However, if circulation to the hand is insufficient, as evidenced by poor capillary refill and cold skin, the vessel should be repaired. Repair of the blood vessel involves joining together the two severed parts of the artery so that blood can flow as it did before the injury. Blood vessels in the distal forearm are quite small, and repair requires microsurgical equipment and expertise. Transfer to a specialist is vital to save the hand.

Ulnar Artery

The ulnar artery is the dominant artery to the hand in most people. Thus, if it is injured, it should be repaired or reconstructed. Repair requires microsurgical expertise, because the ulnar artery is even smaller than the radial artery.

The vessel should be tied off only if no one with microsurgical skills is available or if the patient is actively bleeding. In addition, some patients have sufficient circulation to the hand even if the ulnar artery is injured. In these few patients, the vessel can be safely tied off. In general, however, it is not recommended to tie off the ulnar artery permanently if specialists are available for referral.

Bibliography

1. Modrall JG, Weaver FA, Yellin AE: Diagnosis and management of penetrating vascular trauma and the injured extremity. Emerg Med Clin North Am 16:129–144, 1998.
2. Watchmaker GP, Mackinnon SE: Advances in peripheral nerve repair. Clin Plast Surg 24:63-73, 1997.

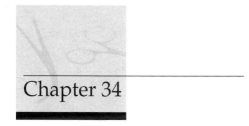

Chapter 34

HAND BURNS

KEY FIGURES:
Neglected hand
Escharotomy

Severe hand burns are especially problematic injuries because of their propensity for causing long-term disability. Proper treatment of the burned hand may mean that the patient can return to work and a normal lifestyle.

Unfortunately, if a large portion of the body is burned, the importance of the hands in terms of overall functional outcome is often overlooked. But if not properly treated, burns of the hand can result in severe dysfunction and significant morbidity. Simple interventions can make a huge difference in final outcome.

This chapter discusses specific interventions for treatment of a hand burn. A thorough discussion of the treatment of the "whole patient" with a burn injury is found in chapter 20, "Burns."

Initial Treatment

- Cleanse the burned hand with a gentle soap and cool water. Saline-moistened gauze also may be used for cleansing. Remove any clothing or other material attached to the burned tissues.

- Grease embedded in burned tissues often can be removed by gently wiping with a petrolatum ointment. If tar is stuck onto the skin, leave it alone; it will separate as the tissues heal. If you pull the tar off, you probably will remove healthy skin, making the injury worse than it needed to be.

- Make sure that the patient's tetanus immunizations are up to date.

- Pain medication is important; intravenous administration of morphine is the most useful approach.

- Apply an antibiotic ointment, such as silver sulfadiazine, to the burned areas, and cover lightly with gauze.
- Gentle cleansing with saline and application of antibiotic ointment optimally should be done twice each day, but daily is acceptable.
- The hand should be kept elevated (on a pillow or folded sheet) to minimize swelling.
- Oral or intravenous antibiotics should be used *only* if signs of infection are present.

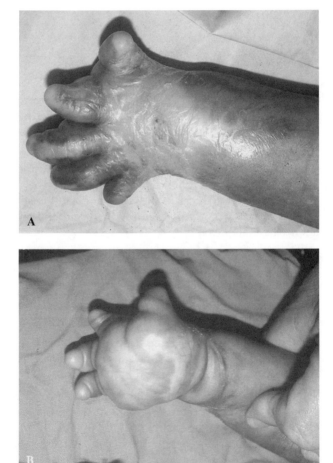

Severely burned hand of a child who did not receive proper care. The hand is essentially nonfunctional and will not grow properly. *A*, Dorsal surface. *B*, Volar surface.

Blisters

A blister is a collection of fluid beneath a layer of burned skin. It represents a partial-thickness injury (see discussion of depth of burn on the following page). In general, a blister serves as a useful biologic dressing because it allows the deeper tissues to remain in a sterile environment. Blisters promote healing and decrease pain.

Leaving the blister alone is often the best initial treatment. However, some blisters become very tight, to the point that blood flow to the hand is diminished. Ischemia can lead to further, unnecessary tissue loss. Tight blisters also interfere with hand and finger motion. Therefore, when a blister feels very tight, it should be opened and the outer skin layer should be removed. The top skin layer also should be removed from blisters that have burst or look as if they are about to burst.

How to Debride a Blister

Debridement of blisters is not a painful procedure if done properly:

1. Clean the area with Betadine or some other cleansing solution.
2. Use a knife or scissors to make an opening in the outer layer of the blister.
3. Remove the outer layer of the blister by cutting it off a few millimeters from the point where it attaches to the surrounding nonblistered skin.
4. The fluid in the blister has a high protein content and may be almost gelatinous. Completely remove the fluid and gel-like material, and gently wipe the area with saline-moistened gauze.
5. Apply antibiotic ointment to the area, and cover with gauze.

Prevention of a Stiff and Useless Hand

A severe burn to the hand poses significant risk for long-term morbidity. The injured hand tends to assume a flexed posture, which can lead to stiffness of the interphalangeal (IP) and metacarpophalangeal (MCP) joint ligaments. Without aggressive treatment during the time required for the burn to heal, the hand may become permanently stiff with limited function.

- **Occupational therapy** is a vital component in the treatment of severe hand burns. If a therapist is available, make the referral.

- **Encourage the patient to move his or her hands and fingers often**, especially at dressing changes. The nurse or family can move the fingers and hand for the patient if the patient is unable to do so. Active and passive range-of-motion exercises should be done.

- **Pain control** is important because movement hurts.

- **Place the hand in a splint** to prevent it from assuming the flexed position that ultimately may limit function. The splint should keep the wrist in 20° of extension, the MCP joints in 70° of flexion, and the IP joints as straight as possible. The padding for the splint should be changed if it becomes soiled. At a minimum, the patient should wear the splint at night; critically injured patients should wear the splint at all times until the burns have healed.

- **Careful tangential excision of the burn and split-thickness skin grafting** should be done relatively early (within days of the injury if possible) for full-thickness burns. This will prevent the development of tight scars, which can lead to severe movement limitations. Only health care providers with surgical expertise should undertake these procedures. See the discussion of surgical treatments for more information.

Determining Depth of Burn

As explained in chapter 20, "Burns," it is often difficult to determine the severity of the burn at the first examination. Reevaluate the burn once it has been cleansed and regularly thereafter. Burns are described as first degree (superficial), second degree (partial thickness), and third degree (full thickness).

Table 1.   Burn Wound Classification

Burn Depth	Appearance	Pain	Sensation
Superficial (first-degree)	Erythema	+	Yes
Partial thickness* (second degree)	Blisters, hairs (if present) stay attached	+++	Yes
Full thickness (third degree)	Thick, leathery feel Pale color Hairs (if present) do not stay attached Thombosed veins may be seen	0	No

* Partial-thickness burns can be superficial or deep. A superficial partial-thickness burn may have a thin blister, and the skin will be soft and pink. A deep partial-thickness burn appears white and feels softer than a full-thickness burn; some hair follicles are still attached. A deep partial-thickness burn often behaves like a full-thickness burn.

The skin of the hand has a wide range of thickness. The skin over the dorsum of the hand is much thinner than the skin over the palmar surface. A more severe burn injury is required to cause a full-thickness burn to the palmar vs. the dorsal surface. Because the extensor tendons are so close to the surface, full-thickness burns to the dorsal surface of the hand can be especially problematic.

Estimating the depth of the burn is important to approximate time to healing. First- and superficial second-degree burns should heal within 2 weeks, whereas deep second- and third-degree burns can take 3–4 weeks or longer to heal.

If the burns do not show significant evidence of healing after 7–10 days or if a full-thickness burn occurs in an area where tight scarring is likely, consideration should be given to early surgical intervention (see Tangential Excision).

Surgical Treatments

Escharotomy

Severe, circumferential full-thickness burns of the hand and fingers require extra precautions. The burned skin becomes leathery and loses all elasticity. As the underlying tissues swell (from a combination of the burn injury and from the fluid that the patient receives), the burned skin cannot "give," and pressure builds up in the tissues. Pressure build-up can lead to decreased circulation, which can result in further loss of tissue.

In all patients with severe burns, check for palpable pulses at the wrist. If they are not present, blood circulation to the tissues probably is inadequate because of the tightness of the burned tissues. An escharotomy must be done emergently to prevent further tissue loss.

Escharotomy is the placing of incisions into the burned tissues to release the tightness. Do not extend the incisions into the deeper tissues; *cut through the burned tissue only*. Incisions must be placed with care to prevent injury to the important underlying nerves, tendons, and vessels.

Escharotomy can be done at the bedside. **Caution:** Escharotomy can be a bloody procedure. Be sure that blood is available, along with gauze, clamps, and an electrocautery device.

Although the eschar itself has no sensation, the procedure can be quite painful. Intravenous morphine or intravenous sedation/general anesthesia is required.

To Treat the Fingers

An incision is made along the side of the finger. Usually only one incision is needed on each finger. Try to avoid placing the incisions on the radial borders of the fingers. Placing the incisions along the ulnar surfaces of the fingers will prevent future problems with scar sensitivity when the patient attempts to grasp objects.

To Treat the Hand

Four dorsal, longitudinal incisions should be made between the metacarpal bones. Place a clamp into the deeper tissues, and spread open the jaws of the clamp to relieve the pressure over the underlying interosseous muscles.

To Treat the Forearm

The incision starts at the radial side of the wrist and proceeds proximally along the radial side of the forearm. The incision should be extended onto the upper arm (staying along the radial border of the arm) until the tight burn has been released completely.

If the above incision does not completely relieve the pressure in the arm, an incision along the ulnar aspect of the arm and forearm should be made. Take care around the elbow. Keep the incision anterior to the medial epicondyle at the elbow to prevent accidental injury to the ulnar nerve.

Incisions should be left open; do not try to close them. The purpose of escharotomy is to relieve pressure and prevent further tissue loss. Perform the same type of dressing changes in these open areas as you

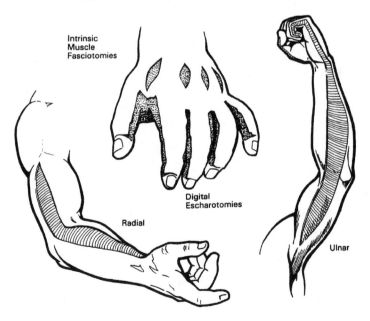

Escharotomy incisions should be placed to minimize risk for injury to nearby nerves, tendons, and vessels. (From Achauer BM: Burn Reconstruction. New York, Thieme Medical Publishers, 1991, with permission.)

perform to the burned skin. Alternatively, you may apply saline-moistened gauze to the incisions.

Be sure to keep the hand elevated and in a splint to minimize swelling. Split-thickness skin grafts will be required for final wound healing.

Tangential Excision

Tangential excision is a method to remove burned tissue. See chapter 20, "Burns," for specific details. Care must be taken to avoid removing uninjured tissue. To perform this procedure you must have technical expertise to avoid injury to underlying tendons, nerves, and blood vessels.

The excision should be done with a tourniquet on the extremity. The tourniquet allows you to excise more accurately only the burned tissue. It is important to leave the thin layer of tissue surrounding the tendons (peritenon) intact, if it is not burned. This tissue is vital for successful skin grafting. If the peritenon is burned, skin grafting is not possible. A distant flap is required for wound closure.

When the tourniquet is released, the area will bleed uniformly, letting you know that all burned tissue has been removed.

The wound is then ready for split-thickness skin grafting. See chapter 12, "Skin Grafts," for details.

Postoperative Care after Tangential Excision and Skin Grafting

Keep the hand elevated (on a pillow or folded sheet) to minimize swelling.

Keep the hand in a splint, as previously described.

The splint should be worn at all times for the first 2 weeks. As the grafts heal, the patient can wear the splint only at night. Critically injured patients should wear the splint at all times.

Once the grafts have begun to "stick" (5–6 days), start gentle active and passive range-of-motion exercises of the hand and fingers.

After a few weeks, as the grafts heal and the patient begins to use the hand more, the splint can be worn only at night. The splint should be used at night for at least 1–2 months.

Care after Burns or Skin Grafts have Healed

Once the tissues have healed, it is important to start treatment to prevent the scars from becoming thick and tight:

Scar massage is a useful modality that requires no special equipment.

Gently rub the fingers and hand with a mild moisturizing cream 2–3 times/day to soften scars, diminish itching, and improve functional outcome.

The best way to prevent hypertrophic scarring is to fit the patient with a pressure garment (if available). The pressure garment should be worn for as many hours of the day as the patient tolerates for several months.

For further discussion of these and other useful treatments, see chapter 15, "Scar Formation."

Bibliography

1. Achauer BM: The burned hand. In Green DP, Hotchkiss RN, Pederson WC (eds): Green's Operative Hand Surgery, 4th ed. New York, Churchill Livingstone, 1999, pp 2045–2060.
2. Robson MC, Smith DJ: Burned hand. In Jurkiewicz MJ, Krizek TJ, Mathes SJ, Aryian S (eds): Plastic Surgery: Principles and Practice. St. Louis, Mosby, 1990, pp 781–802.

Chapter 35

HAND CRUSH INJURY AND COMPARTMENT SYNDROME

KEY FIGURES:
Volar forearm fasciotomy incisions
Hand/dorsal forearm fasciotomy incisions
Finger fasciotomy incisions

The previous chapters about the hand have discussed easily identifiable, individual injuries to the upper extremity. A crush injury is more complex and may affect all of the tissues of the hand and forearm. It is, therefore, more difficult to treat. The risk of long-term disability after a crush injury is quite high.

Initially, the affected hand and forearm may appear to have suffered only minor damage because external wounds are few. Significant damage to the skin and underlying tissues may not become appreciable for hours or even days after the injury. Initial care plays an important role in final functional outcome.

Most of the necessary interventions require surgical expertise. However, the initial examiner must be aware of all of the potential problems that may develop so that proper specialty help can be obtained. This chapter outlines such problems and discusses specific treatment for compartment syndrome (the most severe complication of crush injury) if specialty help is not available. It may save not only hand function but also the patient's life.

Crush Injury: Definition and Examples

A crush injury occurs when a compressive type of force is applied to the tissues. At the site of injury the tissues experience several forces simultaneously, including shearing, contusion, and stretching in addition to pressure. This scenario is much different from what the tissues experience when injured, for example, with a knife.

Examples of crush injuries include the following:

- Getting the fingers, hand, or forearm caught in a wringer or roller machine.
- A motor vehicle accident that occurs as the patient is resting an arm along the window sill on the outside of the car. The car flips over onto that side, crushing the extremity.
- Getting the hand or forearm caught between two heavy objects that are compressed together.

Effects on the Tissues

Skin and Subcutaneous Tissue

The skin may be seriously injured with multiple lacerations and contusions. Foreign material may be embedded in the wounds. Alternatively, the skin may look largely intact. However, large flaps of skin may have been created by the injury. If the skin is detached from the underlying fascia and muscle (**degloving injury**), the circulation to the skin is greatly compromised. The result can be significant skin loss.

In addition, blood and serum may collect in the tissue plains between skin and muscle. Build-up of pressure may cause further tissue damage and possibly a **compartment syndrome** (see below).

Muscle

Direct pressure injury and shearing forces lead to overstretching and tearing of the muscle. The results are bleeding and swelling within the muscle itself. A compartment syndrome with potentially devastating consequences may develop (see below). In addition, disruption of muscle-tendon connections may result in loss of function.

Tendons

Although a crush injury probably will not tear a tendon completely, the stretching forces may create small, partial tears. During the healing process, scar tissue forms to heal such tears and may cause the tendons to adhere to surrounding tissues. Adhesions may interfere significantly with the tendon's ability to glide smoothly, resulting in loss of joint motion and hand function.

Nerves

Usually, nerves are not torn by a crush injury. However, the nerve's ability to conduct electrical impulses may be temporarily or possibly permanently disrupted. It may take weeks to even months to determine whether the loss of nerve activity is permanent.

With damage to sensory nerves, the patient may experience tingling and numbness (paresthesias) or even painful hypersensitivity to touch. With damage to motor nerves, weakness or complete loss of function may result.

Blood Vessels

Blood vessels can be injured by direct compression (depending on how long the extremity was crushed) or shearing forces, which may injure the inner layer (the intima). Either mechanism can cause the vessel to clot.

If the injured vessel is an artery, the surrounding tissues lose their blood supply and ischemia results. If the injured vessels are veins, diminution of venous outflow from the damaged area leads to a build-up of pressure in the tissues. This pressure may contribute to the formation of compartment syndrome (see below).

Injury to a major artery or to the veins of the extremity can result in devastating tissue loss if appropriate intervention is not forthcoming.

Bone and Joints

Joint capsules and surrounding ligaments may rupture, resulting in joint dislocation or joint instability. Fractures may occur, and often the bone is broken into several pieces (comminuted fracture).

In children, the growth plates of the bones may be disrupted. Disruption of growth plates interferes with subsequent bone growth, and the bone may not grow to its proper length.

Initial Approach to Patients with a Crushed Hand or Forearm

The key is to get a good history and do a thorough exam. You should have a high index of suspicion so that you do not miss a potentially devastating underlying injury.

History

It is important to know the nature of the injury as well as background information about the patient to guide your physical exam and treatment options. Information that you should obtain includes:

- Extent of injury (e.g., fingers, hands, forearms)
- Mechanism of injury
- Force of crush (some pieces of equipment have known compression forces)

- Duration of crush forces (seconds, minutes?)

- History of previous injury or chronic hand problems (e.g., symptoms compatible with carpal tunnel syndrome)

- Smoking history (encourage patients *not to smoke* because smoking may worsen the injury to the tissues)

- Tetanus toxoid status (be sure tetanus immunizations are up to date)

Physical Exam

The injured extremity must be thoroughly examined. Particular attention should be paid to the following factors. An asterisk indicates that positive findings may indicate a compartment syndrome.

- Appearance of skin (look for blisters, open wounds, elevated areas, foreign material, other abnormalities)

- Circulation to the hand (palpable pulses in the radial and ulnar arteries, capillary refill in the fingers)

- Palpation of forearm and hand (significant swelling, tissue tightness)*

- Neurologic exam (e.g., complaints of tingling or numbness, ability to differentiate between sharp and dull objects, ability to move fingers)*

- Pain out of proportion to injury (e.g., additional pain when you passively move fingers or wrist)*

- Deformity indicating possible bone or joint injury

- Radiographic studies to document a fracture

* Finding may indicate the presence of a compartment syndrome.

What to Do Next

1. If you find evidence of **arterial compromise**, exploration and vascular reconstruction are needed. A specialist is required.

2. **Fractures or dislocations** should be reduced and treated appropriately. See chapter 30 for specific information.

3. If the patient has no evidence of a compartment syndrome (see below) but reports numbness and tingling of the hand consistent with **compression of the median nerve**, a carpal tunnel release should be done. This procedure decreases the pressure on the median nerve and may prevent permanent neural damage. See chapter 38 for details about surgical release of the median nerve.

4. **Lacerations** to the skin should be cleansed thoroughly and examined carefully. If the tissues are soft and the skin is still attached to the underlying muscle, the wounds may be loosely closed. If you

are concerned about swelling in the tissues, leave the wounds open. You do not want to do anything that may increase pressure in the tissues. Once the swelling resolves, you may want to close the wounds or leave them to heal secondarily.

5. If you note **evidence of a degloving injury**, a plastic surgeon (if available) should evaluate the patient. It is quite likely that much of the degloved skin will die, even if it looks viable at the initial examination. If no specialist is available, wash out the wound to ensure that no blood has collected under the skin. Then reposition the skin on top of the muscle. Do not try to suture the skin together, because sutures place added tension on the skin flaps and may further compromise the circulation. The skin will demarcate gradually over the next several days. Skin that turns purple and dies should be excised.

6. **If the patient has a swollen and somewhat painful extremity but the forearm and hand tissues still feel soft**, the patient should be watched closely. Splint the hand in neutral position, and gently elevate the hand. Give pain medication (avoid aspirin and nonsteroidal anti-inflammatory agents), and reexamine the patient several times over the next 48 hours for evidence of a compartment syndrome. After a few days of splinting, as the swelling and pain resolve, the patient should start moving the hand and fingers to prevent stiffness.

7. If the patient has signs and symptoms of a **compartment syndrome**, urgent surgical intervention is required.

Compartment Syndrome

A compartment syndrome develops when increased pressure builds up within a fixed, well-defined space (such as the tissues of the forearm). The increase in pressure prevents venous and lymphatic outflow, which leads to a further increase in tissue pressure. Without appropriate intervention to relieve the pressure, a vicious cycle develops. High tissue pressures also prevent oxygen and nutrients from getting to the tissues. Muscle and nerve are the tissues most prone to injury.

If a compartment syndrome remains untreated, even for a few hours, the result is tissue death. For the patient, tissue death translates into tissue loss and permanent disability.

Muscle death can be a serious problem from more than just the functional standpoint. A byproduct of the dead muscle, myoglobin, can injure the kidneys and lead to permanent kidney damage. Compartment syndrome endangers not only the normal functioning of the hand but also the patient's life.

Signs and Symptoms

It is important to be aware of the potential for development of compartment syndrome and to educate the patient about the early warning signs. The key is early diagnosis so that you can intervene before permanent damage has occurred. An untreated compartment syndrome can lead to severe morbidity and extremity loss and even endanger the patient's life.

- **Severe pain** in the affected extremity, out of proportion to the injury
- Significant **swelling and tightness** in the forearm or hand tissues
- **Pain with passive stretch of a muscle group** (e.g., passive extension of the fingers or wrist stretches the flexor muscles and causes pain in the volar forearm, whereas passive flexion of the fingers or wrist stretches the extensor muscles and causes pain in the dorsal forearm)
- **Tingling or numbness in the hand**, along the median, ulnar, and radial nerve distributions

Note: Pulses at the elbow and wrist may be completely *normal* even with a significant build-up of pressure in the forearm and hand.

Compartment pressure can be measured, but results are highly unreliable without proper equipment and an experienced clinician. In general, if the patient has the above signs and symptoms, treatment should be instituted.

Treatment of compartment syndrome is a *true surgical emergency*. You must get help early. If you have no access to a provider with surgical expertise, the following information will be useful.

Treatment

Fasciotomy

The key to treating a compartment syndrome is to open the involved tissue compartments to relieve the pressure before permanent tissue damage has occurred. This procedure is done in the operating room under general anesthesia.

Skin incisions are made to access the underlying muscle fascia. The fascia must be opened (hence the term *fasciotomy*) to relieve the pressure in the muscles; opening the skin alone is not sufficient.

The need for this procedure is *emergent*. It should not be delayed for days until a specialist is available.

Forearm

The forearm has three compartments: volar (flexor), dorsal (extensor), and mobile wad (upper forearm muscles on the radial side). The compartments of the forearm are somewhat interconnected. Opening (i.e., releasing) the volar compartment *may* relieve the pressure in the other two compartments. However, if the forearm still feels tight after release of the volar compartment, an additional incision should be made to release the dorsal compartment. When making the incisions, take care to avoid injury to the superficial veins.

The **volar compartment** is opened by making a curvilinear incision that starts in the palm (to release the carpal tunnel), then crosses the wrist transversely to the ulnar side of the forearm. The incision then is extended up the center of the forearm in a large arc.

The **dorsal compartment** and **mobile wad** are released by a straight, longitudinal incision on the dorsal surface of the forearm (see figure on next page).

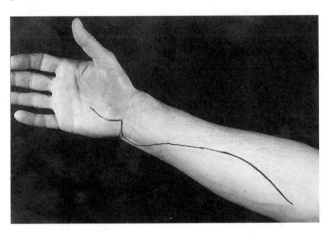

Markings for an incision to decompress the volar forearm. The incision begins in the hand for full decompression of the carpal tunnel.

Hand

On the **volar surface** of the hand, the carpal tunnel should be opened to relieve the pressure, which can injure the median nerve.

On the **dorsal surface**, the interosseous muscles are released by placing the first longitudinal incision over the index metacarpal and another over the ring finger metacarpal. Slide to either side of the underlying bone to release the fascia around the surrounding muscles.

The **thenar muscles** are released through an incision along the radial side of the thumb metacarpal.

The **hypothenar muscles** are released through an incision along the ulnar side of the little finger metacarpal.

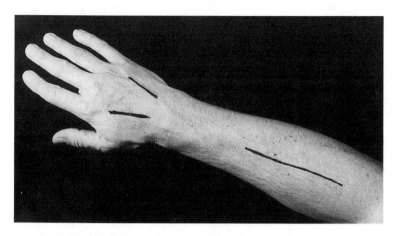

Markings for the incisions needed to decompress the dorsum of the hand and the dorsum of the forearm.

Fingers

If the fingers are very swollen and tight, they must be opened. A mid-axial, lateral incision is used to release each finger. The incisions are positioned along the ulnar side of the index, middle, and ring fingers and are made along the radial side of the thumb and little finger. Be careful to avoid injury to the underlying neurovascular bundle.

When the fascia around the muscle is opened, the muscle "bulges out" dramatically. Initially, the muscle may look purple and nonviable. Wait several minutes; often the muscle becomes redder and healthier looking. Only muscle that remains dusky and purple and obviously looks dead should be excised.

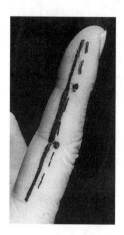

Proper incision for decompression of a finger. The course of the digital nerve is illustrated by the dashed line.

Postfasciotomy Care

1. The incisions should be left open. Saline dressings or antibiotic gauze may be placed over the open wounds. Be sure that the dressings are applied loosely. Daily dressing changes can be started 24–48 hours after the operation. The patient may require anesthesia for the initial dressing change.

2. A splint should be used to keep the hand in neutral position.

3. The hand should be gently elevated (higher than the elbow) to promote venous return and decrease swelling.

4. Further surgery is needed for wound closure. In general, wait at least 3–4 days for the swelling to decrease. A split-thickness skin graft is almost always required for wound closure. If you attempt to close any of the incisions primarily, make certain that there is *no tension on the skin.*

5. Adequate stabilization is required for all fractures. Usually, temporary stabilization can be attained with a splint. If an orthopedic surgeon is available, more definitive bone stabilization can be performed at the time of fasciotomy or wound closure.

Prevention of the Vicious Cycle the Leads to a Compartment Syndrome

Elevate the hand and forearm. The patient must keep the injured hand and forearm gently elevated and not let them dangle in a dependent position The dependent position promotes swelling of injured tissues. The hand should be higher than the elbow.

Use a splint instead of a cast for immobilization of broken bones until the swelling has decreased. A tight cast can contribute to an increase in tissue pressure. If there is a fair amount of swelling in the forearm or hand or if you do not have much experience making a cast, consider putting the extremity in a splint for the first few days. Although a splint does not immobilize the fracture as well as a cast, it is worth taking this precaution initially to prevent the development of a compartment syndrome.

Be sure that the splint is held loosely in place. It is possible to secure the splint too tightly with an Ace wrap—be careful.

If you have placed the patient in a cast: If the patient complains that the cast seems too tight or reports numbness in the fingers, bivalve the cast immediately. Make cuts in the cast along the medial and lateral sides, and separate the underlying padding. If this maneuver does not relieve the symptoms, the cast should be removed and the extremity examined closely for signs of a compartment syndrome.

If an open wound is present: Do not close the skin if it seems at all tight. It is better to have an open wound that heals with an ugly scar than to risk the development of a compartment syndrome by closing the skin tightly.

Keep a high index of suspicion. A compartment syndrome can occur even with an open wound and even when the patient has normal pulses.

Bibliography

1. Buchler U, Hastings H: Combined injuries. In Green DP, Hotchkiss RN, Pederson WC (eds): Green's Operative Hand Surgery, 4th ed. New York, Churchill Livingstone, 1999, pp 1631–1650.
2. Rowland SA: Fasciotomy: The treatment of compartment syndrome. In Green DP, Hotchkiss RN, Pederson WC (eds): Green's Operative Hand Surgery, 4th ed. New York, Churchill Livingstone, 1999, pp 689–710.

Chapter 36

HAND INFECTIONS: GENERAL INFORMATION

KEY FIGURE:
Elevation and splinting

Hand infections are relatively common problems. Seemingly minor injuries can sometimes lead to significant infections. Proper treatment is vital to prevent long-term disability.

Cellulitis vs. Abscess

Cellulitis is a diffuse infection of the soft tissues. No localized area of pus can be drained. The affected area is described as indurated (i.e., warm, red, and swollen). The hand is also painful. A component of lymphangitis (infection involving the lymphatics) may be indicated by red streaking in the tissues, progressing proximally up the arm. The treatment of cellulitis centers on the administration of the appropriate antibiotic regimen.

An **abscess** is a localized collection of pus, often with a component of cellulitis in the surrounding soft tissues (with the above signs). One sign of an abscess is an area of fluctuance. When you apply gentle digital pressure over the area of the presumed abscess, you feel a "give," indicating the presence of fluid beneath the skin. Another sign is that an abscess often seems to "point"; that is, the skin starts to thin from the pressure of the fluid underneath. The primary treatment of an abscess is incision and drainage (I & D)—cutting open the roof of the abscess to allow the pus to drain. Antibiotic therapy may be needed, but the infectious process will not resolve with antibiotics alone.

From the above information, you can see that the distinction between the two entities is important because their treatments are different. I & D is indicated for an abscess, whereas cellulitis does not warrant this intervention.

Gangrene

The term *gangrene* is used to describe tissues that are dead. There are two subtypes of gangrene, wet and dry. The distinction is important.

Dry gangrene describes tissues that are generally black and dried out. There is a distinct border between the dead tissue and surrounding healthy tissue. Sometimes the dead tissues fall off on their own; dry gangrenous fingertips can fall off with minimal manipulation. However, debridement usually is required, but it is not emergent. Dry gangrene usually places the patient at no health risk as long as it does not become infected (see below).

In contrast to dry gangrene, **wet gangrene** can be a significant health risk. Wet gangrene connotes active infection (noted by pain, swelling, redness, and drainage of pus) in the tissues surrounding the obviously dead tissue. Urgent debridement is required to prevent further tissue loss and worsening of soft tissue infection.

Necrotizing Fasciitis

Necrotizing fasciitis is a serious, potentially life-threatening infection of the fascia (the thin connective tissue overlying the muscle under the skin and subcutaneous tissue). The popular press calls it the disease of flesh-eating bacteria.

Necrotizing fasciitis is not common. However, it must be considered in the evaluation of patients with a hand infection that seems to be rapidly progressing proximally up the forearm. Necrotizing fasciitis should also be considered when the patient is sicker than you would expect for simple cellulitis.

The skin is swollen, but often without the typical signs of cellulitis. The skin simply does not look "right." You may be able to feel subcutaneous air in the soft tissues of the arm, or you may see air in the soft tissues on x-rays (normally, no air is present in soft tissues on x-ray).

The patient is often quite ill (high fever, low blood pressure, general weakness, and even shock may be present). The infection can spread quickly up the arm and into the chest. Radical debridement and even amputation may be necessary to save the patient's life.

Treatment requires aggressive operative debridement (opening up the soft tissue spaces, as with an abscess) to remove diseased tissue, intravenous antibiotics, and close monitoring for aggressive treatment of septicemia. Hyperbaric oxygen also may be indicated but does not replace aggressive operative treatment. Patients with necrotizing fasciitis should be treated by a surgeon with critical care expertise.

Evaluation of an Infected Hand

History

Ask the patient about events that may have led to the development of the infection. This information may help to guide your treatment.

Antecedent Trauma

A history of being cut by glass or sustaining a puncture wound should raise concern about the presence of a foreign body in the soft tissues.

Ask whether the patient was bitten by an animal. An animal's canine teeth, especially those of a cat, may penetrate much deeper into the underlying tissues than you expect. Find out what type of animal was involved; different animals have specific bacterial organisms that may require a particular antibiotic. Ask about the possibility of rabies exposure (see chapter 6, "Evaluation of an Acute Wound," for information about rabies prevention).

If the patient has a wound over a metacarpophalangeal knuckle, you must ask specifically whether the wound is due to human teeth. People are often embarrassed to admit that they have been in a fight. Ask point-blank: Did you punch someone in the mouth? Did someone bite you? This information is important because the human mouth has strong pathogens that can lead to significant soft tissue destruction. Choice of specific antibiotics is based on the usual organisms found in the human mouth.

Recent History of Swimming

Well-managed swimming pools usually are treated adequately with chemicals, and the ocean has such a high salt content that neither venue is associated with specific organisms that cause infection. However, streams, ponds, lakes, and aquariums are associated with specific bacteria that can cause significant infections. In addition, ask whether the injury occurred while the patient was working on a boat or fishing.

Medical Issues

Patients with diabetes often develop infections that are unexpectedly difficult to treat. You must treat such infections aggressively and ensure that blood sugar is well controlled.

Ask about the patient's tetanus immunization status.

Physical Examination

1. The classic signs of a hand infection are redness, warmth, swelling, and pain. The swelling associated with a hand infection is often quite pronounced.

2. Look closely for puncture wounds and other signs of trauma.

3. Determine whether the patient has a localized collection of pus that requires drainage or diffuse soft tissue infection.

4. Look for induration extending proximally up the forearm.

5. Look for red streaks extending up the arm.

6. If the forearm is involved, palpate for crepitus or subcutaneous air in the forearm tissues (signs of necrotizing fasciitis). To test for crepitus, press on the soft tissues. If air is present under the skin, it will feel as if you are pressing on crinkled layers of cellophane or popping air bubbles beneath the skin.

7. Look for signs of systemic illness (fever, chills, low blood pressure, generalized weakness, and malaise).

8. Look for evidence of enlarged lymph nodes in the armpit or back of the elbow.

Additional Studies

The basic studies include complete blood count with a white blood cell count and x-ray evaluation of the infected area. Include the forearm if the induration extends proximally up the forearm. Blood cultures should be done if the patient is febrile or looks ill. If there is an open wound present, culture it.

What to Assess on X-rays

1. Foreign bodies

2. Unsuspected fractures or dislocations

3. Evidence of joint contamination: air in the joint, destruction of joint surfaces, foreign material in the joint. Any of these findings warrants operative exploration.

4. Underlying bone infection: the bone edges appear irregular if bone is involved with the infectious process. If bone is involved, 4–6 weeks of antibiotic therapy are needed.

5. Air in the soft tissues strongly indicates necrotizing fasciitis. Localized air may be present in the soft tissues at the immediate vicinity of an I & D site, but diffuse air in the tissues is a sign of necrotizing infection.

Importance of Key Elements in the History and Physical Examination

Foreign Bodies

If a foreign body is located in the infected tissues, the infection will not resolve unless it is removed. However, a foreign body in soft tissues without cellulitis does not have to be removed unless it is causing symptoms.

Animal Bites

Pasteurella multocida and *Staphylococcus aureus* are associated with cat and dog bites. Treatment with an antipseudomonal and antistaphylococcal antibiotic (amoxicillin/clavulanate, cefuroxime) is required. Cat bites often penetrate more deeply than you expect and may involve underlying joints or tendons. Exploration and washout of the joint and tendon may be required. Cat bites have a much higher incidence of subsequent infection than dog bites (80% vs. 5%, respectively).

Human Bites

Eikenella corrodens, other anaerobes, and *Streptococcus viridans* are associated with infections caused by a human bite. If the patient is seen early after the injury, before signs of infection have developed, treat with amoxicillin/clavulanate. Once signs of infection are present, intravenous antibiotics, such as amoxicillin/sulbactam or ticarcillin/clavulanate, are indicated. Operative exploration also may be required if the underlying joint is affected. In addition, abscess formation is common after a human bite.

Seawater and Shellfish-related Injury

If the infected tissues are swollen and red but not particularly hot or tender, the causative organism may be *Mycobacterium marinum*. Treatment requires long-term (3 months) administration of doxycycline or rifampin/ethambutol. An infectious disease specialist should be involved in the treatment of such patients.

If the infected area has all of the typical signs of cellulitis, treatment should cover bacteria of the *Vibrio* species; tetracycline or an aminoglycoside may be used.

Freshwater Injury

Aeromonas hydrophila is associated with freshwater infection. A fluoroquinolone or trimethoprim/sulfamethoxazole should be used for treatment.

Red Streaking

Red streaking is a sign of lymphangitis, which means that the infection is traveling through the lymphatic system. Staphylococcal infections are most commonly associated with this physical finding.

Enlarged Lymph Nodes Around the Elbow or Armpit

The presence of enlarged lymph nodes may indicate cat-scratch disease, a *Mycobacterium marinum* infection, sporotrichosis or nocardial infection. An infectious disease specialist should be consulted because these unusual infections can be difficult to treat.

General Initial Treatment

The infected hand is often diffusely swollen. Initially it may be difficult to determine whether the patient has an abscess in need of drainage. If the patient otherwise looks well and has no signs of flexor tenosynovitis (see chapter 37, "Specific Types of Hand Abscesses"), underlying joint infection, or necrotizing fasciitis, treat conservatively. Do not make cuts in the skin looking for an abscess; you may well find nothing.

Conservative Approach

1. Start the appropriate antibiotics.
2. Splint the hand in neutral position (see chapter 28, "Hand Splinting and General Aftercare"), and elevate the hand. These two interventions are the cornerstone of treatment for all hand infections. Splinting and elevation significantly reduce swelling, thus making it easier to determine whether an abscess is present.

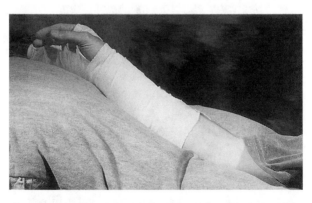

The proper way to elevate an injured hand. The hand should be higher than the elbow to promote drainage and decrease swelling in the hand.

3. Warm (not hot) compresses applied to the inflamed area of the hand may be useful.

4. After 24 hours reevaluate the hand.

- Significant improvement may be seen. If there is no evidence of an abscess, continue splinting, elevation, and antibiotics. The splint should be removed once pain and swelling have resolved. Regular exercise then becomes important to prevent stiffness. Continue the antibiotics for 7–10 days until the infectious process has resolved completely.

- Alternatively, a localized collection of pus in need of drainage may be identifiable. The following chapter discusses specific types of hand abscesses and their treatment.

Bibliography

1. Gilbert DN, Moellering RC, Sande MA (eds): The Sanford Guide to Antimicrobial Therapy, 29th ed. Vermont, Antimicrobial Therapy, Inc., 1999.
2. Lampe EW: Clinical Symposia: Surgical Anatomy of the Hand. 40th anniversary issue 40(3):31–36, 1988.

Chapter 37

SPECIFIC TYPES OF HAND INFECTIONS

KEY FIGURES:
Felon
Paronychia
Collar button abscess

Felon

A felon is an abscess of the fingertip along the volar skin pad. The fingertip is swollen and quite painful. Without proper treatment, the infection can progress and cause serious complications. Necrosis of the fingertip skin, osteomyelitis (infection of the underlying bone), and even flexor tenosynovitis (see description later in this chapter) may result.

If the infectious process is caught before abscess formation, it can be treated with antibiotics alone. If no improvement is observed with antibiotics or if fluctuance is present, incision and drainage are necessary.

Incision and Drainage

1. Anesthetize the finger with a digital block using lidocaine, bupivacaine, or a mixture of the two.

2. Clean the fingertip with some type of antibacterial agent.

3A. If the "point" (i.e., area of maximal tenderness and fluctuance) is on the volar fingertip pad, make a longitudinal incision over this point. Take care to keep the incision distal to the distal interphalangeal (DIP) flexion crease.

 B. If the "point" is on the lateral surface, make a longitudinal incision on the ulnar side of the digit (radial side for the thumb or little finger) parallel to the expected position of the digital nerve. Take care to keep distal and dorsal to the DIP flexion crease to prevent injury to the digital nerve and artery.

4. Use a clamp to open the incision and thoroughly drain the space.

5. If you have access to a microbiology lab, send a specimen of the pus for culture to identify the causative organism.

6. Irrigate the abscess cavity with sterile saline.

7. Pack a small piece of gauze into the cavity, and cover the fingertip with dry gauze.

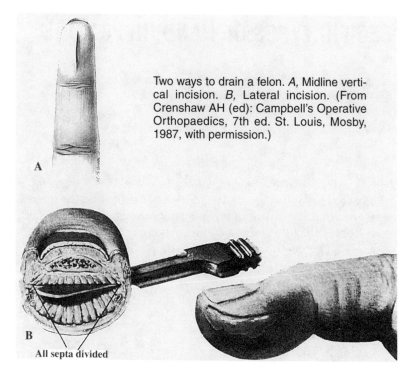

Two ways to drain a felon. *A*, Midline vertical incision. *B*, Lateral incision. (From Crenshaw AH (ed): Campbell's Operative Orthopaedics, 7th ed. St. Louis, Mosby, 1987, with permission.)

All septa divided

Aftercare

- Keep the hand elevated.
- Remove the packing the next day, and clean the finger with gentle soap and water or saline.
- If possible, repack the cavity with saline-moistened gauze. Change this dressing 1 or 2 times each day.
- Once you cannot pack the cavity with gauze, simply apply antibiotic ointment to the area and cover with a dry gauze 1 or 2 times each day.
- Be sure to wash the finger with gentle soap and water or saline twice daily.

- Encourage active and passive range-of-motion exercises to prevent the finger from becoming stiff.
- Continue the oral antibiotics for several days, until the tenderness and redness resolve.

Paronychia

A paronychia is an infection around the fingernail, in the surrounding skin fold (eponychial fold). It usually is caused by *Staphylococcus aureus*. The skin around the proximal portion of the fingernail is swollen, and the finger is quite tender.

If the infection is caught early, the finger can be successfully treated by soaking it in warm, soapy water several times a day and giving oral antibiotics. If pus is present around the base of the nail, drainage is needed.

Drainage

1. Anesthetize the finger with a digital block using lidocaine, bupivacaine, or a mixture of the two.

2. Soak the finger in warm, soapy water for 5–10 minutes.

3. Place the tips of a closed clamp under the skin fold around the nail to open the abscess. Wash the space out with saline, and then pack it with a small piece of gauze.

4. Remove the gauze the next day. Instruct the patient to continue the warm soaks and cover with antibiotic ointment and dry gauze 2 or 3 times/day.

Treatment of a paronychia. *A*, Elevation and removal of one-fourth of the nail to decompress the paronychium. *B*, Incision of the paronychial fold with the blade directed away from the nail bed and matrix. (Illustration by Elizabeth Roselius © 1998. From Green DP, et al (eds): Operative Hand Surgery, 4th ed. New York, Churchill Livingstone, 1999, with permission.)

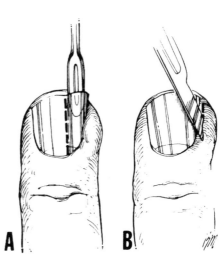

5. If this approach does not lead to resolution of the infection, the skin fold may need to be incised and formally opened. The proximal part of the nail may need to be removed as well.

Caution: Be wary when a patient presents with an infection around the fingernail that does not seem like a "typical" infection. The finger may be swollen but not very tender, and small vesicles (blisters that are not pus-filled) are around the base of the nail. This presentation indicates a *herpetic* (viral) infection, which is seen most commonly in medical and dental personnel and people whose hands are often in water.

Do *not* incise and drain. Leave the vesicles alone. Incision and drainage carry a high risk for secondary bacterial infection, which can be quite difficult to treat. Herpetic infection is self-limiting and resolves in 3–4 weeks. If you have access to anti-herpes medications, oral treatment (acyclovir, 400 mg 3 times/day for 10 days) may relieve symptoms.

Acute Suppurative Flexor Tenosynovitis

The flexor tendons of the fingers travel within the confines of the surrounding flexor sheath. This anatomic arrangement allows the smooth gliding action of the flexor tendons, which is responsible for optimal finger flexion and hand function. The sheath around the flexor tendons of the fingers runs from the distal palmar skin crease of each finger to just proximal to the DIP joint flexion crease. It is essentially a closed space.

Acute suppurative flexor tenosynovitis is an infection within the confines of the flexor sheath. It is similar to an abscess and often requires drainage for resolution. Acute suppurative flexor tenosynovitis is potentially a serious infection and must be treated expeditiously. It can lead to the destruction of the gliding mechanism necessary for normal tendon function. If not treated appropriately, it can result in significant permanent limitation in finger and hand function.

History and Physical Exam

This infection is often associated with penetrating trauma to the finger. However, some patients cannot recall any significant antecedent injury.

Cardinal Signs

- Flexed posture of affected finger
- Diffuse swelling of the entire finger, which may extend to the dorsal surface of the metacarpophalangeal (MCP) area
- Significant tenderness along the volar aspect of the finger (where the tendon sheath is located)
- Pain with passive extension of the affected finger

The main area of tenderness, especially when the patient presents early in the course of the process, is over the A1 pulley. The A1 pulley represents the beginning of the flexor sheath, near the volar, distal palmar crease. Tenderness in this area is the most sensitive sign of acute flexor tenosynovitis and may help to differentiate it from other infectious processes involving the finger. For example, a felon or simple cellulitis of the finger does *not* have tenderness over this area.

If you are unsure of the diagnosis, you can treat conservatively with a splint, hand elevation, and antibiotics for 24 hours. You should splint the entire hand in neutral position. If symptoms improve, continue conservative management; if symptoms progress or do not improve significantly, operative exploration is necessary.

Operative Treatment

Because of the potential for long-term disability if treatment is not prompt, drainage should be attempted if no specialist is available. If a specialist is available, refer the patient.

1. General anesthesia is best, but a wrist block may be used.

2. Use a tourniquet to keep blood out of the operating field and facilitate exploration of the finger. The tourniquet also helps to prevent accidental injury to digital nerves and vessels. With general anesthesia, place an upper arm tourniquet. With a wrist block, use a forearm tourniquet. *Do not exsanguinate the arm.*

3. Keep in mind that digital nerves and vessels run along the sides of the fingers.

4. Make a traverse incision in the DIP flexion crease. Use a clamp or blunt scissors to separate the soft tissues gently so that you can identify the distal portion of the flexor sheath. It is grayish and much thicker than normal (a few millimeters vs. < 1 mm).

5. Open this portion of the sheath.

6. Make a transverse counterincision in the palm over the distal palmar skin crease of the finger. It should not be too large (about 1.5 cm).

7. Carefully spread the soft tissues until you identify the sheath. It may appear gray and thick. Take care not to damage the digital arteries and nerves on either side of the sheath. Use blunt dissection, and do not cut *anything* until you are sure of what you are cutting.

8. If you have difficulty in identifying the sheath, extend the incision distally in a zig-zag fashion to improve access to the underlying tissues.

9. Open the sheath. Send a swab of the fluid from the sheath to the microbiology lab for analysis.

10. Place a catheter (20 gauge is best) similar to what you use for intra-venous access into the sheath. Wash out the sheath by attaching a syringe with saline to the catheter and irrigating the sheath until the fluid that comes out is clear and no longer cloudy (cloudiness is due to the presence of pus in the canal). Irrigation fluid should come out of the distal incision by the DIP flexion crease.

11. If you had to extend the palm incision beyond the simple trans-verse incision, close the additional incision very loosely with one or two nonabsorbable sutures. Otherwise do not close either incision; the incisions will heal on their own.

12. The catheter should be left in place to allow irrigation of the sheath every few hours for the first 24 hours after surgery. If possible, attach the catheter to IV extension tubing so that a syringe can be attached outside the dressing.

13. Place a piece of gauze in each open wound.

14. Release the tourniquet, and apply gentle pressure over the incisions to control bleeding.

15. Place dry gauze between all fingers and around the affected finger.

16. Wrap the hand with soft gauze.

17. Splint the hand in neutral position.

18. Secure the IV tubing attached to the catheter in the flexor sheath to the outside of the splint so that it does not dislodge.

Postoperative Care

1. The hand should be kept elevated in a splint.

2. Continue intravenous antibiotics. When the symptoms and signs of infection improve, change to oral antibiotics, and complete a 7–10 day course.

3. Irrigate the sheath with 3–5 ml of saline every 3–4 hours. Pain medication should be given before beginning irrigation.

4. Change the dressing after 24 hours, and remove the gauze packing and catheter at this time.

5. The patient should continue to wear the splint until the swelling and tenderness improve.

6. The patient should start passive and active motion once the swelling and tenderness improve.

7. The incisions heal on their own. The patient can apply antibiotic ointment after a few days and cover each incision with a bandage.

Note: There is no such thing as acute suppurative extensor tenosynovitis because there is no sheath around the extensor tendons of the fingers.

Patients with **rheumatoid arthritis** may develop a noninfectious tenosynovitis, which essentially is inflammation of the tendons caused by the underlying rheumatic disease. Often the tendons are involved more proximally at the wrist, and flexor or extensor tendons may be affected. This inflammatory disorder is quite different from an acute infectious process and does not require antibiotics or urgent surgical intervention. The symptoms are more chronic, and the physical findings are not as dramatic as those due to an infectious process.

Abscess on the Dorsal Surface of the Hand

The patient often presents with a very swollen hand and fingers. At first it may be difficult to appreciate the abscess cavity because of the diffuse nature of the swelling. In the presence of an obvious abscess, proceed to incision and drainage. If you are not certain whether or not an abscess is present, and the patient does not appear ill, treat conservatively at first with splint, hand elevation, and antibiotics for 1 day. Often after 24 hours of conservative treatment, the swelling decreases in areas not involved with the abscess. The abscess cavity is then identifiable.

Incision and Drainage

1. If the skin overlying the abscess is very thin (i.e., the abscess is "pointing"), no anesthetic may be required.

2. If the patient is in too much pain, local anesthetics may not be very useful because they do not work well in infected tissues. However, a block may work, or, if indicated by the extent of the abscess, general anesthesia may be required.

3. Make a longitudinal incision through the most fluctuant part of the abscess. Do not be timid when making the incision. Excise an ellipse of skin so that the opening is large enough to drain the abscess completely and to allow packing of the cavity with gauze.

4. Use the tips of a clamp to explore the abscess cavity. Make sure that the cavity does not extend to the volar side of the hand. If it does, a counterincision should be made over the volar extension of the cavity. This extension allows better drainage of the entire abscess. If you need to make a counterincision on the volar surface, first inject some anesthetic into the area.

5. Pack the wound with gauze.

6. Use a splint to keep the hand in neutral position.

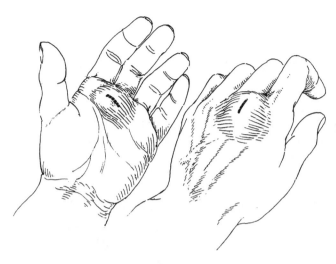

A collar button abscess extends from the volar to the dorsal surfaces of the hand. Both sides of the hand must be drained individually because the two areas are connected by a narrow path. (From Chase RA: Atlas of Hand Surgery. Philadelphia, W.B. Saunders, 1973, with permission.)

Postoperative Care

1. Keep the hand elevated and in the splint until the swelling and other signs of infection have improved.

2. The gauze packing should remain in place for 1 day. Then remove the gauze, and repack the cavity with saline-moistened gauze. Cover with dry gauze. This entire procedure should be done 2 or 3 times/day until the wound has healed.

3. The patient may wash the hand with gentle soap and water at each dressing change.

4. Antibiotics should be continued until the surrounding cellulitis resolves (probably only a few days).

5. Once the infection has resolved, the patient must start regular (several times per day) active and passive range-of-motion exercises to prevent permanent hand stiffness and limitation of hand function.

Bibliography

Neviaser RJ: Acute infections. In Green DP, Hotchkiss RN, Pederson WC (eds): Green's Operative Hand Surgery, 4th ed. New York, Churchill Livingstone, 1999, pp 1033–1047.

Chapter 38

CHRONIC HAND CONDITIONS

Chronic hand pain is a common complaint, especially among people who work with their hands. What initially may seem to be only an annoying pain can turn into significant disability without adequate treatment. This chapter discusses several of the most commonly encountered chronic hand disorders.

Trigger Finger

Anatomic Background

The flexor tendons travel through a connective tissue, synovial-lined tube as they course through the fingers. This tube runs from the metacarpophalangeal (MCP) joint (just proximal to the MCP flexion crease as you look at the palm of the hand) to a point immediately proximal to the distal interphalangeal (DIP) joint.

This tube is highly pliable and thin. The tissue is slightly thicker in several areas, called pulleys. The purpose of the pulleys is to prevent the tendons from bowstringing during finger flexion. This action is important for adequate grip strength and proper hand function. The most important pulleys are A1, A2, and A3, which overlie the MCP joint, the proximal phalanx, and the proximal interphalangeal (PIP) joint, respectively.

The digital neurovascular bundles (digital nerve and vessels) run along either side of the tube in the soft tissue.

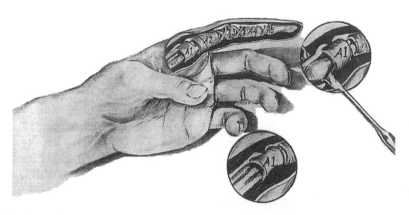

Anatomy of the flexor tendon pulley system. Top inset illustrates flexor digito-rum profundus nodular thickening. Bottom inset illustrates flexor digitorum su-perficialis decussation fraying. (From Zelouf DS (ed): Atlas of the Hand Clinics. Philadelphia, W.B. Saunders, 1999, with permission.)

Definition of Trigger Finger

The technical name for trigger finger is stenosing tenosynovitis. It is postulated that repetitive use of the fingers or thumb causes the A1 pulley to become thick and unyielding. Pathologic thickening in the tendon near the pulley also may occur. As a result of such changes, the tendon is unable to glide properly through the pulley. In extreme cases, the tendon may become stuck outside the entrance of the pulley (just proximal to the MCP flexion crease).

The clinical result is triggering of the affected finger or thumb. Triggering means that the digit assumes a flexed posture. Active straightening of the affected digit is often difficult. Massage of the tissues of the distal palm and passive extension of the finger or thumb may be required. Sometimes the digit cannot be fully extended even with these measures.

Before the development of triggering, patients often complain of chronic pain not only in the area of the MCP joint but also in the area around the PIP joint.

Congenital trigger finger may be seen in infants. Because of the small size of the tissues, this problem should be treated only by a hand specialist.

Diagnosis

The history of triggering is usually the most important finding. Sometimes patients simply complain of a dull pain in the distal palm or the PIP joint of the affected digit(s).

On physical exam, feel the tissue just proximal to the MCP joint at the distal palmar skin crease. This is the location of the A1 pulley. Gently flex and extend the affected digit, and you may feel a small "knot" moving back and forth. This "knot" clinches the diagnosis in a patient with the above clinical symptoms.

Nonoperative Treatment

Steroid injection around the A1 pulley may provide symptomatic relief, which can delay the need for surgery for many months. Betamethasone is commonly used; inject 0.25–0.50 ml around the A1 pulley. Warn the patient that it will take a few weeks to see whether the injection is successful. A second steroid injection can be given 6 weeks after the initial injection if no improvement has been noted. Sometimes the second injection is successful even if the first resulted in little improvement.

How to Inject the A1 Pulley

1. Draw the steroid solution into a syringe. Use a small needle (≤ 21 gauge) for the injection.

2. The landmark for the A1 pulley is the distal palmar skin crease of the affected digit.

3. Starting with an injection of a local anesthetic is not necessary because it will hurt just as much as the steroid injection. But give the patient a choice.

4. Alternatively, 1 ml of lidocaine can be added to the steroid solution to help alleviate the chronic pain temporarily.

5. Stick the needle into the tissues. You need to go deeper than the superficial skin. If the patient reports feeling pins and needles, you are probably in the digital nerve. Back out a few millimeters, and reposition the needle.

6. Draw back on the syringe to ensure that you are not in a blood vessel.

7. Ask the patient to flex and extend the finger with the needle in place. If the needle moves with the tendon, it may be lodged in the substance of the tendon. Back out the needle a few millimeters, and ask the patient to move the finger again. Keep adjusting the needle until the needle tip is no longer in the tendon.

8. Once the needle is in the correct position, inject one-half of the solution in the syringe. Move the needle a few millimeters to another position near the A1 pulley, check for the above positioning concerns, and inject the remainder of the steroid solution.

9. Remove the needle, place a Band-Aid over the injection site, and gently massage the tissues for a few minutes.

Operative Treatment

Operative treatment should be considered when two steroid injections are unsuccessful in alleviating symptoms or when symptoms argue against waiting 4–6 weeks for improvement.

A patient whose finger is locked in flexion also should undergo surgical treatment. Waiting for a steroid injection to work is impractical because of concerns about subsequent joint stiffness due to inability to move the finger for so long a period.

How to Release a Trigger Finger

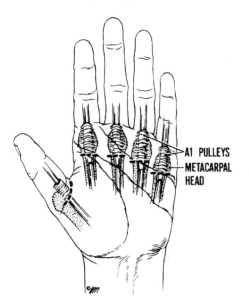

Incisions for release of trigger fingers and thumb. The index is released through an incision in the proximal palmar crease, the ring and little fingers in the distal crease, and the middle finger midway between the two palmar creases. The thumb is approached through its meta-phalangeal crease. (Illustration by Elizabeth Roselius © 1998. From Green DP, et al (eds): Operative Hand Surgery, 4th ed. New York, Churchill Livingstone, 1999, with permission.)

1. Trigger finger release can be done with a **wrist block** or **Bier block**. General anesthesia is used less commonly.

2. The hand should be exsanguinated, and a tourniquet should be used on the forearm or upper arm. It is important to have a bloodless field to prevent injury to the nearby neurovascular bundles.

3. The incision (1–1.5 cm) should be centered over the distal palmar skin crease of the affected digit. It can be made with a vertical or horizontal orientation. The vertical orientation may be more protective

of the neurovascular bundle, but it is somewhat more difficult from an exposure perspective.

4. Using **blunt dissection**—that is, using the scissors to spread the tissues, not to cut them (see chapter 2, "Surgical Techniques")—separate the soft tissues until you see the underlying tendon and A1 pulley. *Do not cut anything until you are certain that the neurovascular bundles are protected.* Use retractors to keep the tissues to the side of the your working area once the A1 pulley has been identified.

5. Use sharp scissors or the tip of your knife to open the pulley. Then open the entire pulley with a scissors. You will know you are at the end of the pulley when the tissue becomes thin and pliable compared with the thickened A1 pulley. The pulley is approximately 1 cm in length.

6. Flex and extend the finger to ensure that the tendon moves back and forth easily and that the entire pulley has been opened.

7. For postoperative pain control, inject a few milliliters of bupivacaine into the tissues that you have been dissecting.

8. Release the tourniquet, and apply pressure to control bleeding. Close the skin incision with a few interrupted sutures. Apply antibiotic ointment over the suture line, and cover with gauze dressing.

9. Alternatively, close the incision with a few interrupted sutures. Apply antibiotic ointment over the suture line, cover with gauze, and gently wrap the hand with an Ace wrap. Once the hand is dressed, release the tourniquet. Continue to hold pressure over the area around the incision for several minutes.

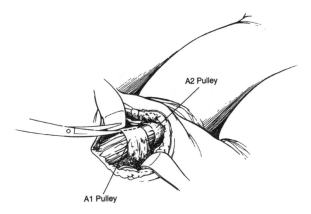

A2 Pulley

A1 Pulley

Trigger finger release. The A1 pulley is divided carefully with either scissors or knife. (From McCarthy JG (ed): Plastic Surgery. Philadelphia, W.B. Saunders, 1990, with permission.)

Postoperative Care

1. Acetaminophen or nonsteroidal anti-inflammatory agents should be adequate for postoperative pain control.

2. Keep the hand elevated to decrease swelling and decrease pain.

3. The patient should be encouraged to use the hand for light activities within 1–2 days after surgery.

4. Remove the dressing the day after surgery, and clean with gentle soap and water daily.

5. Apply antibiotic ointment to the suture line daily for the first few days. Cover with dry gauze as needed.

6. After 10–14 days, remove the sutures. Instruct the patient to increase gradually the activities performed with the hand until the patient has resumed regular activities.

Carpal Tunnel Syndrome

Anatomic Background

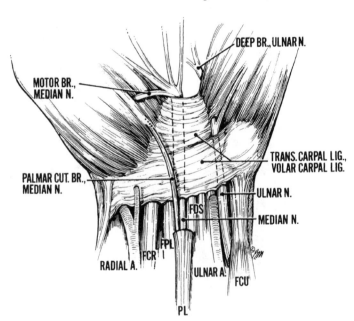

Anatomy of the carpal tunnel. The median nerve and flexor tendons transverse the carpal tunnel, lying beneath the transverse carpal ligament. (Illustration by Elizabeth Roselius © 1998. From Green DP, et al (eds): Operative Hand Surgery, 4th ed. New York, Churchill Livingstone, 1999, with permission.)

The carpal tunnel is essentially the space in the center of the palm just distal to the wrist. The carpal tunnel is bound by bone on three sides, and the transverse carpal ligament is the roof (i.e., the most superficial boundary). It is a relatively tight, fixed space.

The median nerve travels through the enclosed space of the carpal tunnel with the nine flexor tendons to the fingers and thumb. Anything that decreases the size of the tunnel, such as tissue swelling from repetitive hand and wrist movements, can place pressure on the median nerve. Pressure on the nerve causes dysfunction and clinical symptoms.

Although the median nerve at the wrist is primarily sensory, it gives off a motor branch to the thenar muscles responsible for opposition. The motor branch of the median nerve can originate from the main nerve before going under the transverse carpal ligament, in the carpal tunnel, or, most commonly, after leaving the confines of the carpal tunnel. The motor branch also can pierce through the ligament to innervate the muscles. It is important to have a thorough understanding of this anatomy to prevent injury to the motor branch if operative intervention is undertaken.

Definition of Carpal Tunnel Syndrome

The symptoms of carpal tunnel syndrome (CTS) include pain and tingling in the hand and distal forearm as well as numbness along the median nerve distribution of the hand. Hand clumsiness may occur, and the symptoms often are aggravated when the hands are in extension or grasping objects. Examples include reading the newspaper or grasping the steering wheel while driving.

Night awakenings with hand numbness, and pain in the hand or distal forearm are also common complaints. Significant weakness and muscle wasting are late symptoms.

Diagnosis

Gentle tapping on the median nerve at the wrist causes tingling or the feeling of electric shocks. This phenomenon is called a positive Tinel's sign. Development of numbness in the median nerve distribution with flexion of the wrist, called a positive Phalen's sign, is also indicative of CTS.

Special electrophysiologic tests can be done to measure the nerve conduction velocity and the status of the muscles supplied by the median nerve. Although the physical signs and symptoms are often enough to diagnose CTS, these studies are useful when the diagnosis is in doubt. Electrophysiologic studies are also useful for documentation and medicolegal purposes.

Nonoperative Treatment

Often stopping or at least decreasing the amount of time in which the hand performs repetitive movements is necessary for symptom relief.

In addition, splinting the hand in neutral position (immobilizing only the wrist in 10–20° of flexion) during work and sleep may alleviate the symptoms. It often takes several weeks to see improvement. The splint should be used for at least 6–8 weeks before determining that it is not helpful. If symptoms improve, the splint should be worn an additional 1–2 months.

The use of nonsteroidal anti-inflammatory agents (e.g., ibuprofen, naproxen sodium), may help to relieve pain and decrease swelling.

A cornerstone of therapy is evaluation by an occupational or other movement therapist, who can teach the patient how to use the entire upper extremity in a more efficient manner. By incorporating use of the entire arm instead of just the hand or wrist, the patient distributes the strain of work more evenly. This approach should remove some of the stresses on the wrist and hand and may alleviate symptoms.

Another option, which should be used with caution, is to inject steroids around the median nerve. Betamethasone, 0.75–1.0 ml, can be injected in a manner similar to performing a median nerve block (see chapter 3, "Local Anesthesia"). You must take care to avoid injection into the median nerve, which can cause nerve injury and further problems.

Operative Treatment

Carpal tunnel release (CTR) involves dividing the transverse carpal ligament to relieve the tightness in the carpal tunnel and thereby decrease pressure on the median nerve. Worldwide, CTR is performed most often by making a longitudinal incision in the palm and dividing the transverse carpal ligament under direct vision. Alternatively, in areas with access to endoscopic technology, CTR can be done with a small incision near the wrist or in the palm, with use of an endoscope to visualize and divide the ligament.

Although this operation is considered by many to be relatively minor, this writer does not agree. Complications, including injury to the median nerve or its motor branch and incomplete release of the transverse carpal ligament, may occur even when the operation is performed by a clinician with extensive hand surgical training. This procedure should be undertaken only if you have surgical expertise and a thorough understanding of the anatomy in the area. The patient should have significant signs and symptoms of CTS, including denervation of the thenar muscles.

Also, unless there are signs of muscle denervation, conservative treatment, especially movement therapies to teach the patient to use the upper extremity more efficiently, should be fully explored before turning to surgery. Not all hand surgeons agree.

How to Perform Carpal Tunnel Release

1. CTR can be done using a **wrist block**, **Bier block**, upper extremity **regional block**, or general anesthesia.

2. The hand should be exsanguinated, and a tourniquet should be used on the forearm or upper arm. It is important to have a bloodless field to prevent injury to the median nerve and surrounding structures.

3. The hand should be held in a fully supinated position for the operation. It is useful to wrap gauze around the thumb and clamp it to the operating drapes to help hold the hand in position.

4. A slightly curved incision, approximately 3–4 cm in length, is made in the distal palm over the ray of the fourth metacarpal. The incision is immediately ulnar to the vertically oriented palmar skin crease. If the incision needs to be elongated for better exposure, cross the wrist in a zig-zag fashion.

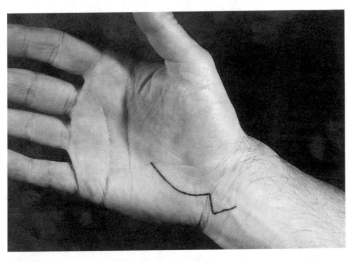

Carpal tunnel release. The skin incision should be made along a line over the fourth metacarpal bone to prevent injury to the motor branch of the median nerve. If the incision needs to be elongated for better exposure, cross the wrist in a zig-zag fashion.

5. If you are not experienced with this procedure, do *not* try to be slick by using a small incision. Make an incision that allows you to see clearly what you are doing.

6. Gently separate the tissues using **blunt dissection**. You need small self-retaining retractors or assistants who can hold retractors to keep the soft tissues out of the way.

7. You will encounter a muscle, the little known palmaris brevis. Gently tease the fibers to get them out of the way.

8. Beneath this muscle layer is the gray/white transverse carpal ligament.

9. Make a small opening in this layer with the tip of the knife or scissors.

10. Carefully extend the opening a few millimeters until you can see the underlying median nerve (it is a smooth, cream-colored structure). Then place a clamp into the opening in the ligament to protect the nerve, and use the tips of the scissors to divide fully the transverse carpal ligament. Dividing the transverse carpal ligament opens the carpal tunnel.

11. The distal extent of the ligament ends just before the palmar arch (an important vascular structure). Take care not to injure this vessel.

12. The ligament extends proximally onto the distal forearm as a fascial layer. Open the distal part of this layer by gently pushing the the barely open scissors from the leading edge of the fascia in the palm toward the distal forearm. You will know that you have divided the fascia thoroughly when you can easily pass your finger into the distal forearm without feeling any tightness. (This step is necessary only if the surgical incision has not crossed the wrist. If the incision has crossed the wrist, the fascial layer will be opened during normal dissection.)

13. For completeness, feel for a mass in the carpal tunnel. A mass is a rare cause of CTS.

14. For postoperative pain control, inject a few milliliters of bupivacaine into the tissues that you have dissected.

15. Release the tourniquet before closing the incision, and be sure that hemostasis is adequate. Close the wound with a few interrupted sutures, and cover with antibiotic ointment and dry fluffed gauze. Wrap the hand gently with an Ace wrap.

16. Alternatively, place a few interrupted sutures to close the incision. Apply antibiotic ointment over the suture line, and cover with fluffed gauze. Wrap the hand gently with an Ace wrap, and apply

gentle pressure to the area around the incision. Then release the tourniquet.

Postoperative Care

1. Acetaminophen or a nonsteroidal anti-inflammatory agent should be sufficient for pain control.

2. Keep the hand elevated as much as possible.

3. An ice pack placed on the volar aspect of the hand helps to alleviate some of the pain and swelling.

4. The soft dressing can be removed the day after surgery. The suture line should be cleansed with gentle soap and water each day. Keep the suture line covered with a gauze, and wrap the hand gently with an Ace wrap. The hand can be used for light activities, and gentle range-of-motion exercises should be done with the fingers.

5. Remove the sutures after 14 days.

6. Once the sutures are removed, gently massage the scar for several months to keep it from getting tight.

7. Gradually increase the use of the affected hand until the patient has resumed regular activities.

8. Occupational therapy is quite useful in the postoperative period.

Osteoarthritis

The most common joint disease of the upper extremity is osteoarthritis (OA). Although there are several other types of arthritis, OA is the only form discussed because of its high prevalence. Approximately 70% of people over 65 years of age have changes consistent with OA.

OA is caused by loss of joint cartilage and growth of new bone at the joint edges. The joints primarily affected are the finger DIP joints and the thumb carpometacarpal joint. The PIP and MCP joints are involved less often.

Symptoms include pain with hand use, joint enlargement and deformity, and joint stiffness with loss of motion.

The primary goals of treatment are relief of pain and maintenance of adequate hand function. Acetaminophen and nonsteroidal anti-inflammatory agents are the most useful medications. Several homeopathic remedies (e.g., arnica) also can be quite useful.

Occupational therapy or other movement therapy to encourage efficient use of the entire upper extremity is an important adjunct to treatment.

Surgery usually is done only for intractable pain and joint destruction that leads to significant loss of hand function. The most common procedure is fusion (arthrodesis) of the affected DIP joint. Arthrodesis or arthroplasty (joint replacement) may be indicated for a severely symptomatic PIP joint. These highly technical procedures should be done only by a hand specialist.

Bibliography

1. Kozin SH: The anatomy of the recurrent branch of the median nerve. J Hand Surg 23A:852–858, 1998.
2. Palmer AK, Toivonen DA: Complications of endoscopic and open carpal tunnel release. J Hand Surg 24A:561–565, 1999.
3. Taras JS, Miskovsky C: Nonoperative management of trigger digits. Atlas Hand Clin 4:1–8, 1999.

Chapter 39

EXPLORATION OF AN INJURED HAND OR FOREARM

KEY FIGURES:

Tourniquet
Midlateral finger incisions
Brunner zigzag incisions
Volar surface incisions

Dorsal incisions
Proximal and distal
  extension of wound

When exploring an injured forearm or hand, you must be aware of the surrounding tendons, nerves, and blood vessels. You do not want to injure one of these structures accidentally. This chapter explains basic principles about how to operate safely on an injured hand or forearm. It is not intended to qualify you as a hand specialist; it is intended for rural health care providers who have no access to hand or reconstructive specialists. The chapter also provides important background information for all health care providers.

Anesthesia

To operate on an upper extremity properly, you must provide adequate anesthesia. Either general anesthesia or some type of nerve block must be given so that the patient feels no pain and is able to stay completely still during the operation. (See chapter 3, "Local Anesthesia.")

Tourniquet Use

The hand has an excellent blood supply. Thus, any incision into the tissues will ooze blood continuously throughout the procedure, making it difficult to see exactly what you are doing. To prevent inadvertent injury to the important nearby structures (tendons, nerves, and blood vessels), it is best to operate in a bloodless field. This means that the circulation to the hand must be temporarily interrupted while you operate.

To interrupt the vascular supply to the hand, a tourniquet is placed proximal to the site where you are working to compress the blood vessels supplying the extremity.

Equipment and Supplies

Before placing the tourniquet, be sure to pad the area where the tourniquet will be placed with two layers of web roll (soft cotton wrap).

A pneumatic tourniquet is the best equipment to use because you can accurately set the inflation pressure as well as a time limit. An alarm will sound when the time limit has been reached.

A regular blood pressure cuff also can be used as a tourniquet. It is best used for short procedures because the pressure in the cuff often gradually decreases, and the bloodless field is lost. It is helpful to have someone available to monitor the cuff pressure and pump up the cuff before the pressure decreases too much.

An alternative is to wrap an Esmarch (wide rubber wrap) tightly around the upper arm 4–5 times and tape it in place. This technique is effective, but should be used only as a last resort.

Placement of the Tourniquet

For procedures that will take longer than 30 minutes to complete, it is best to place the tourniquet on the upper arm. Because such procedures usually are done with a Bier block, an axillary block, or general anesthesia, pain control should not be an issue.

For short procedures (less than 20 minutes) that involve the hand or wrist, a forearm tourniquet can be used with a digital or wrist block as appropriate. For this short period, most patients can tolerate the discomfort associated with the inflated tourniquet on the forearm.

When you are working on a simple, isolated finger injury, a digital tourniquet can be used. (See chapter 29, "Fingertip and Nail Bed Injuries.")

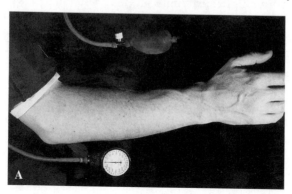

A blood pressure cuff can serve as a tourniquet to allow the procedure to be done in a bloodless field. Note the padding beneath the tourniquet. *A*, Upper arm.
(Figure continued on next page.)

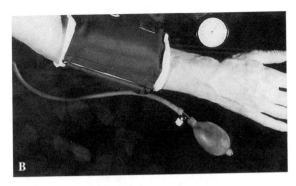

A blood pressure cuff can serve as a tourniquet to allow the procedure to be done in a bloodless field. Note the padding beneath the tourniquet. *B*, Forearm.

Exsanguination of the Extremity

Before the tourniquet is inflated, the extremity should be exsanguinated (i.e., all blood should be removed from the extremity). For this purpose, a large rubber wrap (Esmarch) can be wrapped around the extremity before the tourniquet is inflated. Start at the fingertips, and proceed proximally. The Esmarch should be stretched as you wrap it around the extremity to squeeze blood out of the tissues. You should allow a few centimeters of overlap with each turn of the wrap. Once you have reached the tourniquet, inflate the tourniquet and remove the wrap.

An alternative method is to have several assistants use their hands to apply pressure to the patient's elevated extremity. In this way, they manually squeeze the blood from the tissues. Inflate the tourniquet while their hands are still in place. This method requires several assistants.

You should *not* exsanguinate the hand if infection is present. Exsanguinating an infected extremity may spread the infection proximally and have serious consequences.

Inflation Pressure

Amount

The tourniquet should be inflated to a pressure approximately 100 mmHg higher than the patient's systolic blood pressure—usually 250–300 mmHg. This pressure level applies to the pneumatic tourniquet and blood pressure cuff. The pressure of a rubber wrap cannot be measured.

Duration

A pneumatic tourniquet can stay in place for 2 hours before it is necessary to let down the tourniquet (release the pressure).

If you are using an Esmarch wrap as a tourniquet, I recommend removal after 1–1½ hours.

If necessary, the tourniquet can be reinflated after the extremity is given a few minutes of uninterrupted blood flow.

Tourniquet Release

When the tourniquet is released, circulation returns to the extremity. For the first 5–10 minutes, the blood flow is greater than usual and the hand becomes very red. This increase in blood flow is due to the effects of ischemia on the tissues. The vessels dilate for the first few minutes after blood flow returns. The initial effect is increased bleeding from the incision, which can be a little scary if you are not expecting it.

To prevent blood loss, place saline-moistened gauze in the wound before deflating the tourniquet and apply gentle pressure while the tourniquet comes off. Continue the pressure for several minutes.

Of course, the bleeding may be due to an injured vessel. If it is particularly brisk and does not decrease after several minutes of direct pressure, the wound should be checked thoroughly to rule out vascular injury. If you have any concern that you may have accidentally injured a blood vessel during the procedure, the tourniquet should be deflated before the incision is closed.

Make sure that all pulses are intact after the tourniquet is released. The tourniquet can cause a blood vessel to clot, although clotting is unusual and occurs only in severely diseased blood vessels.

If you are reasonably sure that you have not accidentally injured a blood vessel during the procedure, you may close the wound *before* releasing the tourniquet. Be sure to use a secure dressing and to apply gentle pressure to the area before deflating the tourniquet.

Incisions

Depending on the reason for exploration, you may not have much choice about where to place the incision. If the patient has a laceration or an abscess, its location dictates the placement of the incision. Even in these situations, however, you may need to extend the incision for adequate exploration and treatment. Thus you should know the basics about proper placement of incisions on the hand.

Proper placement of incisions is important for several reasons. One reason is to prevent injury to underlying structures. Another is that improperly placed incisions can result in poor wound healing, tight scarring, and, ultimately, limitation in hand function. You do not want to worsen the problem because of a lack of understanding about the proper way to position an incision.

It is always best to draw out your planned incisions before cutting the skin. This technique allows you to think carefully about the design and to make changes *before* you create the incision.

Fingers

Volar Surface

An incision that crosses the joint flexion crease incorrectly often heals with a tight scar. A tight scar on the volar surface of the finger can result in permanent flexion of the finger and limitation of finger movement.

There are two correct ways to make incisions for access to the volar tissues of the fingers. Both avoid crossing the joint flexion creases incorrectly. The choice depends on the area in which you need access to underlying tissues.

Midlateral incisions can be placed on either side of the finger, volar to the digital vessels. They can extend from the metacarpophalangeal flexion crease to the distal phalanx.

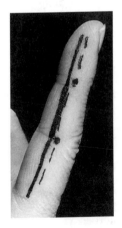

The midlateral incision is one approach to the volar side of the finger. Note the position of the digital nerve *(dashed line)* in relation to the planned incision *(solid line)*.

Brunner zigzag incisions go on a diagonal from the lateral edge of the joint crease to the opposite lateral edge of the next crease. They give the best exposure to the central aspect of the digits.

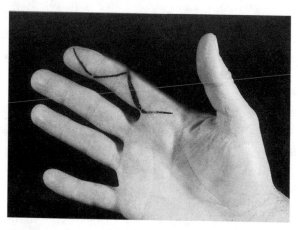

Brunner zigzag incisions provide another approach to the volar side of the finger and allow access to the center of each finger. To prevent tight scarring, the volar skin creases should not be crossed at a 90° angle (as would occur with a straight longitudinal incision through the central volar aspect of the digit.)

Dorsal Surface

On the dorsal surface of the finger, there is less concern about crossing the skin creases. Simple longitudinal incisions usually provide the best exposure and heal well.

Hand

Volar Surface

Straight incisions on the volar surface of the hand often result in tight scars that may prevent full opening of the hand and thus lead to decreased function. For this reason, diagonal incisions that zigzag across the palm are recommended.

Brunner zigzag incisions. Using a nearby flexion crease as a starting point and guide, make incisions that follow a diagonal and zigzag across the palm. On the average, each incision should only be 2–2½ cm in length. The incisions should be placed at a > 30° angle to one another.

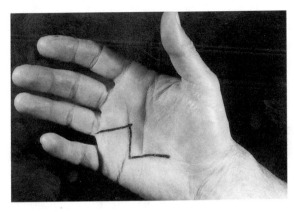

Incision for the volar surface of the hand. The palmar skin creases should be incorporated into the incisions. The incisions then should be extended in a zigzag fashion.

Dorsal Surface

As on the fingers, a tight scar on the dorsal surface of the hand may interfere with hand function. Longitudinal incisions usually provide the best exposure.

Alternatively, to prevent the need for multiple longitudinal incisions if you need access to a large area of the dorsal surface, a transverse incision is acceptable.

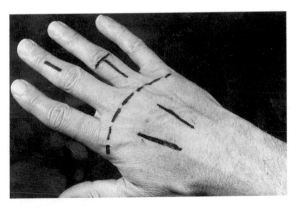

Incisions on the dorsal surface of the hand and fingers. Multiple choices are available depending on where exposure is needed. Placement is not as critical as on the volar surface.

Forearm

Volar and Dorsal Surfaces

Longitudinal incisions can be used on the volar and dorsal surfaces. If a wound from an injury is already present, simply extend it in a curvilinear manner parallel to the long axis of the forearm.

At the Elbow

Do not cross the flexion crease of the elbow (the antecubital fossa) in a straight line. Such incisions can lead to tightness about the elbow when the wound heals. It is best to use a zigzag technique.

Alternatively, make a transverse incision at the antecubital crease and then extend the ends of the incision in a curvilinear fashion down the forearm or up the upper arm as needed.

When a Laceration is Present

Often the patient with a hand injury in need of surgical exploration already has an open wound. It is best to incorporate the wound into your incision by extending the edges of the wound, using the above mentioned principles for proper incision placement.

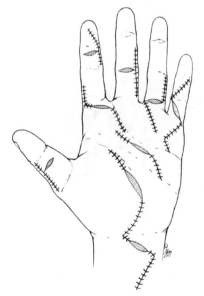

When exploring a hand with a traumatic laceration, use the wound incision whenever possible. If more exposure is needed, try to extend the traumatic wounds in a zigzag fashion. The original wound should be entended only as far as necessary, using proper incisions. (Illustration by Elizabeth Roselius © 1998. From Green DP, et al (eds): Operative Hand Surgery, 4th ed. New York, Churchill Livingstone, 1999, with permission.)

Bibliography

Conolly WB: Atlas of Hand Surgery. New York, Churchill Livingstone, 1997, pp 29–32.

Index

Page numbers in **boldface** type indicate complete chapters.